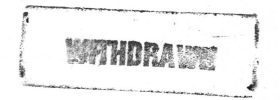
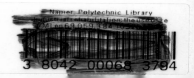

INDUSTRIAL REHABILITATION
The use of redundant buildings
for small enterprises

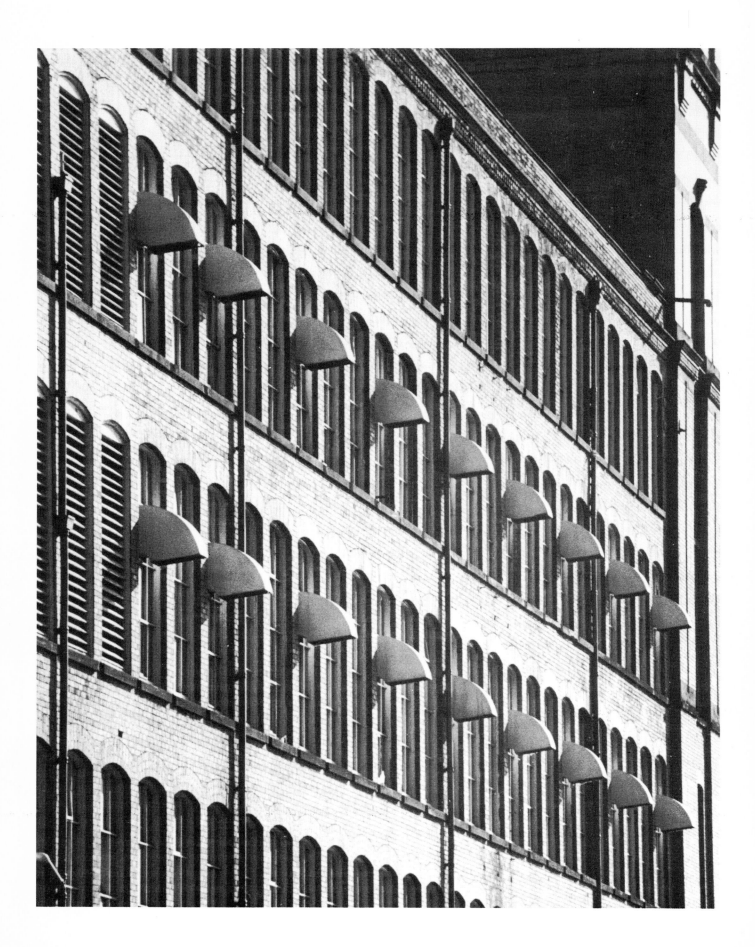

INDUSTRIAL REHABILITATION

The use of redundant buildings for small enterprises

Peter Eley and John Worthington

The Architectural Press: London

First published 1984 by
The Architectural Press Limited
9 Queen Anne's Gate, London SW1H 9BY

Based on a series of articles which appeared in *The Architects' Journal* between 22 March 1978 and 21 November 1979.

British Library Cataloguing in Publication Data

Eley, Peter
    Industrial rehabilitation.
      1. Industrial buildings—Great Britain—Remodeling
      I. Title   II. Worthington, John
      690′.54′0288   TH4511

    ISBN 0-85139-862-6

Frontispiece: Bright's Mill, Rochdale, retained for re-use

Typeset in 10 on 12 Plantin by Phoenix Photosetting, Chatham
Printed in Great Britain by Mackays of Chatham Limited

Contents

Preface

When in the early 1970s we began to advocate the re-use of redundant industrial building stock to provide accommodation for embryo entrepreneurial enterprises, the idea was seen as trivial in itself, and irrelevant to the main thrust of professional endeavour, that of undertaking comprehensive redevelopment and catering for the large blue-chip manufacturing concerns. Nearly ten years later, attitudes have changed dramatically. Today comprehensive planning is unrealisable, local economic initiatives with small firms as their lynch pin are acceptable, and large organisations are diversifying into smaller independent and more practicable entities. The architectural profession has realized that it is unrealistic to expect to be able always to provide new buildings on greenfield sites, and that economical uses must be found for the huge stock of deteriorating buildings left marooned in the inner areas of our cities.

Industrial Rehabilitation was originally conceived in 1977 as a series of articles and published in the *Architects' Journal* during 1978–79. At that time the articles were opening up new horizons and new professional roles. Five years later, with a considerable body of experience available, one can be assured that building reuse and the diversification of employment to smaller firms in both the manufacturing and service fields was not a fad, but is an essential ingredient in sustaining a healthy economy. This book, then, is addressed to all those concerned with the nuts and bolts of improving local employment opportunities: planners, industrial development officers, building professionals, community groups and building owners.

Part one presents a typology of firms, the redundant buildings available, tenancy arrangements, and agencies for development. Part two provides a step by step approach to the development process, with particular emphasis on the assessment of financial viability. Part three describes twenty-six schemes, the majority of them catering for new patterns of work on the bottom rungs of the premises ladder, which would have been inconceivable ten years ago; the restructuring of the UK economy is placing greater emphasis on individual initiative, small innovative firms, and the husbanding of existing resources. *Industrial*

Rehabilitation is a simple technical handbook in support of such initiatives.

Many of the concepts and attitudes expressed in this book were conceived in our work with URBED: a non-profit-making research and consulting organisation whose main work is directed at fostering small enterprises in the context of local economic development, and at finding new uses for empty buildings. In 1976 the URBED Research Trust (funded by the Gatsby Charitable Foundation) supported John Worthington in a study tour of America to review the experience of building re-use and of Community Development Corporations. The outcome of this study tour was the conviction that an enhanced service could be provided to users, enabling joint public/private ventures, local economic initiatives, and the reuse of discarded buildings to have a major impact on economic regeneration. Our studies showed that with flair and commitment a solution could be found to inner city decay.

The message from America that "Reusing buildings is not just a nice idea" and "preservation means business" became the cornerstone of the *Architects' Journal* articles and has since been accepted by both central government, local authorities and the private sector.

We would like to express our very real thanks to all those who contributed articles to the original series, especially to Nicholas Falk of URBED, who contributed so much of the thinking about small firms and local economic development, and the original article on assessing financial viability. Also to Bernard Williams and John Desmond of Bernard Williams Associates, who provided all the information on costs; to Dr Martin Symes of the Bartlett School of Architecture, University College London, who wrote the original article on meeting statutory requirements, and provided case study material for the chapters on planning and equipping the space; to Michael Bussel of Ove Arup and Partners who wrote on structural aspects of the building fabric, and to Ronald Hurst who wrote on mechanical and electrical services; to Brian Stout from 5 Dryden Street, who wrote on the management of working communities;

and to our colleagues at Duffy Eley Giffone Worthington (DEGW), who gave continuing support to the project and especially to Colin Cave, who wrote the original article on managing projects.

Finally, our very real thanks are due to such pioneers in the field as David Rock, Mike Franks, Michael Murray, Mike Franklin and Jake Stafford, and to Malcolm Allan, Industrial Development Officer at Hammersmith and Fulham. Without the commitment and enthusiasm of professionals such as these there may never have been a coherent body of experience to write about.

Peter Eley
London January 1984
John Worthington

Part I
The Context

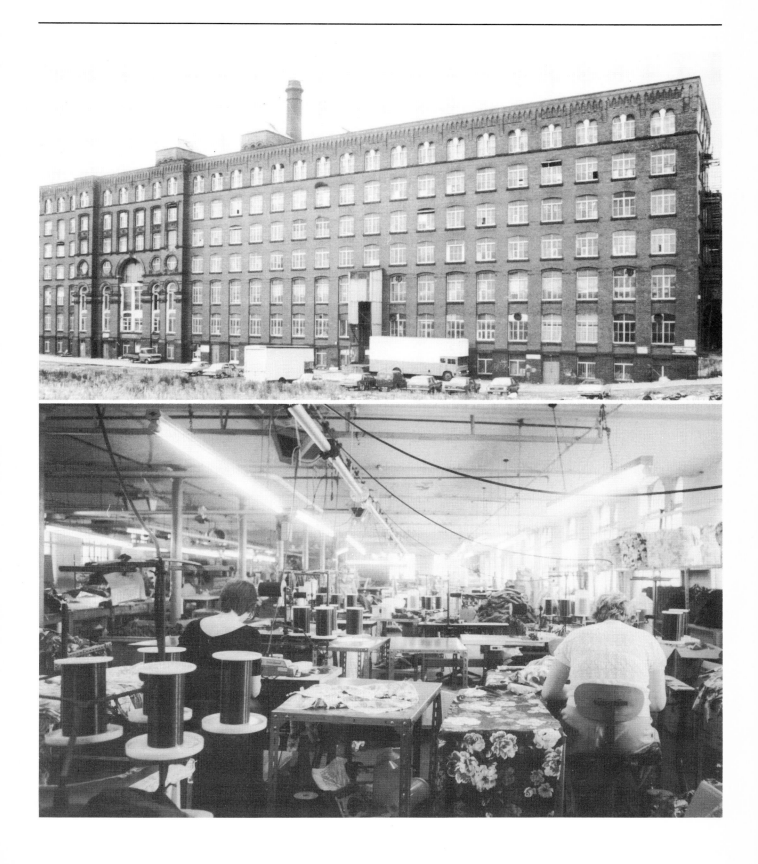

Previous page: Meadow Mill, Stockport, let in multiple units by a developer, and one of the tenant enterprises making upholstery covers.

1 The Challenge Ahead

1.00 Introduction

Reusing redundant buildings is more than just a romantic idea. Old buildings are a potential resource, which if rehabilitated can often provide cheaper and more appropriate premises for new and growing firms. By finding fresh uses decay can be halted and whole neighbourhoods rejuvenated while at the same time maintaining a sense of time and place.

The 1980s are witnessing a major shift in attitude towards the reuse of our decaying inner city building stock. The climate of political and institutional opinion has moved towards the reuse of existing buildings and the support of small firms, which in combination are seen as a means of revitalising the nation's employment base.

The enthusiasm of the late 1960s for comprehensive redevelopment and the desire to make a fresh start dulled our confidence in the potential assets that our existing heritage offered.[1] Pressure groups such as SAVE have focused attention on our industrial heritage and shown new opportunities. HUD (the United States government department responsible for housing and urban development) argues in its publication, *A Future From Our Past*[2] that reusing old industrial buildings can give texture and character to an area, a richer mixture of space than may be provided economically in new buildings, a building stock of solid construction that depreciates at a slower rate and a sense of historical continuity and civic pride.

Rehabilitation rather than wholesale redevelopment is now an established approach. Attractive, well located buildings are being taken up by developers with financial backing from the institutions and renovated for use as office, hotel or industrial purposes and where buildings are lying vacant local authorities are beginning to undertake development directly. In marginal situations where institutional funding is not forthcoming, developments are being undertaken gradually, the rental from the first stage financing the next stage of work.

The concern for revitalising local economies exists. The need now is for a planning policy that:

● Takes stock of the existing industrial space and works towards a plan which creates a mixture of spaces where new units are built to complement what exists.

● Uses all the resources available by combining grants from different sources in a co-ordinated programme and interesting large firms, academic institutions and voluntary groups in participating in the stimulation of the local economy through joint ventures.

Equally important is the upgrading of buildings presently in use. A casual survey of almost any inner city industrial area presents a depressing sight. Sites with poor access, limited car parking and inadequate storage. Buildings with out-worn fabric, and leaking roofs and poor services. Space that is inefficiently used with areas of gross overcrowding, ineffective storage and badly planned layouts which result in under-use of space overall. Many buildings are only in marginal use with upper floors empty due to lack of investment in services, lifts and fireproofing. Since the end of the last war, resources have been poured into the renewal and rebuilding of housing, with minimal investment in the working environment. A healthy economy relies on an efficient working environment. A daunting task lies ahead: not just to bring life back into the empty buildings, but to improve the efficiency of space use and nurture the marginal short-life uses that have sprung up in buildings earmarked for redevelopment so they grow into established enterprises.

The chapters which follow are concerned mainly with the problems of adapting the vast old multi-storied industrial and warehousing spaces which reflect our past economic structure for organisations and working processes more in keeping with our future economic profile.

2.00 What are the problems of the inner city?

Physical decay is a visible and demoralising aspect of our inner cities. The urban landscape is like a Gruyère cheese pitted with empty sites and derelict buildings. The decay of the environment is demoralising not only for those who live and work there, but as a symbol of the waste of the nation's resources.

2.01 Discarded buildings
Our major industrial cities are full of empty industrial

buildings, most of which are too large for the type of tenants attracted to the inner city. London alone has well over 2.2 million m² of vacant industrial space, 40 per cent of which is in buildings over 5,500m². In the London Borough of Hackney and Islington there is approximately 1 million m² of vacant industrial and commercial floor space, some 20 per cent of the total floor space available, or the equivalent of 1 in 5 factory buildings standing empty. The decline of heavy manufacturing and the textile industry in the north west has led to similarly high levels of vacancy. On Merseyside the redundant dock buildings if laid end to end (which many of them are) would stretch for over 3 miles. The once thriving centre for multi-national plants, Kirkby Industrial Estate, has 150,000m² of empty industrial floor space, and the closure of British Leyland's plant at Speke brought 145,000m² of floorspace on to the market. In the West Yorkshire county area where the textile industry was based there is approximately 1 million m² of industrial space on the market of which over 330,000m² is in mill property. Oldham alone has thirteen empty mill buildings which account for 11,000m² of space.

The high rate of vacancy is the most obvious sign of the changes that have occurred in the economies of our inner city areas. Discarded industrial buildings are due largely to three factors.

Changes in planning
Firstly large tracts of the inner city stand in limbo where local authorities compulsorily purchased land for comprehensive redevelopment or road widening schemes, which have now been shelved. The weed-filled open spaces, and isolated industrial shells of Sheffield, Liverpool and Derby are the result of a planning change of heart, not war damage.

Changes in location of large firms
Secondly, large manufacturing firms have moved to green field sites or declined and died. Between 1961 and 1976 employment in London fell from 1.4 million to under 90,000. The decline was caused by large multi-plant firms closing down their older inner city plants and transferring production to more efficient green field sites. Further incentives to move out of the inner city were provided by government grants, and earlier organisations like the Location of Offices Bureau (LOB) which argued that green field locations offered better conditions, lower cost premises, room for expansion, easy communications and access to a skilled workforce.

Changes in manufacturing
Finally, the country's manufacturing base is changing. Britain was the first country in the world to go through the industrial revolution, and is now one of the first to feel the effects of moving into a different era. The country is passing through a period where the scale of manufacturing is changing, and new energy sources and materials are demanding new locations and processes. The impact of these changes has led to the closure of large industrial complexes and a movement of skilled labour, leaving behind the less skilled in areas with declining economies and vacant vandalised buildings. Parallel with the decline in manufacturing have come technological changes in distribution. The rise in imports since

the 1960s has increased the need for modern warehousing facilities. At the same time service industries such as central and local government, insurance and banking have expanded demanding central city office space.

2.02   Declining neighbourhoods
Run down, shabby buildings breed run down economies. URBED (Urban and Economic Development Group) in a study for the OECD described the typical stages in the decline of a commercial area[4]. Decline starts with plant closures and the loss of personal income through loss of earnings and public income through rates. This leads to the decay of the building and environmental blight. These in turn make the area off-putting to those still living or working there, which deters any private investment and conditions continue to deteriorate.

A closer study of the spiralling effect of vacancy shows that:

• Closures lead to higher unemployment, lower disposable incomes and hence a declining trade for shops and other local services.

• A contracting rate base puts increased financial pressures on the local authority, so that those with the most vacant premises may be least able to afford to take action; alternatively rates must be raised and an extra burden is imposed on the firms that remain.

• When buildings are due to be vacated, maintenance ceases; the longer a building is unused the more it deteriorates; vandalism and the elements put up the cost of rehabilitation.

• As buildings decay, so the neighbourhood begins to look dilapidated, and becomes visually depressing; the problem can be aggravated as non-conforming uses such as panel beaters and junk yards appear.

• A run down environment encourages the breakdown of respect for property; crime and vandalism are common, and conflict may occur between the original occupants who have been unable to move as the area changed, and the 'newcomers'.

• Once firms in an area have stopped investing and new firms are not moving in, it soon looks as if the 'economic tide is going out' owners begin to 'milk' their companies if they cannot sell them as going concerns.

• Outside investors are reluctant to invest in a location whose future seems unsure. The more buildings that are vacant, the greater the risks will be for any new investment.

Until fairly recently the problem of isolated empty buildings could be dealt with on an ad hoc basis, through community action or individual enthusiasm. Today the malaise has spread. Decaying areas and declining local economies require more organised initiatives.

2.03   Unbalanced economy
The country's traditional reliance on well-established large companies in heavy manufacturing, is changing. The high cost of labour and overheads had led to:

• The decline of manufacturing and the increase of distribution and assembly functions; imports mainly of manufactured goods rose from 10 per cent of the GNP in 1960 to 25 per cent in 1978.

- A change in skills from heavy manufacturing to light industrial and assembly.

- An increase in service industries and office work; as manufacturing has contracted, large offices have expanded in areas such as banking, insurance and central and local government.

- A move away from old established large scale, hierarchical firms, to smaller more flexible organisations, or decentralised large organisations with greater ability to adapt to changing technology and markets.

Small firms could play a vital part in the revival of both our inner city areas and the economy at large. The city would benefit from the fact that small firms use space and labour intensively and provide a balanced economy, the nation would benefit from the increased innovation and supply of specialised goods which help us to compete internationally. Britain however is lagging behind other western economies in the vitality of its small firms sector. The UK share of the number of small firms per head of population is smaller than that of other industrialised countries. Germany has 40 per cent more small firms per head of population and the USA has two or three times the birth rate and only one quarter the death rate of small firms in the UK. For the tiny firms (below 10 people) the comparison is even more alarming. Why has the UK fallen behind other countries? The reasons often given are government regulations stifling initiative, the UK tax structure and the high cost of finance.

However, we are now seeing a swing in favour of small-scale enterprise. The last two governments have both appointed ministers responsible for the small firm sector. Each budget has made some concessions to small firms' financial problems.

Incentives have been initiated to provide more suitable premises. The growth of the 'alternative society', small-scale technology and the industrial common ownership movement all point towards a concern for individual small working units. Even within large firms there is now a trend towards the growth of small autonomous work units.

Small firms cumulatively make up a large sector of the employment market[5]. In manufacturing 94 per cent of all the firms fall into the small firm category and employ 21 per cent of the total manufacturing workforce. Of the small firms a large proportion are 'very small' firms employing below 50 persons and reusing premises of less than say $1400m^2$. The emphasis in this book is on providing small units of accommodation for firms that have a high density of employment (up to $15m^2$ per person), a relatively low level of servicing and handle small high value added components.

Taken as an aggregate small firms are an essential part of our economy and offer many advantages.

Advantages to the consumer
- Greater flexibility and responsiveness than the larger firm.
- Possibly a cheaper service.
- Great resilience, flexibility and less vulnerability and disruptions. Such as industrial action.

- An important source of innovation, developing new products or services that large companies may suppress or ignore.

Advantages to staff
- The benefits of better co-operation between management and workers.
- An opportunity to learn a trade, take greater responsibility and have direct contact with all aspects of the firm's work.

Advantages to the overall local economy
- The benefits of stability; the economic fortunes of one large firm may have a disastrous effect on an area, whereas the passing of several small firms can be assimilated more easily.
- The diversity created by different types of firm creating a wide variety of products.

2.04 Inadequate premises

Traditionally small firms in the City found accommodation in backyard sheds, mews spaces, underneath railway arches, and in the less attractive floors above shopping streets, (figure 1). With the comprehensive redevelopment of the late 1960s many of the sources of cheap accommodation were obliterated and a great number of small firms either withered away, or the more dynamic moved to factories in the new towns.

At about the same time large firms were finding that their inner city factories were unsuitable for new production techniques, badly located for deliveries, were becoming increasingly isolated from a skilled workforce and did not provide room for expansion. The result has been that during the last 10 years large firms have been steadily moving out of the central and inner city leaving behind large empty buildings, most of which are too big for the smaller tenant.

The main problems
The main problems relating to premises for small firms in the inner city are the size and location of the buildings available for conversion; the reluctance of established commercial developers to provide small units of accommodation; and the cramped and poor condition of existing units of accommodation.

The buildings available are often large and difficult to subdivide, have medium or short term leases and are located in areas of planning uncertainty which makes the financing of conversion work difficult. An in-depth evaluation by URBED[6] of the feasibility of reuse for small units of 13 vacant buildings in Hackney and Islington showed that the main stumbling blocks to conversion were the owners' 'hope value' for a change of planning use; poor access (all but 10 per cent of the sample had over 90 per cent site coverage); and high rehabilitation costs due to the length of time the buildings had stood empty.

Commercial developers are reluctant to provide small units of accommodation, which are seen by financial institutions and developers as:

- More risky, small firms being felt to be more vulnerable to failure, so making poor covenants.

- Less convenient to manage compared with a few large units.

● More expensive to develop.

● Less profitable and attractive than investing in new accommodation for pre-letting to large and reputable organisations.

Finally, the small units of accommodation that are available are cramped, have difficult access and are in very poor condition. The most frequently reported complaint by small firms in an industrial survey undertaken by the London Borough of Southwark[7] was the run-down nature of the buildings, followed by problems of access, delivery space and room for expansion. These attitudes are borne out by a JURUE (Joint Unit for Research on the Urban Environment University of Aston, Birmingham) survey[8] for the DoE of the industrial stock of Birmingham which concluded that '61 per cent of the firms . . . considered inadequate premises to be one of the most important problems they face, mentioning it as often as difficulties with labour supply. The most common criticisms that industry makes of its premises are of lack of space, either in the building (20 per cent of all firms in Birmingham) or on the site as a whole (17 per cent of firms); poor goods vehicle access, insufficient parking; the age of the buildings; and the difficulties of using multi-storey premises'.

3.00 What are the opportunities?

High levels of vacancy are not necessarily an indication of lack of demand. Studies have shown that the high level of vacant buildings is largely to do with the size of units available, planning uncertainty, problems of access and the cost of rehabilitation due to the condition of the building fabric. Recent experience suggests that with the right sized units the demand exists. The URBED survey for the Hackney and Islington partnership recognised a significant decline in the rate of vacancy in the two boroughs. Within one year (1979) the number of vacant buildings of over 2000m² reduced from 50 to 13 buildings. Of these between a half and two thirds had been rehabilitated, many of them for multiple use by small firms, and the remainder demolished.

In Islington between 1976 and 1980 the number of vacant buildings fell by 60 per cent and the amount of vacant floor space by 29 per cent, suggesting a greater demand for smaller properties.

3.01 The potential demand
It now seems apparent that a potential demand for inner city premises exists from:

● New firms, who have traditionally grown up in inner city areas, where they were close to their customers and suppliers, had an available labour pool and could find cheap second-hand premises. The inner city still continues to offer the most attractive environment for embryo and infant enterprises. But suitable sized premises at the right prices are lacking.

● Established firms, who are unable to expand or reorganise due to the cramped conditions of their existing premises. If the right sized and quality premises existed on the market existing firms might move, relinquishing small units of cheap 'second-hand' space for starter firms. A recent indust-

rial survey by the London Borough of Islington of 467 firms showed that 21 per cent of the firms felt their present premises were too small.

● Branch plants, of larger organisations who during the 1960s moved to green field sites. The trend to decentralisation has begun to reverse as large companies have realised the value of a location close to sources of decision making, academic institutions, and centres of international exchange. Several studies have shown a demand for units of accommodation below 250m² for firms in services, assembly or component manufacture.

3.02 Multi-storied buildings
Inner city multi-storey industrial space, compared with the green field single-storey facility, is normally viewed as being inadequate for new efficient firms. It is felt to be constraining for modern factory layouts and efficient materials handling techniques.
The argument propounded against the multi-storey inner city factory is that it does not provide a floor to ceiling height suitable for modern goods handling techniques and large uninterrupted spaces for flow line layouts. Perhaps these criteria are no longer so relevant. The pattern of our industrial base is changing, with a greater emphasis on firms that:

● Produce products with a high value added, and small materials input.

● Are organised for one-off or batch production with small-scale sophisticated machinery in a clean, quiet and well-lit environment.

Typically these firms may be in electronics, instrumentation, or the assembly of high technology equipment. The environment is more akin to an office environment than traditional industry, with less demand for the control of pollution, heavy vehicle access, storage and long production lines. Major concerns will be locational: to find attractive environments, close to amenities and in buildings with a human scale.

An American study[10] on the industrial potential of the central city suggests that for certain industries multi-storey industrial buildings can provide:

● Greater flexibility due to the fact that if a firm is in a multi-occupancy building it can probably expand within the building, whereas in a suburban single-occupancy factory a firm wishing to expand may only do so by building additional space or moving.

● Higher intensity of use; a comparison of firms of a similar industrial type in urban and suburban locations showed a reduction in the space required by the firm with the city location, due to a reduction in storage requirement as a result of a greater frequency of deliveries.

● Reduction in site coverage and therefore balancing out of overall occupancy costs; the urban firm, due to its centralised location, does not rely on the provision of staff and visitors' car parking to the same extent as the suburban location.

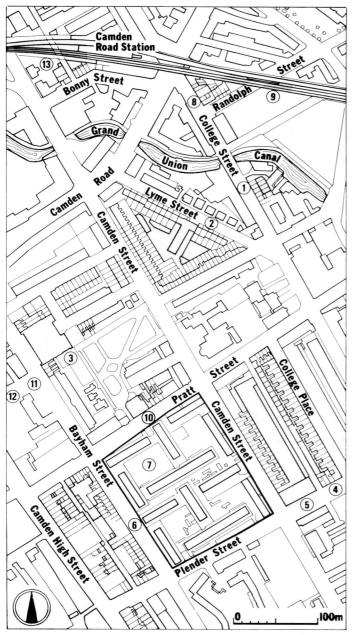

Figure 1 *Traditional accommodation for small industrial firms (Camden, London).*

The traditional type of accommodation used by small industrial firms in the London area is all too often, quite frankly, appalling – damp, cold, cramped, with layout and materials handling problems.

Perhaps most satisfactory is the railway arch. Surprisingly spacious, capable of insulation and generally cheap, with adequate access and yard space: suits car repair firms and manufacturers using noxious processes, such as metal founders. Mews units remain in use (particularly in the clothing district of London's Fitzrovia); but their small size does not allow for expansion by a successful enterprise, and access for delivery vans or essential car-users is notoriously difficult. Backland factories have the same problems and tenants may find the problems of moving goods across different floor-levels, or installing machines in triangular-shaped machine shops, insuperable. For small concerns, requiring up to 300m^2 and employing 20 or so workers, the conversion of large, old, multi-storey buildings may provide the most successful accommodation. For instance, in London's Camden area, former piano factories (once the major local manufacturing industry, but now almost dead) now house a great variety of small manufacturers, warehousemen and repairers. Modern lifts have been installed, services renewed where required and redecoration carried out. The letting rent of £12.50m^2 suits most small firms.
Norman Beddington
Secretary, Camden Industrial Action Group

Examples of re-used buildings in London's Camden area

1 Mid-Victorian terrace houses with associated buildings:	Craft joiners, silkscreen printers, shop and interior decorators, joinery contractors.
2 Victorian piano factory:	Let off floor by floor to clothing manufacturers.
Miscellaneous out buildings in mews:	Hospital contractor, pipe manufacturers, metal sculptor.
3 Purpose built factory (1940s):	Precision engineers employing 140; foundry (entrance at rear).
4 Mews workshop buildings (turn of the century):	Some let individually or in pairs. Clothing manufacturer, fabric printers, piano reconditioners. About half refitted and used as offices by Camden Council.
5 Turn of the century depository:	Divided along its length into units for clothing manufacturers. Largest unit (including corner building and impressive frontage to Camden Street) let to theatrical costumiers.
6 Miscellaneous mews buildings; some still connected through shops onto Camden High Street:	Mainly car body repairs but also: laundry, small precision engineers, clothing manufacturers.
7 Curnock Street Estate, circa 1965, displaced 16 small firms (mostly manufacturing):	1 or 2 firms relocated in the area.
8 Victorian shop (flats above):	Clothing manufacturer.
9 Railway arches and adjoining yards:	Car body repair shop, coach works.
10 Late Victorian factory:	Dress model manufacturers or stockists.
11 Victorian warehouse:	Mostly empty (advertised for offices). Part taken by office/warehouse for bookshop headquarters.
12 Three-storey Victorian workshop mews building:	Mainly clothing manufacturers, small (original) glazing contractor.
13 Under railway arches and assorted buildings behind Surrey Street:	Garage for taxi firm, repair garages, small contractor, clothing manufacturer.

● Optimum production line layouts on each floor of a very large multi-storied building in effect creating a number of single storey factories in the air.

A relevant review[11] of 14 buildings successfully converted for multiple use in the boroughs of Hackney and Islington showed all of them to be over two storeys, 75 per cent of them being above three floors.

3.03 Mixed use developments
Old buildings grow and mature with time. Unlike new buildings which tend to have simple forms, the old industrial stock is more complex in form, with varying shaped spaces. The Covent Garden area in London where small-scale residential buildings have expanded on the lower floors to provide larger workshop or commercial spaces is typical of such developments[11]. The buildings consequently have become complex in section, with different depth spaces on each floor (figure 2).

The potential asset of an inner city location is the complexity of its building stock, which provides a variety and character that seems impossible to recreate in slab blocks where each building contains one one space type and form is constrained by a multitude of statutory requirements. To maximise this asset mixed uses may be developed, where the requirements of each use are matched to the character of the space available. Imagination and sympathetic rulings by planners could allow for new combinations, such as:

● Marts, where the role of display, education, manufacture and selling are integrated.

building types	form	%age of buildings	%age of buildings with ground floor over 130m²
simple (single type of space)		66	34
complex (variety of types of space)		34	61

Figure 2 *Sectional form of Covent Garden buildings*

● Working and living communities where the workshop, the residence, the outlet and training become combined.

● Community centres where recreation, education, social welfare and work merge.

● Job training centres and new enterprise workshops.

American examples
Perhaps due to planning conditions, imaginative mixed use developments are still rare in this country[13]. In North America recycled buildings have provided the home for existing mixed use schemes such as Ghirardelli Square in San Francisco and Trolley Square, Salt Lake City that have become the cornerstone of downtown revitalisation programmes. Redundant buildings have also provided the physical setting for new organisational forms such as the 19th century factory in Utica which has been converted into a factory outlet mall – a collection of manufacturers' outlets sell consumer goods at discount[14]. In Boston, the Piano Craft Guild is a combination of housing, studios and community uses in an old piano factory. Perhaps the increasing interest of housing associations in industrial and commercial development will provide a way of developing similar opportunities in the UK.

4.00   What new initiatives exist?

The case studies of revitalised individual buildings and local industrial areas (in part III) present a picture of initiative and imagination often despite the constraints of bureaucracy and institutional attitudes. An analysis of the schemes shows a trend towards community initiatives, a more flexible approach to the provision of space and a concern for local economic issues.

4.01   New uses of space
Making the most effective use of vacant buildings and converting them economically has stimulated new thinking about the way that space can be subdivided. Initial conversion costs have been greatly reduced and flexibility increased by the use of moveable screens and storage units to define boundaries between firms with compatible activities which do not create noise or disturbance. In many cases the minimum space to be let may be the use of a desk with the support of secretarial services, conference room and telecommunications.
Empty buildings are frequently complex in section due to the fact that they have developed through additions over a period of years. The combination of both shallow and deep space may suggest a mix of users, and a number of successful schemes have combined office, workshop, display space and, in some cases, residential units. The Side Gallery in the Quays of Newcastle is a mixed use development in a complex of space off a public stair which includes living accommodation, a gallery and studio workshops.
Other schemes have achieved financial viability by providing a mix of both large and small units with varying levels of specification and access, marketed at different rentals. Westminster Bunting's development in the old AEI (Associated Electrical Industries) complex at Woolwich is a typical example of such schemes. Within one complex they provide a variety of rehabilitated or new accommodation for firms at different stages of development.
Finally, new approaches to the use of space have been generated by the necessity of finding viable ways of using buildings with short-life tenure. The demand to minimise building work, has forced tenants and building owners to accept different standards and rely on self-help. Waterside Workshops at Rotherhithe London, on a short-life lease from the Greater London Council, is communally managed by a dedicated group of craft firms who pay a flat rent independent of the amount of space used, have a corporate decision-making structure and undertake all the building work themselves.

4.02   Community enterprise
Recent experiments such as the Home Office's Community Development project have led to a growing awareness of the importance of a healthy local economy which allows people to earn a wage commensurate with their needs. With the use of funds available through Manpower Services Commission programmes, a number of community enterprise projects have arisen (table I). The objectives of such enterprises are to:

● Recycle profits either into the development of new enterprises (and so additional jobs) or into benefiting the local community.

● Create a trading organisation owned and controlled by the residents of an area, which can provide permanent jobs for local people in viable enterprises.

Such firms in their initial years will be fragile and need every assistance that can be provided by central and local government and the established business community.

4.03   Grass roots developers
Local economic planning has stimulated the desire for communities to develop the use of their major assets – land and buildings. Early experiments included the Bury St. Edmunds Town Development Trust[16] created in 1977 to redevelop a redundant hospital site and the North Kensington Amenity Trust which grew out of the fight by local residents in the late 1960s against motorway proposals. Today the Trust activities are varied and the prospects include the provision of new industrial units, a training trust and a £2.5 million project for shop and workshop units and community spaces. Much of the success was generated by the trust developing its only asset, wasteland blighted by the high level expressway.
Recently a number of local enterprise trusts have arisen

Table I   Community enterprises

Name	Product Service	Legal structure	Initiated by	Finance from	Other help from
Govan Enterprises	Multi-functional company: foodshop, cleaning, local market, home produced crafts.	Company limited by guarantee; controlled by residents; charitable status.	Study group of local people on unemployment brought together by Govan Area Resource Centre (GARC is a local community work agency).	Grant from British Shipbuilders to pay Business Development Manager; small grants from Gulbenkian and Rowntree Foundations; loan from GARC; local fund-raising.	Marks and Spencers (through Scottish Action Resource Centre) and Local Enterprise Advisory Project (an advisory agency established to help promote local and community enterprise in the West of Scotland).
Craigmillar Festival Enterprises Ltd	Multi-functional company: general building and contracting.	Company limited by guarantee with charitable status.	Employment working party of local tenants association (Craigmillar Festival Society).	Lothian Regional Council (grant for General Manager's Salary); Scottish Development Agency (loan); bank (overdraft); Craigmiller Festival Society.	Esso Petroleum (donation of site of disused petrol filling station); Bank of Scotland; Scottish Action Resource Centre.
Goodwill Incorporated Ltd	Renovation and sale of second-hand furniture and other goods.	Company limited by guarantee with charitable status.	Glasgow Council of Voluntary Service.	Urban Programme (Strathclyde Regional Council and Scottish Office); Manpower Services Commission (JCP and STEP); Local Industry.	IBM; Marks and Spencers; British Petroleum) Scottish Action Resource Centre; Strathclyde Regional Council; other companies in the West of Scotland.
Highlands and Islands Development Board	Government Agency which sponsors community cooperatives in the Highlands and Islands. Nine co-operatives so far set up include fish-farming, general stores, horticulture, knitwear, sheepskin rugs, building, plant-hire.	Community Co-operative (Industrial and Provident Societies Acts).	HIDB policy working through specially appointed field workers.	Locally raised capital matched £ for £ by HIDB; grant to pay General Manager plus administration (100% for three years, 50% for years 4 and 5); other grant and loan capital assistance for approved projects.	Local Community Education Project; local community leaders.
Telegraph Textiles Ltd	Clothing manufacture.	Workers' co-operative (using model rules of Industrial Common Ownership Movement).	Local people with support from Telegraph Hill Neighbourhood Council.	Lewisham Borough Council for feasibility study; Urban programme through Docklands Joint Committee for capital expenditure and wages costs.	URBED (Urban and Economic Development Ltd.); Lewisham Borough Council.
A Touch of Glass	Manufacture of tiffany (stained glass) lampshades.	Company limited by shares.	A businessman and a designer.	Manpower Services Commission (STEP Enterprise Workshop); personal loan; bank overdraft.	Local MP; British Overseas Trade Board.
House of Lambeth	Manufacture wood products.	Company limited by guarantee.	Lady Margaret Hall settlement.	Manpower Services Commission (STEP).	Rank Xerox; PA Management Consultants; Action Resource Centre; Lambeth Borough Council.
Kennington Office Cleaners Co-operative	Office cleaning service.	Worker's co-operative (using model rules of Industrial Common Ownership Movement).	Group of local women with support of community worker from Lady Margaret Hall Settlement.	Lambeth Borough Council (loan).	General and Municipal Workers Union.
Lambeth Industries Ltd	Provision of small scale workspaces for local enterprise, together with advisory and other services.	Company limited by guarantee.	Lady Margaret Hall Settlement and Lambeth Council Employment Promotion Officer.	Lambeth Borough Council (Inner City Partnership funds); Manpower Services Commission (STEP).	British Petroleum, London Enterprise Agency.

under the guidance of the Centre for Alternatives in Urban Development.

4.04   New patterns of building management
The provision of small units of accommodation has traditionally been frowned upon by institutional developers as creating undue problems of management. In the vacuum new forms of developers have arisen, and with them, new forms of building management.

The working community
David Rock, an architect looking for space in central London in 1972 for his small but growing architectural practice took over a derelict printing works of 2,000m^2 at 5 Dryden Street, Covent Garden[15] (figure 3) which he converted for multiple use for his practice and several other small firms with the idea they could collaborate on larger projects. From this proposal stemmed the concept of the 'working community' or compatible firms who through a limited

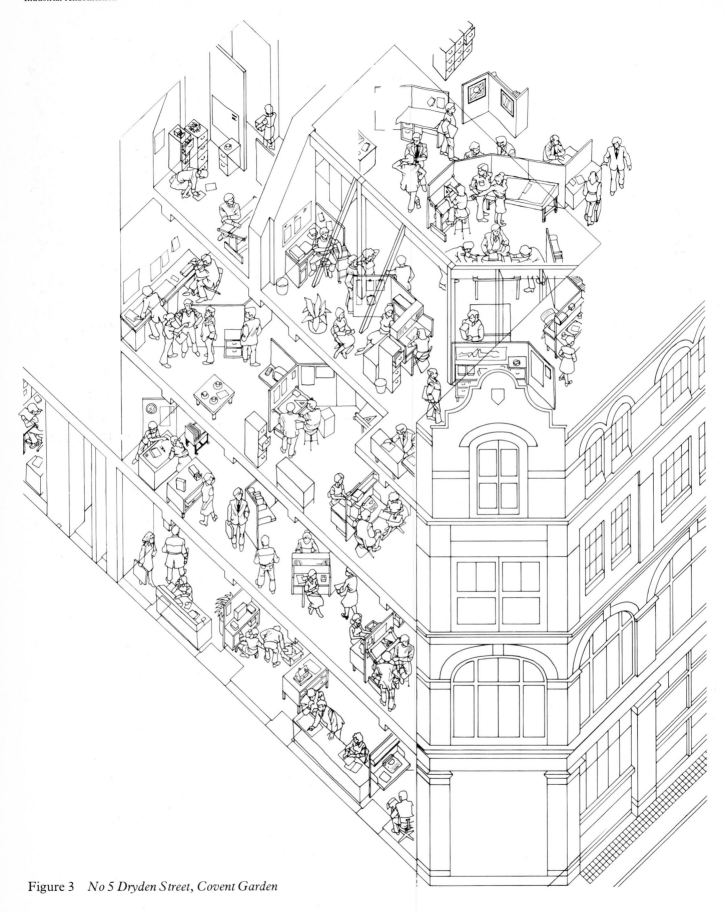

Figure 3   *No 5 Dryden Street, Covent Garden*

company manage a building and joint services. The participating firms take joint responsibility for the scope and quality of the scheme, and make sure that vacancies are kept to a

minimum. The success of 5 Dryden Street led to a more
ambitious project, the Barley Mow workspace, in the original Sanderson wallpaper factory at Chiswick. The scheme,

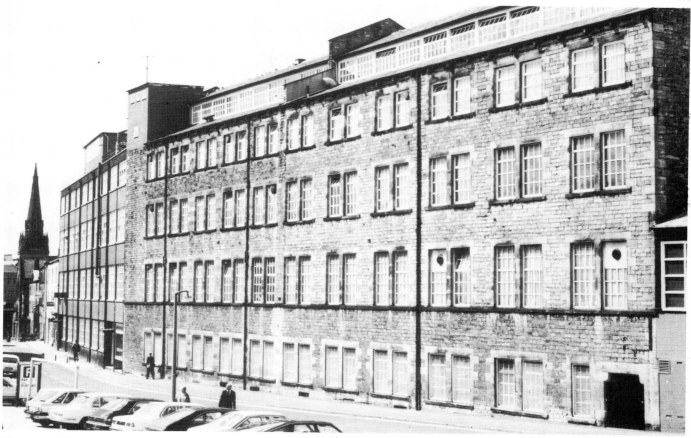

Figure 4 *Enterprise Lancaster*

with the potential to house over 250 people in a combination of offices and workshops includes as its common services a canteen, exhibition area and printing facilities.

Vertical industrial parks
In America the conversions of some of the larger redundant industrial buildings have been conceived as vertical industrial parks, each floor being leased as a site, with the marketing, management and servicing undertaken with the professionalism and dedication of a well-managed modern industrial estate.

Additional initiatives
Simply providing small premises may not be sufficient to foster new enterprises. To help the infant firm, and so indirectly assure the success of a multi-let venture, there are a number of additional initiatives that can be taken such as:

● Setting up a 'new enterprise network' where individuals with ideas, skills or products to offer can meet those with the necessary roles and management abilities; the concept is to provide an exchange for experience or under-utilised resources.

● Opening up markets; a central sorting house function that introduces the services and products of small firms opening up markets to large firms in the area.

● Providing training and assistance, in association with local academic institutions.

In a number of schemes local authorities have combined with large institutions such as voluntary organisations to provide space and support for new ventures. Enterprise Lancaster (figure 4) is a joint venture between Lancaster borough council and the university. The scheme is conceived as an incubator environment for high technology firms developing out of academic research, and provides management and technical support.

The community of St. Helens Trust Limited initiated by Pilkingtons is now well established. In areas suffering from steel closures, the British Steel Corporation (BSC) through an associate company BSC Industries has striven to create small industrial units to provide opportunities for their redundant employees.

5.00 What role can the professional play?

All these initiatives demand commitment from individuals to help themselves, and the support of the business community, government and the voluntary sector.
The professional designer who wishes to work in this field requires skills that are more those of the community worker, fund raiser, manager and space planner and he or she should be prepared to:

● Look for buildings with fresh eyes, tailoring architectural solutions and the organisation of building work to the limited budget of his client, and the local resources that may be available.

● Produce advice sometimes outside his architectural knowledge but based on his commonsense and experience;

11

as a designer he should have the ability to see strategic possibilities, as well as the short-term tactical demands, and clearly define and express these issues for decision taking.

● Work directly with those involved with the project, transferring his experience to the site layout and project management team while at the same time learning from them.

● Become the initiator of conversion projects, involving himself with finding the finance, attracting tenants and setting up a constituency as the project continues.

● Reappraise his methods of working and contractual procedures to more accurately reflect his clients' needs. With limited funds and time available the client may wish to do as much for himself as possible, looking to his architect to define the issues and provide the technical support.

Three areas in which the architect may contribute are:
1 by becoming directly involved with setting up and managing a project for the multiple use of an old redundant building.
2 the architect can provide direct support and professional advice to local community groups and undertake feasibility studies. A number of chambers of commerce and voluntary associations are now beginning to explore ways they can help the small firm.
3 architects may become actively involved with the running of building preservation trusts. In the same way that professionals were instrumental in starting the first housing associations, so the same role could apply to the development of industrial accommodation through 'industrial housing associations'.

The role of the architect is not obvious. The majority of the examples of conversions included in this book have been done on a shoestring, without professional advisers. The success of a project relies more on the correct choice of location and building, and a viable scheme for financing, than on attractive details. However, there is scope for professional input in understanding the regulations, and making correct strategic decisions so as not to close off future options. With limited funds and time available the client may wish to do as much for himself as possible, looking to his architect to define the issues and provide the technical support.

2 The Nature of Small Enterprises

1.00 Introduction

1.01 The importance of the small firm
The importance of the small firm sector to our economy is its diversity. Very small firms have within their ranks newly formed firms some of whom might grow to become flourishing organisations, others of whom might not survive; firms who rely on innovation and speed of response to stay in the market place; and craft-orientated enterprises whose satisfaction is gained from providing a good product. The needs of small firms are notoriously difficult to assess. It is common to think of offices and factories as distinct building types, and manufacturing and service industries playing distinct roles, yet anyone who has had dealings with firms employing less than say 10 people will know that they are extremely hard to categorise.

2.00 Different types of small firm

Until recently, most data on small firms came from the report of a Committee of Inquiry on Small Firms chaired by John Bolton and presented in 1971 (The Bolton report, 1971, HMSO)[1]. However, the present emphasis on regenerating inner city areas and creating jobs has led to the publication of several surveys (see bibliography) which enable one to be far more precise on the nature and needs of small firms. The Bolton report characterised firms in terms of employment, eg, under 200 employees in manufacturing, or in terms of turnover (see table I). It also defined the characteristics of small firms as follows:

- Their share of the market is usually relatively small.

- They are usually managed by owners, or part-owners, in a personalised way.

- They are independent, in the sense of not forming part of a larger combine that dictates policy.

Within this broad category, some important distinctions can be made in terms of the *type of industry*, the *function*, and the *size* of the firms concerned. The term industry can be used to refer to the stage in the production or distribution of wealth which starts with mining or quarrying (primary)

through manufacturing (secondary) and finally ends in wholesale and retail distribution, including service (tertiary). Other business services such as insurance (quaternary), construction and transport provide support at all stages, (figure 1).

2.01 Differences in terms of industry
According to the findings of the Bolton Committee the majority of small firms are engaged in the manufacturing (secondary) and retailing (tertiary) sectors of industry. About 55 per cent of the firms employing less than 200 are in five main manufacturing sectors, (table II).

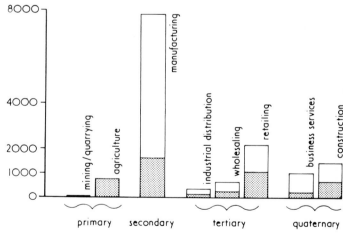

Employment (private sector) in the four stages of activity

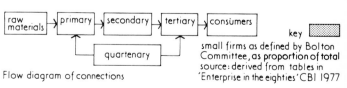

Flow diagram of connections

key

small firms as defined by Bolton Committee, as proportion of total
source: derived from tables in 'Enterprise in the eighties' CBI 1977

Figure 1 *Distribution of enterprises into primary, secondary, tertiary and quaternary industry in the UK. The graph indicates the number of enterprises in each and the number which are small enterprises – shown by the dot tint. Small firms employ most people in manufacturing and retailing.*

Table I   Small firm sector as defined by Bolton Committee

Industry	Definition adopted by the committee	% of firms in the industry* 1963	% of total employment 1963	1971	Average employment 1963
Manufacturing	200 employees or less	94	20	21	25
Retailing	turnover £50 000 pa or less	96	49	48	3
Wholesale trades	turnover £200 000 pa or less	77	25	37	7
Construction	25 employees or less	89	33	44	6
Mining/ Quarrying	25 employees or less	77	20	49	11
Motor trades	turnover £100 000 pa or less	87	32	32	3
Road transport	5 vehicles or less	85	36	40	4
Catering	All excluding multiples and brewery-managed public houses	96	76	75	3

Source: Reports on the Censuses of Production and Distribution and other official inquiries (and Research Unit Estimates). 1971 figures from *Enterprises in the eighties*, published by the CBI.
*For instance, 94 per cent of all firms in the manufacturing industry employ fewer than 200 people.

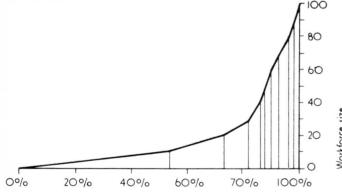

Figure 2   *Most small firms are very small, employing under 25 people, (Thus in Southwark over 50 per cent of the firms employed under 10 people, well over 75 per cent employed under 50 (source: Southwark Industry Survey).*

Manufacturing industries where small firms are dominant are:

● Those producing relatively simple semi-durable consumer goods where tastes vary or change often, eg clothing, furniture.

● Those producing specialist capital goods or components eg mechanical engineering, metal goods.

The most common opportunities for the new firm in manufacturing are:

● Where a large firm can no longer supply a product or component for which there is a small but assured demand eg very specialised applications.

● Where demand and technology are changing faster than large firms can adapt eg micro-electronics.

● Where the economies of scale are small and the barriers to entry low eg clothing.

● Where the entrepreneur applies a craft skill on his own rather than being part of a company.

● Where the entrepreneur can obtain key resources more economically than established firms eg employing his family, or taking over a bankrupt firm.

● Where the entrepreneur can perform a specialised service which increases the manufacturer's efficiency eg warehousing or stock-holding.

2.02   Differences in terms of function
It is also possible to distinguish between functions within industries. Firstly, the individual firm may carry out all or any of the following activities under one roof: manufacturing, storage, distribution, retail and office functions. Secondly, firms vary according to the market segment they are in; for example, ladies' fashion goods are hand-made in small East End workshops, whereas underwear may be mass-produced in large Northern factories. These distinctions, however, do not describe very precisely the functions carried out in a set of premises by a particular firm. Hence for planning purposes a different set of categories is

Table II   The five main manufacturing industries employing fewer than 200 people

	% of output of all small firms*	% of total output of sector accounted for by firms with less than 200 workers†	Floor space per worker (m²) in Southwark	in Sheffield	Labour intensity man-hours per £ of output
Mechanical engineering sector	15.0	24.5	57.3	23.9	0.67
Metal goods not specified elsewhere	12.3	37.7	84.3	23.9	0.58
Paper, printing, publishing sector	11.0	25.3	50.4	15.1	0.52
Timber and furniture sector	10.0	54.3	43.1	54.4	0.59
Clothing and footwear sector	6.0	35.4	24.1	97.7	0.63
All manufacturing	100.0	18.8	52.0	34.3	0.59

* For instance, small firms in the 'clothing and footwear' sector account for 6 per cent of the total output of all small firms. Only the five leading manufacturing sectors are listed here and their aggregate output adds up to 54.3 per cent of the total – the remainder is account for by sectors not included in the table.
† For instance, firms of fewer than 200 people in the 'timber and furniture' sector produce 54.3 per cent of the total output in timber and furniture.

required, which takes some account of the use made of the premises. These include:

Office (administration)
Industry (processing goods or materials)
Warehousing (storage)
Showroom (display)
Commercial (sales).

The problems arise when one then tries to relate these functional categories to small firms in a specific way. For to survive, small firms have to be both versatile and specialised. Some small firms want to combine nearly all the possible functions in one place, while others will specialise in different functions with the street acting as a conveyor belt.
It is hard to deduce accommodation requirements simply from functional category, without knowing more about the businesses concerned. For example, small warehouses may employ as many staff per square metre as manufacturing (as a survey carried out by the London Borough of Hammersmith revealed), while even the same industry, such as furniture, can vary enormously from the traditional craftsman carving with hand tools to the production line factory.

2.03 Differences in terms of size

A further distinction we need to make relates to *size*. There is an important difference between firms with a management tier and those without. Within the small firm sector there are important differences between:

● Very small firms (below 50 employees, where the office will typically be a separate but integral part of the factory).

● Tiny firms (below 10 employees, where the distinctions between activities are blurred).

Analysis of the employment returns available to local authorities can provide a useful review of the profile of small firms in a given area. For instance in the London Borough of Southwark[2] there are 2550 manufacturing firms of which only 100 have more than 100 employees (figure 2). Within the small firm category nearly 90% of firms are very small and over half are tiny.
Though the larger firms will of course employ proportionately more of the population and occupy more of the space, they concern us less than the smallest firms, some of whom have the greatest growth potential (most large firms started small), the greatest problems and are most suited to being accommodated in old buildings. (table III).

2.04 Classification of work

Differences in type of work
Companies may be classified into groups according to the finished goods that they produce. This is termed the Standard Industrial Classification (SIC) Table IV lists the SIC industrial categories with a high proportion of small firms and ranks them according to density of employees. Within one SIC category firms may vary greatly[3] in their demands depending on size and degree of mechanisation. For example, within the clothing sector, a small firm may have a high density of employees each working at an independent machine, on small batch orders which are collected daily. In

Table III Types of small firms that may be found in converted premises (based on inquiries received by Stockport industrial liaison officer).

Employment Sector	Typical uses	Accommodation type	Average density of employment
Offices	Branch bank Professional offices Brokers Agents Research groups Consultants Pressure groups	Professional suites Studio 'Shop front'	11.5m² per person
Service industry	Car repair Electrical repair Builder Engineering contractor Shoe repairer Appliance repairer Instrument repairer Reprographic	Workroom Workshop 'Shop front'	15.0m² per person

Manufacturing	Engineering
	  Metal fabricators
	  Forgers
	  Anodisers
	  Sheet metal workers
	  Blacksmiths
	  Polishers
	Optical goods manufacturers
	Furniture fabricators
	Jewellers
	Clothing manufacturers
		'Shop front'
		Workrooms
		Workshops
		Factory
			28.0m² per person

Distributive trades	Components Builders merchants Timber yards Publishers (Book distributors) Antiques Electrical suppliers	'Showroom' Warehouse Depot	80m² per person

contrast the large clothing manufacturer may be highly automated on a 'production line' both manufacturing and storing orders for weekly delivery. Each firm will have different premises requirements.
Density of use may vary according to the number of employees or amount of machinery or storage. Uses with a high employee to floor ratio have critical demands for means of escape, wc provision etc, whereas firms with fewer employees but more machinery may create specific demands on floor loading, fume extraction and servicing. Density of use significantly affects the match between usage and building. Shallow depth buildings (10–15m deep) are most suitable for firms requiring small cellular spaces and having a high density of staff, whilst deep spaces (20m and above) are best suited for organisations which require the minimum separation between activities or have a high proportion of machinery or storage which does not require natural light.

Table IV Industries with a high proportion of small firms ranked according to density of employees

Standard Industrial Classification category / Description	Density (Average area per worker m²)	15 to 30m²	30 to 50m²	50 to 100m²	100 to 250m²	250 to 500m²	500 to 1000m²	Work organisation (Unit/Batch/Process manufacturing; Individual/Group office)	Demand on building (Noise/vibration, Smell, Fumes, Heating, Lighting, Water and waste, Ventilation, Power)	Demand on site (Site coverage, Parking, Deliveries, Storage, Work area)
XV [Clothing and footwear] 442 Men's and boy's tailored outwear; 445 Dresses, lingerie, infants wear; 446 Hats, caps and millinery; 450 Footwear	11		●			●	●	Unit and Batch	Noise, heat and smell from presses. Artificial lighting at workplaces	100 per cent coverage. Deliveries. Refuse
XXI [Insurance, banking, finance] and business services] 860 Insurance brokers; 862 Financial brokers; 864 Advertising and market research; 865 Business services	13				●	●	52	Group	Normal office demands. Access for visitors	100 per cent coverage. Parking
XXV [Professional and scientific] 876 Research and development; 879 Other professional services	15.75	●	●	●	●			Individual Group	Normal office demands. Lab/bench services and waste disposal	100 per cent coverage. Parking. Deliveries
IX [Electrical engineering] 364 Radio and electronic components; 365 Sound reproducing equipment; 367 Radio radar and capital goods	17·5		●	●				Batch	Artificial light needed. Sedentary work	100 per cent coverage. Deliveries. Parking
VIII [Instrument engineering] 352 Watches and clocks; 353 Surgical instruments and appliances; 354 Scientific instruments	19.25		●	●				Batch	Artificial light at workplace. Sedentary work	100 per cent coverage
V [Chemicals and allied industries] 271 Manufacturing chemicals; 276 Synthetic resin, plastics and rubber	20.50							Process	Smells or fumes produced. Special services needed	40 per cent coverage. Deliveries. Storage of goods. Refuse
XIX [Other manufacturing] 491 Other rubber goods; 493 Brooms and brushes; 494 Toys, games, children's carriages; 496 Plastic products; 499 Musical instruments	23.50				●	●		Batch, Process	Smells and dust produced. Special services needed	50 to 100 per cent coverage. Deliveries. Refuse
XIV [Leather goods and fur] 432 Trunks, handbags etc	24.00			●				Unit, Batch	Smells dust produced. Natural light needed. Refrigeration needed	100 per cent coverage. Parking. Deliveries
XII [Metal goods] 390 Small tools; 392 Cutlery, spoons, etc; 396 Jewellery; 399 Forgings, pressing, stamping	24.25				●	●	●	Batch	Smells, fumes, dust heat, waste disposal. Special loadings	60 to 100 per cent coverage. Deliveries
XIII [Textiles] 418 Manufacturing lace products; 422 Made up textiles (canvas bags)	28.75									
XVIII [Paper, printing, publishing] 482 Packaging products; 483 Manufacturing stationery; 489 Printing and publishing of periodicals	32.50				●			Batch, Process	Heavy floor loading. Smells, noise, waste disposal problem	100 per cent coverage. Deliveries. Storage. Parking
XVI [Pottery and glass] 462 Pottery, china and earthenware; 463 Glass blowing	36.75				●			Unit	Heat, dust produced	60 per cent coverage. Deliveries. Parking
XXVI [Miscellaneous services] 894 Motor repairs; 895 Repair of boots and shoes; 899 Reprographic services	46.50	●	●	●	●			Unit	Smells, noise produced. Artificial light	100 per cent coverage. Parking
XVII [Timber and furniture] 471 Joinery work; 472 Manufacturing furniture upholstering; 474 Shop fitting; 479 Wood manufacturers	46.75	●					●	Batch	Dust, noise, power. Vibration. Heavy loading	60 per cent coverage. Deliveries. Storage

Table IV   Industries with a high proportion of small firms ranked according to density of employees—*continued*

Standard Industrial Classification category	Description	Density — Average area per worker (m²)	Size of unit						Work organisation — Unit (Manufacturing) / Batch (manufacturing) / Process (manufacturing) / Individual (office) / Group (office)	Demand on building — Noise/vibration / Smell / Fumes / Heating / Lighting / Water and waste / Ventilation / Power	Demand on site — Site coverage / Parking / Deliveries / Storage / Work area
			15 to 30m²	30 to 50m²	50 to 100m²	100 to 250m²	250 to 500m²	500 to 1000m²			
VII 349	[Mechanical engineering] Manufacturing machinery parts	62.50			●			●	Batch	Special services, power required Heavy loading	40 to 100 per cent coverage, Storoage Deliveries
XXIII 821	[Distributive trades] Wholesale distribution Retail distribution Bespoke tailors Repair of clothes and shoes Repair of electrical appliances Repair of cycles, watches etc	74.50	●	●	●	●	●			Heavy floor loading Mechanical handling may be required	40 to 100 per cent coverage Deliveries Storage Parking

Note on Table IV

Table IV shows a selection of industries with a high proportion of small firms. The industries are described by the Standard Industrial Classification and ranked according to the density of employees to floor area.

The Standard Industrial Classification provides a list of industry headings, and each of these are sub-divided into categories (minimum list headings). Repair work is either classified under manufacturing or distribution depending on where the bulk of the repair work is carried out. In special cases, such as motor and shoe repair which are regarded as services, these are classified under miscellaneous services.

When selecting probable uses for a building, table IV may be a useful guide in selecting a suitable range of tenant uses. For example, uses with a high employee to floor-space ratio (shown as density) will have critical demands for means of escape and numbers of WCs; while those with fewer employees but more machinery may create special requirements of floor loading, extract of fumes and servicing.

Density of use. The figures based on the Greater London Development Plan report of studies are the average gross floor area required per worker. They are an average for each industry and wide variations may be experienced between different sub-classes of activity. For instance within the timber and furniture sector the density of employment will vary widely between wood-turning firms producing small items and veneers and upholsterers.

Size of unit. These figures are based on returns to a number of industrial development officers and our own observations. The unit size refers to the floor area required per tenant, which may in turn be sub-divided into a number of enclosed spaces.

15 to 50m² units	Workrooms, studios, shops
30 to 250m² units	Workshops, office suites
100 to 1,000m² units	Factories, warehouses, offices, showrooms.

Work organisation. The way small firms use space and organise their work process is reflected in the density of employment and the amount of equipment they use.

Demand on building The firms being discussed have been limited to those without complex servicing requirements. This column gives a rough guide to the considerations that may apply when selecting suitable uses at the preliminary planning stages. Heating may vary from minimal background heat of 13°C for active uses to a heating level 20 to 22°C required for sedentary activities.

● Lighting, either natural or artificial, may be required with levels of up to 700 lux task lighting for precision work.

● Water and waste may vary from centralised facilities (wc and kitchen) to sinks at each workplace for firms dealing with chemicals.

● Ventilation may vary from the use of natural ventilation through requirements for local mechanical extract to full air conditioning without the use of central plant.

● Power through normal electric outlets or three-phase electricity.

● Special requirements, eg piped gases, overhead gantry, fume boxes, special floor loadings, disposal of 'effluents'.

● Demand on the site. Most small industrial firms have a demand for external space.

● Parking. Depends on the location, skill of labour force and importance of attracting visitors.

● Deliveries. Even the smallest manufacturer may have to take deliveries from large trucks, which will be improved by off-street parking and an adequate turning circle.

● Storage. Goods, raw materials or refuse.

Organisation of work

Work in the small firm may be organised in two ways:—

Workbench orientated, where each employee has his own desk or workbench, eg office work, component assembly, garment trade or jewellers

Equipment orientated, where employees move between a number of shared items of equipment, eg glass blowing, joinery shop, printing works.

For firms in the office sector, we adopt two classes of work-organisation types (table V):

Individual: where most employees work separately, and have small support staff.

Group: where employees work together in groups, often re-forming for each project.

Table V   Office firms classified in terms of work organisation

Staff work method	Key characteristics	Notes
Individual	Hierarchical Maximum sub-division Cellular offices	Individuals work separately with small group of supportive staff (eg law practice). or: Individuals work separately and come together to share information (eg research organisation).
Group	Non-hierarchical Open plan Interactive Changing groups	Staff work in project groups, which may change as new projects arise. Outside visitors.

Typically inner city industrial space is in multi-storied building with 75 per cent or more of the available space above ground level. Measured against today's modern concepts of flow line processes, bulk storage, and heavy goods vehicle deliveries, upper floors are seen as being inefficient. This argument tends to be borne out by the crude categorisations suggested by the SIC industrial categories. However, a more precise look at the nature of furniture manufacturing for example shows that in the small firms sector each part of the process involves a separate firm. This means that a turner of legs may operate on an upper floor whilst the veneerer requires ground floor premises.

3.00   Age of firm

The type of premises required depends not only on the particular industry or business involved, but also on its stage of development and expectations.

3.01   Evolutionary stages in a firm's needs
A useful distinction to make is the degree of control that a firm wants and can afford to exercise over its environments. A research project undertaken for the URBED Research Trust[5] distinguished a number of stages in the business life cycle, which were dubbed embryonic, infant, growing, established and institutional. As firms grow so they become more independent and can afford a wider choice of premises. If certain rungs on the premises ladder are missing (see chapter 4) businesses may become constrained or overstretched.

Embryonic stage
The embryonic stage is when the business is still an idea or a hobby. Most people start without much capital or confidence and want to minimize their commitments and obtain maximum support and encouragement. Where residential accommodation is plentiful, people often start in their garage, a spare room, or on the kitchen table. Their existing job provides security, while they try to establish the basis of a new business through 'moonlighting'.

Infant stage
The infant stage is when the business develops from a hobby or part-time interest into a venture that supports one or more self-employed people. It begins to own equipment, which takes up space, and a separate address may be required. A supportive environment close to other related firms is particularly important at this point. The infant can grow very quickly, and scope for expansion is important. This is often best provided in old buildings in run-down areas.

Growing stage
The growing stage is one where the supportive environment becomes less important, as the firm is more independent. Instead of sharing resources, the firm wants to be able to own them. The firm now wants self-contained rooms with its own entrance. It may start employing people on production, instead of sub-contracting the work, and will require better quality premises if it is to attract and retain staff.

Established stage
The established stage is the point where a certain level of inertia has been reached, and repeat orders enable the business to consider longer term questions, like owning their own premises. The need for easier access and a better image become important.

Institutional stage
The institutional stage is usually reached when the business becomes part of a group. At this point production often becomes divorced from administration, and the building begins to take on a symbolic as opposed to a functional purpose.

The definition of a series of stages does not mean however, that businesses necessarily pass from one to another. Many businesses, particularly those run by 'craftsmen' tend to remain personal enterprises and avoid taking on greater obligations. Others may try to grow and overstretch themselves.

4.00   Organisational style

4.01   The role of the entrepreneur
The growth of new firms is dependent on the presence of entrepreneurs prepared to take on the responsibility and risk. The entrepreneur is extremely hard to define, but is probably best explained by one of Britain's leading furniture makers, who described the true entrepreneur as someone with ideas and a lively high spirited nature, that leads to other people wanting to do things. He or she acts as a go-between, taking the risks involved in overcoming the credibility gap that any new enterprise must face.

Potential entrepreneurs
Potential entrepreneurs may come from a wide variety of backgrounds, and may include:

●Women who have spare time, or are frustrated by the limitations of conventional 'female jobs'.

●Redundant executives, particularly those who no longer have children or mortgages to support.

●Business graduates or those with advanced degrees who cannot obtain work with sufficient challenge or merit.

●Immigrants, particularly from East Africa and the USA, who are able to rely on networks of ethnic businesses.

●Idealists, such as teachers, community workers, architects and planners, who want to demonstrate the value of alternative life styles.

●Skilled craftsmen who have experienced redundancy and want to become independent.

●Employees in relatively safe jobs who see opportunities to make extra money.

●Inventors or designers who have developed a prototype which they cannot get anyone to manufacture.

4.02   Craftsmen and Opportunists
Entrepreneurs can generally be divided into two broad cate-

gories; *craftsman* (who may be an accountant or an architect and not just someone who works with his hands) is concerned primarily to employ himself or herself. The aim is for independence to practice a particular life-style, and so the craftsman avoids taking on responsibilities that might involve risks. By working with a partner, often a spouse, the craftsman can survive the ups and downs of the trade. In contrast the *opportunist* wants the satisfaction of having put together a deal, and the sense of achievement that comes from growth, whether in turnover, customers, employees or premises, as well as the usual trappings of business. The opportunist is much more likely to take risks.

Within the same industrial sector firms may be either opportunist or craft orientated, each requiring a difficult environment and location. Table VI analyses the accommodation requirements of three different industries at the early stages of their life cycle according to their style of organisation.

Table VI   The accommodation requirements of three different business activities in clothing, furniture and electronics according to their motivation and style of development

Type of Firm	Embryonic	Infant
Clothing		
Craft	Hand knitting, bespoke clothes with design input, screen printed fabrics, costumes	
	Work at home, adult education classes, community workshop, craft workshop	Working community Independent small studio
Opportunistic	Short runs of garments, fashion garments, silk screening on sweat shirts, and distribution	Garment batch production Distribution and co-ordination of outworkers Separate space in flatted factory.
	Spare room, garage, subleased space in established firm. Outworkers	Short life industrial building.
Furniture		
craft	Individual designed pieces, cabinet work and repair. Antique sales and repair.	
	Back yard, community workshop, new enterprise workshop, skill centre.	Independent workshop Working community
Opportunistic	Batch production of simple pieces. Second hand furniture.	
	Back yard. Short life shop.	Starter unit. Shop front.
Electronics		
Craft	Production of prototypes or components.	
	Adult education classes, technical college, front room	Flatted factory Working community
Opportunistic	Assembly and distribution of parts. Co-ordination of outworkers and mail order distribution.	
	Space in larger organisation. Innovation centre.	Warehouse. Starter units. Separate space in larger organisation.

5.00   The impact of firms on the local economy

5.01   The multiplier effect

If we consider the contribution to employment that each firm makes, we can see that the further down the production process the firm is, the smaller its own contribution to the total value of its product. The shop, for example, is an outlet for many people's labour. Hence what matters is not simply direct employment, but the indirect effects on trade through what economists call the local multiplier. This depends on how far the new business creates extra markets for local suppliers. For example, a self-employed designer might do no more than work under contract to a large firm outside the area, in which case the local multiplier would be small as all the spending power he influenced would go elsewhere. But if the designer developed prototypes, which he then had made locally, or helped existing firms improve their products, then the multiplier effects would be considerable. Each firm that he used would in turn spend extra money on goods and services which were in part supplied locally. It is therefore useful to distinguish between the direct employment and the turnover that results from a new business (see figure 3).

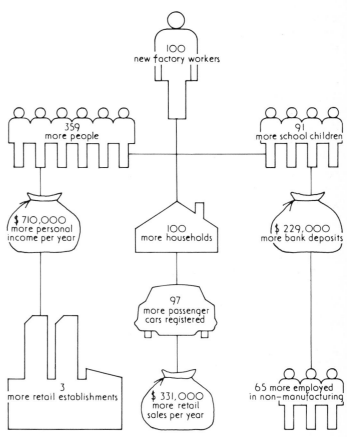

Figure 3   *An American interpretation of the local multiplier effect*

3 The Nature of Redundant Buildings

1.00 Alternative uses

1.01 Changing technology and the building stock
Our physical surroundings are built to last, but society and organisations are continuously changing. Britain in the 1980's is faced with a shift from the work ethic to the leisure ethic, from the world of mechanical power to that of microprocessors, and from a stratified to a classless society. As the technology and organisation of work changes, so do its locational, servicing and spatial demands. The result is that different building types are continuously becoming redundant as markets, cultural values and technology shift. With increased uncertainty planning becomes concerned with predicting future building types that may become redundant, and proposing alternative uses. Table I outlines the life cycle of a building, and the process of redundancy.

1.02 New uses for redundant buildings
When buildings historically become associated with specific functions, it is difficult to envisage alternative uses. Buildings become synonymous with users – the railway station, barracks, school or church. The cultural symbolism of the shape of a church may preclude its use as a warehouse. Preconceptions may be reduced and new opportunities exposed by publishing precedents of alternative uses.
Table II lists a range of possible new uses for building types where the original use has become inappropriate. The data was compiled by circulating local planning authorities in England for examples of buildings in their area where new uses had been accommodated.

1.03 Multiple tenancy conversions for small firms
As large manufacturing companies move out of their original inner city locations, they leave behind empty premises, often on restricted sites and with difficult access problems. The inner city continues to provide a stimulating environment for small firms, many of whom are new and may later grow large. These firms have a high density of employment (up to 15m^2 per person) and relatively unsophisticated production processes. Their accommodation demands are:

Small units (between 30–250m^2)
Low level of servicing
Access for medium sized and lightweight components or products.

An analysis of 14 successful conversions in Hackney and Islington suggests that buildings that are most attractive for use as multiple-tenancy conversions for small firms should have the following physical characteristics (turn to page 22):

Table I Typical life cycle of building

	Stage	Process	Results
1	Birth	New activity or new process is housed by building shell Degree of flexibility provided in design of building may vary	building user is accommodated
2	Expansion	Uses expand to meet new requirements New services introduced; Interior layout adapted	strain placed on fabric possible extensions adaptation
3	Maturity	Uses continue to fit building Or current needs exceed capacity	periodic maintenance and minor adjustments new space taken elsewhere or more extensions and re-planning
4	Redundancy	Change in: sources of power societies' cultural values market needs technology catchment areas	no maintenance; building in limbo application for permission to redevelop attempt at letting vandalism; fire or other damage decision to demolish
5	Rebirth/ demolition	Motivation to reuse. Variety of acceptable uses are matched with the building	building refurbished (whole/part) cycle continues

Table II   Redundant building types and possible new uses

Use category	Building type	Period	Characteristics Location	Configuration	Construction	% Site coverage	Possible new uses
1 Industrial Located near to markets, key sources: raw materials components labour energy	Foundries	C18-19	Urban	Complex	Brick and Timber	90	Light industrial units
	Mining and mineral workings	C17-20	Rural	Uneven ground	Mixed small and large buildings	40	Light industry, distribution haulage and building contractors, waste disposal
	Textile mills	C18-19	Urban and rural, sited near water	Multi-storey structures	Brick, stone, timber	60	Multiple light industrial units, crafts, offices, labs
	Breweries, maltings, oast houses	C18-19	Urban, semi-rural Water supply needed	Complex different processes Irregular profile	Brick, timber	60	Offices, light industrial units, craft centres, residential
	Factories	C19-20	Urban, town, rural	Irregular bays	Bricks, timber, steel, concrete	40 80	Light industrial units, polytechnic
2 Power production Located near centres of population and industrial activity	Water mills	C17-19	Mostly rural, towns by water	Complex irregular profile	Brick, stone, timber	50	Crafts and local centres residential
	Engineering houses, pumping stations	C18-19	Rural, urban,	Large, small and tall single-storey	Brick, timber	70	Theatre, concert halls, museums
	Gas works	C19	Urban + fringes	Complex mixed structures	Brick, steel	40	Industrial, distribution
	Power stations	C20	Inner city, urbanised areas	Large structures	Concrete, steel and light cladding	40	As above
3 Storage Located near transport facilities, primarily points of production and distribution	Warehouses	C18-20	Docks, rivers, canals, railways, produce	Regular bay, multi (and single) storey structures	Brick timber, steel	90	Very varied: crafts, light industrial units, arts centres, offices, residential, museums
	Depositories	C18-20	Cities + fringes	Regular bay, multi (and single) storey structures	Brick, timber, steel	90	Multi-light industrial units, craft workshops, distribution
	Barns	Medieval, modern	Rural (towns), farms	Single or two-storey	Brick, timber, concrete, asbestos	40	Crafts, light industrial, leisure, residential, community centres
	Sheds	C19-20	Urban and rural	Simple usually single storey	Brick, metal	70	As above
	Cold stores	C19	Urban	Heavy walled		90	Industrial
4 Transport Changes in technology have great physical effect	Railway viaducts, bridges	C19	Cities towns (Rural)	Regular compartments under arches	Brick	80	Light industrial units, storage, retailing
	Road viaducts, bridges	C20	Towns, rural	Regular compartments	Concrete	50	Light industrial community and leisure uses
	Railway stations	C19	Urban rural	Complex simple	Brick, stone, timber	80 40	Offices, workshops, light industrial, retailing
	Locomotive sheds Omnibus garages	C19 C20	Urban	Regular bay structures	Brick, timber, iron	80	As above
	Parking, garages (especially on residential estates)	C20	Urban	Single or two-storey structure	Concrete	60	Industrial units, additional residential (flats)
	Goods yards	C19	Urban, rural	Sprawling	Small structures	20	Industrial units
5 Military Emerge and grow during periods of military activity, national expansion, unrest Intermittent use over time	Ordnance factories	C18-20	Semi-rural	Variable	Mixed small and large buildings	40	Industrial units and redevelopment
	Barracks	C18-20	Town, rural	Cellular structures	Brick timber	60 30	Industrial units, storage distribution
	Forts	C18-19	Rural (urban)	Complex irregular	Massive:stone/ natural rock	50	Industrial units
	Airfields	C20	Rural (rural fringe)	Light structures	Brick, metal	20	Industrial units and redevelopment

continued on page 22

Table II Redundant building types and possible new uses—*continued*

Use category	Building type	Period	Characteristics Location	Configuration	Construction	% Site coverage	Possible new uses
6 Social Institution Emerge to suit needs and resources of current social and cultural values	Schools	C16-20	Urban, rural	Complex, simple	(Stone) brick, timber steel, concrete	80 30	Industrial units, arts centres, craft workshops, residential
	Churches	Medieval C20	Urban	Irregular profile large space	Stone (brick), timber	60	Storage, retailing, community centres, light industry, offices,
Increase with population growth, higher standards and services	Halls		Rural	Simple structure		30	Museums, arts centres, residential (if small)
Changes due to centralisation or larger catchment areas	Hospitals	Medieval C20	Urban, rural	Complex	Brick, timber	80	Residential, hostels, industrial
	Prisons	C18-20	Urban, rural	Complex	Stone, brick	60	Industrial
	Town halls	C19	City, town	Large space + smaller	Brick, timber	80	Showrooms, offices, higher education
7 Residential Living patterns change, related to social and cultural values	Tenements	C19	Urban	Cellular, multi-storey	Brick, concrete	70	Craft workshops and industrial units, other social groups
	Town houses	C17-20	Urban	Cellular, 3-4, storeys	Brick, timber	60	Very flexible: social institutions, offices
	Country houses	C17-19	Rural	Cellular, cluster	Brick, timber	30	Training centre, residential community/research centres
	Tower blocks	C20	Urban	Cellular	Concrete, brick, light cladding	50	Other residential groups eg student hostel

Access

Off-street parking and delivery
60 per cent site coverage or less
Good site access. Off main road, with two way street, with sufficient width for parking
5 minutes distance from tube and bus routes
Goods lift and wide stairways
Three or less floors.

Configuration

Three or four-way aspect
18 meters deep or less
(to allow natural light and ventilation)
Floor to floor height of 8–14ft (2.440–4.270m) on ground floor and 8–12ft (2.440–3.660m) on upper floors.

Structure

Frame construction
Concrete or brick.

Condition

Sound structural condition, wind and watertight, with only internal upgrading of finishes required.
Comply with statutory requirements (fire, public health etc.).

2.00 Matching uses to spaces

2.01 Mismatches can be expensive
There is a tendency to believe that a skilled designer can adapt almost any existing building to almost any new use, by judicious alterations to the fabric and services.
This is a dangerous assumption. Some spatial/structural types can be inherently unsuitable for certain categories of use and if designer and client become committed to adapting an existing building to uses it cannot naturally accommodate, costs will rise beyond target levels and an unhappy (perhaps unworkable) solution will result.
It is therefore necessary to identify, at feasibility stage, the true nature of the redundant building under consideration, in terms of the kinds of spaces it contains and the kind of fabric it comprises.

2.02 Classification of types
Tables III–VI will assist the designer by identifying key spatial/structural characteristics of existing buildings, which can be recognised and noted at the very outset of the feasibility investigation. Without a framework of ideas of this kind, it is easy to become preoccupied by incidental characteristics of the building under study, and to miss some of the fundamentals. The spatial and physical categories identified in these tables will be used throughout this study. Figures 1–4 show practical examples of how these classifications can be applied.

2.03 A conceptual framework for matching users and buildings
Firms may be described either by the work that they undertake or by the way that they use space. The way that a firm uses its spaces is dependent upon:

The density of occupancy; the amount of space provided for each member of staff

The amount of space provided for special equipment and storage

The amount of separation required between activities or users

The demand for natural light and ventilation.

Table III   Classification of sites according to location and site coverage, and listing of characteristic types of redundant buildings found in each kind of location

Site coverage		Location of site in relation to surrounding development	
		Isolated site	**Site surrounded by development**
		Advantages: Ease of expansion Ease of access External storage and workspace No conflict with neighbours May be adjacent to main routes Image, location may attract customer Space for parking and deliveries Disadvantages: Difficult to attract female labour Planning constraints Accessibility; may be isolated from main routes	Advantages: Easy to attract female labour Accessible to markets, suppliers and services Large stock of vacant buildings Close to workforce Disadvantages: Noise and fumes conflict with neighbours High land values Limited expansion Difficulties of vehicular access (narrow streets) Planning constraints
100 per cent site coverage	Advantages: effective use of land ease of communication within site Disadvantages: unloading off street limited expansion access storage no parking	Not applicable	Multi-storied large spaces Two to three storied small spaces Mixed small and large spaces eg brewery depository factory hospital town hall
60 per cent site coverage	Advantages: off-street loading and parking expansion common meeting space Disadvantages: definition of entrance maintenance	Up to three storeys mixed small and large spaces eg farm buildings mill barracks	Multi-storied repetitive large spaces Mixed small and large spaces eg brewery depository factory hospital town hall
40 per cent site coverage (single building)	Advantages: car parking, and storage expansion security image	Single or two storeys repetitive small spaces; repetitive large spaces; mix of small and large spaces eg railway station chapel/church house mill school house	Up to three storeys, mixed small and large spaces eg school backland factory
40 per cent site coverage (several buildings)	Advantages: ease of subdivision incremental expansion identity Disadvantages: maintenance	Single or repetitive large spaces eg mill complex hospital military establishment	Large spaces eg school depot hospital goods yard

Buildings may be described according to their configuration, the number of floors, frontage, depth, construction and aspect. Each of these variables affects how the building may be used, its ease of sub-division and cost of conversion. The critical attribute of a building in meeting the demands of different uses is its dimension from front to back (referred to as building depth). Shallow buildings (10 to 15m deep) are most suitable for firms where users are undertaking individual tasks and require separation. Medium depth buildings (15 to 20m) are suitable for a combination of cellular and more open plan areas, while deep buildings (20m or above) are most suitable for organisations which require a great deal of interaction, the minimum of separation, or have a high proportion of machinery or storage which do not require natural light.

Table VII presents a means of describing different types of firms and relating them to different depth buildings.

2.04   Internal subdivision

Within the building, floors may be subdivided in a variety of ways depending on the depth of the space. The sequence of subdivision options may range from small cellular rooms (workrooms or individual offices) to an open-planned layout (table VII).

Table IV   Morphology of sites and buildings, based on four basic types of site; and two basic spatial types of building

Site types	Building spatial types and typical example of each				
	Single space (small)	Single space (large)	Repetitive (small)	Repetitive (large)	Combination of spaces (small and large)
Island sites	chapel	pump house	undercroft	mill	market
Corner sites	pub	cinema	shops	warehouse	newspaper (office and production)
Courtyard sites	schoolroom	barn	mews	maltings	brewery
Street frontages	station	church	houses	factory	town hall
	40 per cent site coverage	60 per cent site coverage	100 per cent site coverage	100 per cent site coverage	100 per cent site coverage

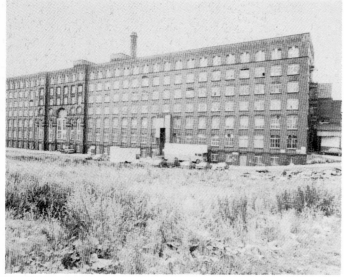

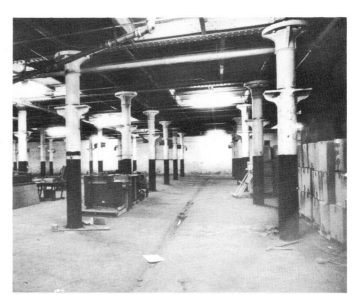

Figures 1 and 2   *Exterior and interior photos of 'large repetitive space' with 'loadbearing perimeter wall and internal columns' (table V). Both photographs are of mill buildings; due to the original manufacturing use, these will often have goods lift and means of escape.*

Table V Classification of buildings according to spatial type; and factors affecting the reuse of each type

Building type	Typical existing use of building	Characteristics	Factors affecting reuse
Small single space	chapel gatehouse stables/coach house	single storied detached load bearing walls size max 100m²	Advantages: • space with character for specialised use Disadvantages: • insufficient space
Large single space	barn hangar warehouse goods shed engine house factory	single storied detached frame or frame and perimeter wall construction size 100m² + floor to eaves height 5m +	Advantages: • flexibility of use • ease of movement of goods Disadvantages: • heating • sub-division • servicing
Small repetitive spaces	house housing workshops lock-up garages	up to four storied terraced narrow frontage up to 100m² on each floor	Advantages: • sub-divided for small units of accommodation Disadvantages: • means of escape • accessibility • loading on upper floors • fire protection
Large repetitive spaces	railway arches warehouse factory mill	multi-storied deep space frame and perimeter wall structure size up to 3000m² on each floor	Advantages: • flexibility of use • suitable for open plan multiple use Disadvantages: • difficulty of sub-dividing into small units • means of escape • access • natural light • fire protection
Small and large spaces	church town hall hospital school industrial complex exchange	up to four storied detached mixed structural system varying floor to ceiling heights	Advantages: • falling vacant in key inner city sites • well serviced, range of spaces provided (suitable for mixed uses) Disadvantages: • complex building forms • heating • internal circulation of goods

(eg factory)

(eg town hall)

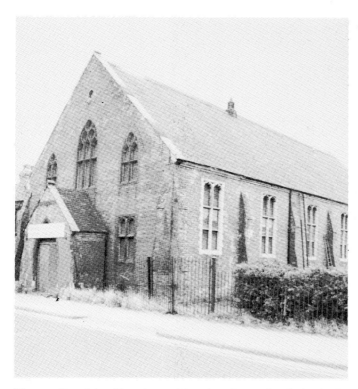

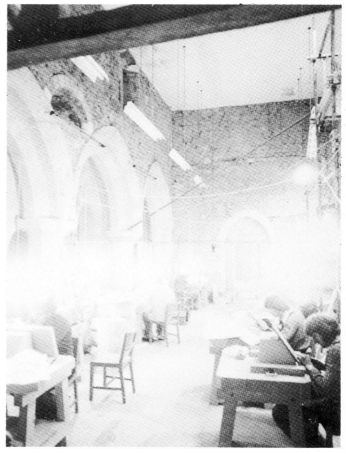

Figures 3 and 4 *Exterior and interior photos of ecclesiastical buildings. In terms of table V these contain both large and small spaces, and in terms of table VI the configuration is narrow frontage/deep space, loadbearing wall construction, single storey. Problems of heating and maintenance likely.*

Table VI   Classification of buildings by height, depth/frontage ratio, form and aspect

Rise
Height affects requirement for goods and passenger lifts, and therefore type of use which may be accommodated.

single storied

2–4 storied

4 storied and above

Configuration
Depth of building affects the amount of natural light and ventilation available. Depths and frontages are classified not in terms of absolute dimensions, but in terms of proportion (ie related to floor site).

depth of building

	shallow	medium	deep
narrow			
medium			
wide			

frontage of building

Structural form
Structural system affects ease of sub-division and flexibility of use.

frame construction

load bearing perimeter wall and internal columns

load bearing walls

Aspect
Aspect affects amount of natural light and ventilation, and ease of access.

one way

three way

detached

two way

Table VII Amount of equipment and storage space

		Amount of equipment and storage space	
		low	high
Degree of separation	high	brokers lawyers research jewellers — shallow space	newspapers — deep space
	low	precision instruments — medium space	printing warehousing & distribution — deep space
	low	clothing insurance architects & advertising electrical engineering instrument engineering — deep space	pottery furniture mechanical engineering — deep space
		high	low

Dependance on natural light for workspaces: high / high / low

Number of people employed

key   ▪ individual rooms   • open space   ▨ equipment and storage space   ▨ circulation & w.c's

4 The Nature of the Premises

1.00 Multi-let premises for small firms

1.01 Categories of accommodation

The different types of premises available for accommodating small firms differ in the:

Type of units provided (size, access, and enclosure)
Management approach and method of leasing.

An analysis of a cross-section of projects for multiple-letting suggests the following categories of accommodation: (See part III chapter 17).

Community workshop
Aimed at the encouragement of embryo enterprises by developing skills and providing equipment, support and training. Community workshops may include:

● Educational workspaces, provided by the local authority, or a government agency and attached to an educational institute or community centre, where individuals can gain experience, use equipment and have skilled support on the basis of a few hours.

● Community enterprises, where a local community group or voluntary trust, with the support of grant aid and central government training schemes, has set up a firm to make and sell products, develop skills, and provide a supportive environment.

● Innovation centres, aimed at full time individuals who have an idea or a process but need support to develop it to the production stage.

Working community
Multiple tenancy building where complimentary small firms share space and common services.

Starter space
May be in individual or multiple-let units. Small, cheap, accessible units with the minimum of communal support. Basic shell which the tenant can upgrade to his own needs.

Flatted industrial units
Multiple-tenancy, conversion of large buildings to provide a variety of different sized units, at different rent levels. A vertical industrial estate, with a caretaker, common security and centrally organised access and frequent deliveries.

Table I summarises the characteristics of the different types of premises.

2.00 Types of units

2.01 Variations in user types
The activities to be accommodated in a building will reflect the type of user and the characteristics of the building.
A building may be required for an individual user – one firm in one or several buildings – or for multiple users, eg several firms in one building. The user or users may undertake one type of function, ie single use, or a variety of functions, ie mixed uses. Table II provides examples of each of these categories and relates them to the appropriate building type.

2.02 Variations in tenancy types
Where a building is planned for multiple use a decision will be required on the type and size of tenancies to be provided. Tenancy types vary according to the form of access, degree of separation between tenancies, services provided, and size (floor area). (Table III).

Types of access

● Direct access Units have a street (or yard) frontage, may receive visitors directly, extend vertically within the building and have their own stairs and/or lifts. This is an expensive solution but has few fire escape problems (since tenancies are small) and is very attractive to service organisations frequently dealing with outside customers. Examples: lawyers' chambers, arcade shops.

● Indirect access Units are reached through internal stairs or corridors which form an intermediate space having to be maintained and policed. This is the most common arrangement and is inexpensive if fire protection is already good. Examples: unit workshops, flatted factories, speculative office buildings.

● Open plan Units as such do not exist but tenants take spaces within an envelope having a single front door. This is

Table I   Types of multi-let premises for small firms (source URBED)

	Types of users	Basic facilities	Type of building	Location
Community workshop Where individuals can use equipment to learn or develop a skill.	Individuals who wish to develop a skill and may consider starting a business.	• Workshop • Equipment • Instruction (adult education).	Part of education or community building or a working community.	Residential area or local centre.
Technology centre Where investors can secure support.	Innovative individuals who require the encouragement to turn a good idea into a marketable product.	• Advice and support from university. • Shared specialist facilities. • Well serviced units.	Well serviced building close to university.	Industrial area close to technological university.
Working community Where complementary small firms share space and common services.	Mainly craft-based firms who would benefit through collaboration, a sympathetic environment, and having experience on tap.	• Individual workrooms or screened space that can be rented without bother. • Shared support services. • Association of tenants.	Old building with little redevelopment value.	Inner city location close to potential customers.
Flatted industrial units Where a number of small firms can rent small units.	Small firms, who want to establish their own identity. A proportion of tenants will be opportunistic and interested in growth.	• A sound shell adaptable to individual requirements.	Redundant multi-storied factory despository or warehouse. School/hospital.	City fringe location or industrial estate close to potential customers.

still usually considered to have social and security risks but there are many advantages: building work can be cheap, tenants can share services and positive interaction may lead to a stronger business environment. Examples: working communities, office 'hotel'.

Degree of separation
• Self-contained unit. Each tenancy has a secure wall and lockable door. Tenancies may be designated by separate floors with access off a common stairwell, or be self-contained units off a common gallery or corridor.

• Shared space. Each tenant's territory is designated by screens or storage units within an open planned space.

Services provided
• Individual services. Each tenancy would have its own toilet and wash facilities.

• Shared services. Tenancies would share common toilet and wash facilities. This solution provides great flexibility and savings for very small tenancies.

Size of units
There is a general shortage of premises of below 230m^2. A 1979 study by the College of Estate Managements Centre for Advanced Land Use Studies at Reading University found that 46 per cent of respondents were in premises of less than 45m^2. For the purpose of this study rentable units have been described as:

• Tiny units (15–75m^2). Best provided in shared space as a workdesk or as an individual room off a corridor.

• Very small units (75–150m^2). Floor of a shallow depth terrace building self-contained unit off a stairway.

• Small units (150–500m^2). Floor of a medium depth building.

• Medium units (500–1000m^2). Complete small building or floor of a large planned building.

Table II   Appropriate buildings for user types

	Single use	Mixed Use
Individual user	Industrial manufacturing firm	One organisation including many functions: (eg publisher including: office, studio, display, warehouse)
	▯ Small single space	▭▭▭ Small repetitive spaces
Multiple users	Similar sized firms manufacturing similar products (eg jewellery). Different sized firms manufacturing similar products	Number of firms with different functions co-operating on end product (eg printer, bookbinder, artist, photographer)
	▢ Large single space	
	▭▭▭ Large repetitive spaces	▤ Large and small spaces

3.00   Building management options

3.01   Styles of management

The character of premises provided will vary depending on the style of management. The traditional management approach is to provide the minimum of support services, with an on-site caretaker responsible for security, cleaning of common areas, and the maintenance and running of central building systems (eg heating). In contrast the working community approach provides an on-site manager, with staff who can give administrative support to the tenants. Through an association of users the tenants can influence the quality and type of services offered, the mix of occupants and the running of the building. Table IV summarises the various building management approaches.

Table III   Range of tenancy types

Configuration and tenancy type	Type of building	Type of management	Type of user
Direct access 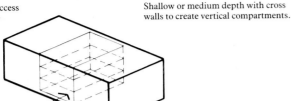 Self contained space rented in a large building. Own stairs/lift(s).	Shallow or medium depth with cross walls to create vertical compartments.	Individual firm's name displayed and each has unit with own services. Management could take one unit over for own use.	Small well-established firms requiring own identity.
Indirect access 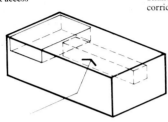 Each unit enclosed and lockable with access from common corridor.	Shallow or medium depth with central corridor on each level.	Common receptionist. Lifts/stairs/corridors from an intermediate space to be maintained. Otherwise as direct access type.	Small firms requiring some security but less concerned with presenting individual identity.
Open plan 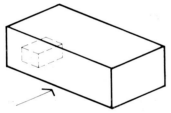 Individual firms areas defined by screens or storage within open plan area.	Deep plan.	Tenants share services and facilities. Tenants participate in management of accommodation.	Small expanding firms with compatible uses. Allows for rapid changes in size and personnel.
Shared space 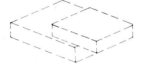 Workplaces rented within another firm's work area, eg sublease on 'gentleman's agreement'.	Any building type.	Head lessee relinquishes no responsibility for space. May provide telephone, secretarial services on time-sharing basis.	Newly founded tiny firms (1 to 5 persons) requiring low overheads and minimum commitments.

4.00   Business growth and working environments

4.01   Need for a premises ladder

As firms grow, their requirements, resources and aspirations change. Like human beings, a firm passes through different stages in its life cycle (as described in chapter 2). This suggests the need for a premises ladder in every local economy (table V).

The small firm sector in the inner city is concerned primarily with the first two steps on the ladder:

• The embryonic stage where a one man band operates part-time or full-time from home.

• The infant stage where the firm has a full-time owner and up to five full or part-time employees. Accommodation may be within a multiple-let building.

Within the early stages of growth, accommodation requirements will also depend on whether the firm is organised along opportunistic or craft-based lines, as discussed in chapter 2.

Table IV   Building management approaches to multiple-use buildings

Manager	Type of developer	Type of development	Management structure	Services provided	Legal structure/type of terms
External management company	Institutional Private developer	Flatted workshops	External manager and caretaker	Minimal shared services	Public or private limited company Lease
Local management company	Local developers Building owners Local authority	Flatted workshops	On-site building manager	Minimal shared services	Public or private limited company Lease
Service company	Charity or trust Local authority Industrial developer	Working community Community workshop Technology centre	Manager and support staff	Full range of shared services	Company limited by guarantee Lease, licence on *per diem* rental
Association of occupants	Neighbourhood group Local authority Common interest group	Working community	Manager and support staff responsible to forum of occupants	Full range of shared services	Common ownership lease, licence or *per diem* rental

Table V   The premises ladder for two types of manufacturing firms

Stage Types of business	Typical premises		Typical requirements		
	A Modern opportunistic	B Traditional craft	Quality	Image	Tenure
5 Institutional Professional management	Specialised new factory	Custom conveerted building	Purpose designed	Corporate	Freehold or lease back from financial institution
4 Established Basic work routinized	Industrial client with front offices		High grade conversion	Own car park and entrance	Owner occupation or long lease
3 Growing Some employees with a basic management structure	Industrial unit	Converted warehouse	Upgrade services finishes	Separate entrance	Short lease (3–7 years)
2 Infant Independent firm supporting a handful of people	Advanced unit Flatted factory Technology Centre Short-life industrial building	Converted railway arch Working community Flatted workshop Studio	Minimum cost conversion	Name on door	Licence or short lease (under 3 years)
1 Embryonic A hobby or pastime	Garage Subleased space from established firm Working community Technology centre	Work at home Workshop Community workshop	As found	Shared entrance Subordinate to larger organisation	Shared space

5 Agencies for Development

1.00 Introduction

1.01 The problem of marginal developments

The problem with most redundant industrial stock is that in the eyes of development agencies it is of marginal value. Such buildings may be too large for small founding firms, and yet inefficient for the large well established firm due to poor access, or cramped sites which reduce the opportunities for expansion. These buildings tend to be sited in secondary or tertiary locations, where there may be a high level of uncertainty concerning demand, building condition and local authority expectations. These locations and buildings will seldom look viable if assessed against institutional criteria to provide returns on investment normally applied to primary locations. One of the reasons why it has been hard to attract finance for marginal projects, is that they are difficult to evaluate from an investor's point of view. Faced with competing demands for finance, any large organisation, whether private or publicly owned, tends to 'stick to the mainstream' and invest in conventional proposals.

1.02 How the public sector could help

Public sector policies could encourage new initiatives on marginal projects by taking action on a number of fronts:

● By inducing owners either to invest themselves or to pass on their property before it deteriorates to the point where reuse is unviable. The costs of holding property empty could be raised and the cost of bringing property back into use lowered.

● By ensuring that local authorities do not stand in the way of private investment, but that in areas where confidence is really lacking they create the kind of environment businesses want.

● By enabling entrepreneurial developers who have relevant experience to take on more projects, and encouraging other bodies, such as prospective occupiers, builders and professionals to undertake small schemes. New types of development bodies are needed to handle complex situations, particularly in areas where the economy is dying.

● By providing both short and long term development finance, involving existing financial institutions as far as possible. This will require the use of new methods of assessment that can judge firstly the real economic potential of an area, and secondly whether the development approach is appropriate.

2.00 Types of development

2.01 Potential developers

Redundant buildings can offer ample scope for a variety of different types of developer as a recent URBED survey revealed.

During the latter part of 1978 URBED undertook a survey of 45 buildings that had been converted for use by small firms. The criterion for the choice of schemes was that they should have at least three firms who were undertaking general or light industrial activities in less than 500m^2 of space.

The buildings analysed fell into four categories according to size (table I). Due to the number of tenancies most of the buildings were effectively industrial estates. The average

Table I Summary of current conversions (areas in m^2)

	Size (actually in use)	Number of examples	%	Occupied floor space	%	Known employment	%
Giant	over 5000	15	33	297 900	84	4074	71
Large	2500 to 5000	9	20	31 700	9	798	14
Medium	100 to 2500	11	24	17 650	5	610	11
Small	under 1000	10	23	6 160	2	252	4
Total		45	100	353 410	100	5734	100

Table II Summary of types of developer according to size of building

		Private developer	Public bodies Local authorities	Voluntary trusts Social enterprises
Giant	Over 5000m^2	11	5	1
Large	2500–5000m^2	9	4	1
Medium	1000–2500m^2	1	1	1
Small	Below 1000m^2	5	2	4
Total		26	12	7

number of tenants was 28 while 5 buildings had over 75 tenants. Clearly the problem of management which deters institutional developers can be overcome. Of the 45 buildings surveyed 16 per cent were initiated by voluntary groups, 27 per cent by public bodies or local authorities and 57 per cent by private developers. An analysis of the type of developers related to the size of the project (table II) showed that the majority of the giant (over 5,000m^2) and large (2,500–5,000m^2) projects were undertaken by local authorities or established private developers, whilst the medium (1,000–2,500m^2) or small (under 1,000m^2) were undertaken as joint ventures between local authorities and private orga-

Table III Agencies for the conversion of redundant buildings

Agents for development	Type of building	Funding	Method of approach
Property companies A few large private developers have specialised in conversion, eg Westminster Bunting (Industrial), Haslemere Estates (Offices). Most appropriate where there is a profitable mix of uses, with lower rent workshops providing planning again.	Interested in buildings with freehold or long term leases (99 year minimum). Deal with large buildings (above 5480m^2) of complex form.	Long term mortgages or loans from pension funds or insurance companies. Some funding favours schemes which provide a few large units of accommodation, for tenants with good covenants.	Main contractor, full professional service (architect, engineer and qs) with in-house project management. May work in partnership with local authorities, providing project management and access to financial institutions.
Local authorities Play a particularly important role with regard to old buildings due to: • professional resources available • incentive to make investments with social value • ownership of redundant buildings which may be better used for industrial purposes than redeveloped.	Ideally suited to rehabilitating old buildings already in their ownership through compulsory purchase and now vacant and deteriorating while awaiting planning decisions. Can initiate development on buildings that are unattractive to private enterprises, eg buildings that are multi-storey, or short leases, or in uncertain or blighted areas.	Loans and direct central government aid.	May use main contractor or direct labour team. Normally have full professional services in-house, but may supplement with outside enterprise, eg advice on costs. May act in partnership with a developer who provides the expertise on project management and letting. Could act in partnership with outside associations who provided tenants, such as a building preservation trust, or some other equivalent of a housing association.
Landlords May be interested in subdividing empty spaces if the resultant mix of uses increases their rent, or allows them to let a building that has been empty for a long period of time, and where redevelopment prospects are definitely limited. Includes large corporations, financial institutions, and nationalised industries.	Prepared to undertake the major adaptations of large and complex holdings, eg warehouses or textile mill complexes. May act where there are short sub-leases on all or part of the property.	Mortgages and loans from institutions or banks or personal investment. Many large organisations, realising they have a major asset in their redundant properties , have set up separate property subsidiaries.	Main contractor, full professional service, possibly in-house project management. May use outside developer or estate agent to advise on letting policy and project management.
Locally based developers Have an intimate knowledge of local planning requirements, the most appropriate vacant buildings and the demand for premises. With lower overheads than the large property company they are often prepared to undertake a scheme which looks unrealistic to the larger organisation.	Prepared to undertake work on medium sized buildings (930 to 5570m^2). Tend to undertake projects where major structural alterations and a change of planning use are not required.	Loans from banks or investment companies. May try and make the project as far as possible self-financing, doing the minimum work through an overdraft facility and then phasing in tenants, so rentals can cover additional building work.	Sub-contractors, direct labour, with project management and supervision by developer. Partial professional service. Typical of a locally based developer, may be a small building firm initiating work for itself.
Building preservation trusts Development companies with charitable status. The organisation is particularly appropriate for projects which are for the public good or where funding from charitable bodies is being sought.	Particularly appropriate to buildings of historic, environmental or architectural interest. Buildings may vary in size and complexity. Probably require conservation input.	May use bank loans, grants from charities or central government grants for listed buildings, plus local government support, in some cases on a revolving fund basis. Can draw from the *Heritage Fund* administered by the Civic Trust, which provides low-cost finance during the development period. Charitable status exempts project from Corporation Tax. Development Land Tax and may allow half rates.	The management group is voluntary but may include professional advisers. Could set up its own building team with its own project manager, drawing on the Manpower Services Commission's Training Workshop or STEP schemes for labour.
Association of users Like housing co-operatives, work best where fairly few (say less than five) individuals or groups are involved with some underlying common objective and the capacity to pool skills. Small groups of relatively large tenants or a trade or professional association may organise the conversion work, and then sub-lease space off with the small tenants being represented through a tenants' association. A traditional example is the Inns of Court for the legal profession.	A building which is easily divided with no major structural alterations and which does not entail complex planning negotiations. A building of under 930m^2 with each floor let off to a separate firm might be ideal for this arrangement.	Finance may be raised from the landlord, and repaid through higher rents or through individual contributions of rent in advance. Funding may be available for certain sectors of employment (clothing) through Department of Industry grants.	Expertise and workforce can be provided from within the association, or the association could work with one of the other types of agent such as a building preservation trust.
Small firms May invest personal capital and labour into upgrading and subdividing their own properties.	Small narrow frontage buildings where the building is in sound condition but may require an additional fire escape, rewiring, subdivision and up-grading of finishes.	Short term bank loan or personal investment.	Work may be undertaken by sub-contractors and direct labour. Co-ordination of project and some building work done by the firms themselves.

nisations or were initiated by trusts, co-operatives or voluntary organisations sometimes with support from the Manpower Services Commission (as job creation schemes).

Table III lists the alternative agents available to undertake developments, indicates how the project can be organised and matches the method of implementing the project to the scale and complexity of the task.

A relevant URBED report has also shown how different development approaches are required to tackle specific projects[1]. Sometimes an institutional approach is required on a historic building; sometimes the new uses have to be reconsidered to make the project economically viable. The report gives details of 23 classic re-use schemes and how their development strategies are unique.

3.00 Private developers

3.01 New initiatives

Many of the initiatives for reusing old buildings have come from the private sector. Firms have found themselves owning buildings surplus to their needs and have decided to develop them for small units; individuals have seen the opportunity of a specific building and taken on the task of redevelopment or small development companies with low overheads have realised that, by reducing margins and selecting buildings carefully, they could create a viable market. Recently, large organisations and financial institutions have begun to enter the field. Regeneration Ltd, a London developer, has undertaken a study for British Steel Corporation (Industry) Ltd into establishing a multi-tenancy industrial complex in 16 acres of now disued Clyde Iron Works, currently providing 80 unts and job opportunities for 250 people, (figure 1). Clearly as nationalised or large industries reorganise their production and close out-of-date or less productive sectors of their output there will be an increasing need for organisations like Regeneration Ltd to set up ventures of this kind, in an effort to maintain economic activity in depressed areas with high unemployment.

4.00 Local authorities

4.01 Increasing opportunities

Local authorities can increase the opportunities for converting redundant buildings into small units by providing short leases, relaxing standards, giving grants, showing sympathy and in special cases undertaking conversion and management themselves to create a working precedent.

In some cases local authorities have taken on the role of developer. The London Borough of Islington has converted vacant buildings in the Clerkenwell area into small workshop units, while in Scotland two new Enterprise Workshops have been established by the Strathclyde Regional Council at Hamilton and Paisley as part of its industrial development plan. The Hamilton Workshop provides premises, equipment and support for new enterprises working to develop new products.

4.02 Acting as catalysts

In other cases the local authority has acted as the catalyst for

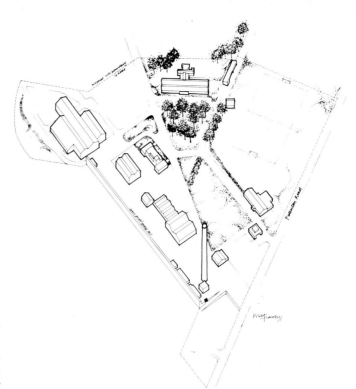

Figure 1 *At Clyde Workshops, 75,000 sq ft of redundant ironworks buildings were adapted to form 80 light industrial workshop units. The development costs, some £250,000, were funded by British Steel Corporation (Industry) Ltd through its subsidiary Clyde Workshops Ltd. Conversion work started in January 1980 under the direction of Regeneration Ltd, which designed the complex and its management procedures. By mid-May 45 small firms had already moved in, and brought 140 new jobs to this depressed area of Glasgow.*

the reuse of exisiting buildings and kept down the inevitable costs associated with bureaucratic organisations by joint ventures. Lancaster Borough Council, in association with the University of Lancaster, runs the old Gillows furniture factory as a very successful incubator environment for new, technologically orientated firms. It provides advice and support to the firms in their early stages of growth and, as they expand, moves them out to larger buildings owned by the borough. The GLC Industrial Centre, in an attempt to harness the expertise and enthusiasm generated in the early multiple-occupancy conversions in the London area, has collaborated with Regeneration Ltd in funding feasibility studies on the re-use of some of the larger vacant buildings in London.

4.03 Offering leases

As an aftermath of the comprehensive redevelopment plans of the late 1960s local authorities are now the owners of large stocks of industrial space, which they have the responsibility to continue to manage or to dispose of. The more adventurous have leased space to local neighbourhood groups on short-life leases, as for example Camden Industrial Action Group and Kingsgate Workshops. Where the buildings are seen to have a longer life, attempts have been made to dispose of the long leases through competitive bids where attention is paid to the quality of the idea, the employment generated and its relevance to the local areas, as well as its financial viability.

4.04   Need for greater encouragement
URBED Ltd, with the help of the Association of Industrial Development Officers undertook a survey of 119 authorities during the latter part of 1978 to find out the objectives of their industrial development programmes, what schemes they were undertaking and how the industrial development function was organised. Under the heading 'What are local authorities doing?', the survey considered five main types of programme which local authorities could use to encourage industry namely planning, premises, finance, personnel and information. Although the survey revealed a marked relaxation of local authority attitudes to industrial development and small firms in particular, it showed that local authorities in general could make an even greater contribution in encouraging industry. Only 37 per cent of authorities were tolerant of mixed uses, 44 per cent were organising advisory services and a mere 32 per cent converting existing buildings. Larger local authorities have taken individual initiatives to provide support to small firms and improve premises.

5.00   Voluntary groups

5.01   Funding
Voluntary groups can use funding from private sources, local authorities or central government. The Pennine Development Trust is a charitable body with support from the Rowntree Trust which has been set up with the objective of utilising the old mills, restoring economic activity and revitalising Pennine villages. Members of the group have converted a mill at Hebden Bridge for craft workshops and a Congregational chapel for office uses. In the London Borough of Lewisham the Telegraph Hill Neighbourhood Group has converted an old factory for use as a garment factory with training facilities and a creche attached.
Much impetus has come from central government (Manpower Services Commission). The Castlecliff Workshops at Edinburgh (figure 3) provide worthwhile work and training for school leavers who would otherwise be unemployed. Located in the old castle barracks, the project provides employment for about 60 with MSC support. The essential characteristics of voluntary groups is that they start with user interests and harness the tremendous energies of local people.

6.00   Development trusts

6.01   Role of development trusts
In areas where the economy is thriving, and high rents are being paid, the private market will eventually develop available space, provided there are not too many constraints. In other cases like much of London's docklands, whole new communities must be built up, and considerable public interest is required. But there is a third category which poses a particular challenge, where private investment could be secured, provided action was taken on a number of

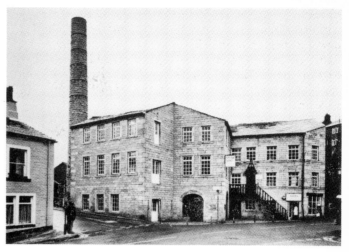

Figure 2   *Bridge Mill, Hebden Bridge, Pennine Development Trust, a classic example of what can be achieved in the way of adapting old industrial premises to new uses. Purchase in 1972 and restored by the Pennine Development Trust it is now one of Hebden Bridge's shopping focal points.*

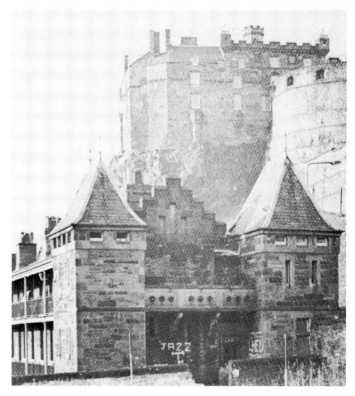

Figure 3   *Castlecliff Workshops, Edinburgh. Craft-orientated workshops help provide employment opportunities for young people.*

fronts. Much of the 3.5 million m² or so of vacant industrial property in London falls in this category, and most cities face similar problems. The obstacles include lack of land assembly, the planning problems associated with mixed use and the uncertainty of renovating old buildings, all of which add to the risks.
The main problems to be resolved are who should take the initiative, who should bear the risk, and who should undertake the development. In such situations, the idea of a

development trust may be helpful. Development trusts can tackle situations which others will not touch, using a combination of imagination, entrepreneurial drive, and social concern to overcome obstacles, fulfilling a role as a 'third force', akin to that of housing associations in the residential field.

6.02 Advantages of development trusts

The advantages that a development trust can bring are basically:

Taking on complex projects with multiple objectives, both commercial and social

Leveraging the initial capital by marshalling resources from a wide range of bodies who share a particular concern

Creating a climate of confidence and overcoming inertia

Securing acceptance by those who might otherwise block development.

Situations where developments trusts can be particularly useful include:

•Pioneering schemes, that initially may not seem commercially viable, but in time can be made self-sustaining. A good example is the sub-division of redundant buildings for letting to tiny firms, where demand will not be evident until a scheme has been implemented. A pioneering experiment can encourage others to follow, or can provide useful lessons. A number of local enterprise trusts such as the Community of St Helens Trust Ltd and Clyde Workshops have been set up to provide space and supporting services to encourage new firms.

•Mixed uses, where a mix of commercial and residential use is appropriate, but where management initiatives may be lacking. Good examples are the use of land under the Westway in London, where development has been co-ordinated by an Amenity Trust. Another is the letting of commercial space under residential units, where various commercial premises associations are being set up.

•Historic areas, including listed buildings and conservation areas where imaginative schemes could attract new uses and keep down the costs of refurbishment. Building preservation trusts can draw on specialised expertise and enthusiasm, obtaining low cost finance from the Heritage Fund. In the St Mary's area, Rotherhithe, the Industrial Building Preservation Trust helped to convert several warehouses for small workspaces.

•Sites awaiting redevelopment, such as small areas of waste land, which often can be transformed into attractive areas, and used for temporary purposes such as community gardens, urban farms, allotments or car parks. Where they are not done for private benefit, such schemes can draw on labour paid for by the Manpower Services Commission's Special Programmes.

6.03 Raising the finance

There are three main problems which limit what development trusts can achieve:

Financing the preparation of feasible schemes

Securing the land or buildings on terms that make reuse viable

Attracting commercial finance without guarantees.

In some cases the development trust may interest a private developer in undertaking the scheme, or may draw together a consortium, in which case no public subsidy would be required. However, there is also a case for the local authority providing development capital in the form of a revolving fund, as this allows some risks to be taken with the incentive of reinvesting surpluses in further schemes. The local authority can then influence the use to which the finance is put.

Alternatively use can be made of grants under the Inner Urban Areas Act for refurbishment schemes. The owner of the building, which may have a negative residential value, should be encouraged to make it available by being offered a share in the income when the premises are occupied.

A development trust could also expect support from companies and foundations, as they can secure tax relief if the trust has charitable status. Finally, a development trust may look for finance from investors by providing them with buildings or sites for which planning permission has been obtained, or selling a development once it has been turned into a safe investment.

6.04 Management councils

Typically these trusts have management councils, representing the various interests involved such as the local authorities or typical occupants, who give their services free. Professional consultants are employed to organise the work. Surpluses from rental income or disposals are reinvested. The legal status is usually that of a company limited by guarantee, and charitable status may be secured in certain situations.

7.00 Central government involvement

7.01 Assistance for inner cities

The Inner Urban Areas Act of 1978 marked an important step forward in providing designated local authorities with powers to assist industrial development, in run-down inner-city areas and also reflected a change of thinking concerning the nature of urban problems, with a new emphasis on the problems of 'economic decline' and 'physical decay'.

Table IV details the ways in which the Act can help in the reuse of redundant buildings.

7.02 The 'Partnership Authorities' and 'Special Areas'

Some local authorities have been designated 'Partership Authorities' which means that part of their administrative boundary is a 'Special Area' for the purposes of the Act. Partnership status enables an authority to make 90 per cent loans for:

Demolition of structures or buildings
Removal of foundations
Clearance of land
Levelling of land.

Neither interest nor capital repayments are required within

Table IV How the Inner Urban Areas Act helps the re-use of redundant buildings

Clause	New power of local authorities	Inner Urban Areas Act: areas within which new power may be used			
		Designated district Part of inner urban local authority, approved by Secretary of State.	**Industrial Improvement Area** Must be in designated local authority, and defined by that authority. Secretary of State can turn down the declaration of an IIA, but cannot create.	**Special Areas** These central/local government partnership areas will be all or part of a designated district and must be approved by the Secretary of State.	**Greater London** Clause enables London authority to claim a grant that has been available to other authorities since the 1972 Local Employment Act.
2	To offer loans for the acquisition of, or works on, land.	•			
3	To offer loans and grants on a) construction of fencing/walls b) landscaping etc c) demolition d) construction of car parking, access roads, turning heads, loading bays, etc, and grants only on e) conversion, extension, improvement of buildings into industrial buildings.		•		
5	To make loans for site preparation: a) demolition b) removal of foundations c) clearance of land d) levelling of land.			•	
6	To pay grants towards rents of industrial buildings including warehouses.			•	
7	To adopt local plan in advance of structure plan.			•	
8	To enable central government to give 100 per cent grants for derelict land in london.				•

two years of mortgage. Partnership authorities can pay grants towards the rents of industrial buildings, including warehouses, and adopt a local plan before the Secretary of State has approved a structure plan. The implications of this latter power are that it is theoretically possible that the 'hope' value attached to many buildings would be brought down by the strict adoption of a land use map.

The partnership arrangement involves a joint committee of central and local government elected members which presides over an officer steering group that comprises of a very wide variety of organisations.

Partnership areas currently include:

1 Liverpool
2 Manchester/Salford
3 Birmingham
4 Lambeth
5 Docklands
6 Hackney/Islington
7 Newcastle-upon-Tyne/Gateshead

7.03 Programme authorities

Programme authorities can give loans of 90 per cent for the acquisition of land or works on the land. They can also designate Industrial Improvement Areas, (see 7.04). Programme authorities do not have a partnership committee, but they do not have to draw up inner area plans. The programme authorities are:

1 N. Tyneside
2 S. Tyneside
3 Sunderland
4 Middlesbrough
5 Bolton
6 Oldham
7 Wirral
8 Bradford
9 Hull
10 Leeds
11 Sheffield
12 Wolverhampton
13 Leicester
14 Nottingham
15 Hammersmith

7.04 Industrial improvement areas

Outside the Special Areas, the district authorities concerned can designate Industrial Improvement Areas, subject to the approval of the Secretary of State. In these areas loans and grants are available for:

Construction of fencing and walls
Landscaping etc
Demolition
Construction of car parking spaces, access points
Conversion, extension, modernisation of buildings for industrial/warehouse use.

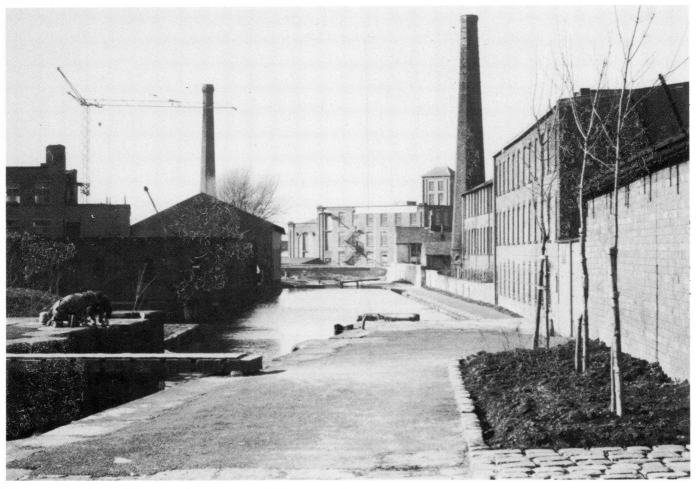

Figure 4 *Rochdale IIA: where the principles of IIAs were evolved and first applied.*

Table V   Appraisal of objectives and improvement policies, Crawford Street, Rochdale

Objectives	Means
1 To improve the conditions at the interface between the residential and industrial areas	Reorganisation of the land use pattern Introduction of buffer zones of open space Landscaping Traffic management Improvements to the appearance of industrial buildings
2 To improve operating and environmental conditions for firms and their employees (and thereby to encourage productive investment by firms)	The creation of space for expansion of off-street servicing and parking Traffic management Landscaping and cosmetic treatment of buildings
3 To create space for new industrial development	Redevelopment of obsolete building, reclamation of derelict land Reorganisation of land uses and landownerships
4 To prolong the life of certain currently obsolescent industrial buildings	Rehabilitation and conversion Expansion of existing buildings
5 To improve vehicular circulation for through traffic on the principal road and pedestrian circulation generally	Limit access and improve junctions onto Oldham Road Create a network of pedestrian routes where traffic is limited or does not exist
6 To improve recreational and visual amenities in the area	Increased provision of open space Improved access to open space General environmental improvement

Grants are limited to 50 per cent of total costs or £1000 per job created, whichever is less.

The overall objective in nearly all IIA's is to restore confidence in the area through a working partnership between the public and private sectors and hence to attract greater private investment.

The Rochdale experiment

The best known IIA is in the Crawford Street area in Rochdale (figure 4) where the local authority pioneered this new planning tool in 1975.

The Crawford Street area, selected for a pilot scheme, was suffering from the usual symptoms of inner city neglect. Predominantly industrial in character, half the area of 49.6 hectares was in active industrial and commercial use, with a large number of small firms engaged mainly in mechanical engineering and textiles; 20 per cent of the area was occupied by housing. The majority of the industrial floorspace was in the large multi-storied textile mills lining the Rochdale canal. There was little new building, less than 2 per cent of the floorspace having been built since the war. Nearly 20 per cent of the industrial and commercial floorspace was vacant and many buildings were derelict. Decline and neglect had attracted scrap merchants and vehicle repairers into the area.

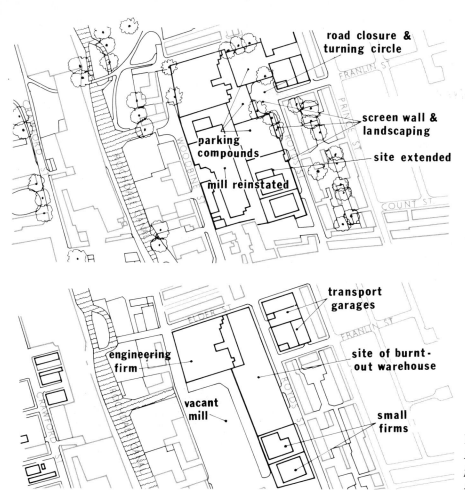

road closure &
turning circle

screen wall &
landscaping

site extended

parking
compounds

mill reinstated

FRANLIN ST

COUNT ST

transport
garages

FRANLIN ST

engineering
firm

site of burnt-
out warehouse

vacant
mill

small
firms

Figure 5 *Royds Street, Rochdale.
Existing plan is lower one: top plan shows
proposals for filling in canal arm and using
site more rationally.*

Rochdale Council's objective in the Crawford Street area was to secure its long term future as a largely industrial area by making it suitable for modern industrial activity and acceptable environmentally to the housing residents. The goal was achieved by following a number of specific objects outlined in table V.

The practical initiatives taken by Rochdale fell into three main categories:

Land assembly and access
Buildings
Traffic management.

By reorganising the land use, rationalising the mangement of existing building stock and introducing a traffic management scheme, the council was able to ensure the area had a viable future (figure 5).

Part II
The Process

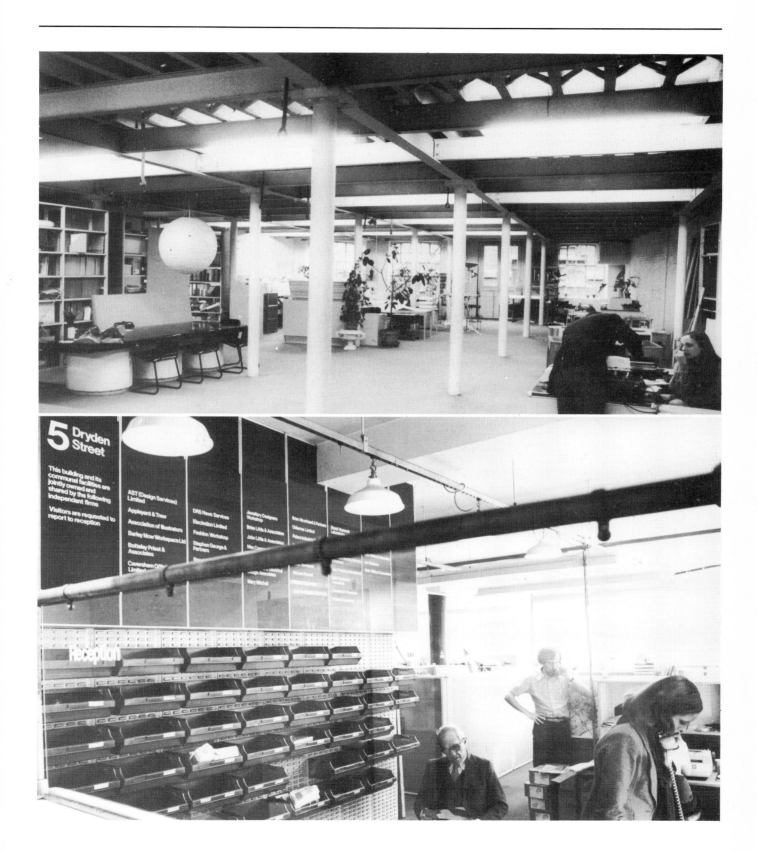

Previous page, top picture: architects' studios in a former warehouse in Earlham Street, converted by the Greater London Council as part of their Covent Garden renewal scheme. Bottom picture: part of the working community's shared reception area in David Rock's conversion of a former printing works at 5 Dryden Street, also near Covent Garden.

6 The Development Process

1.00 Introduction

1.01 Steps in the development process

The development process for reusing existing buildings varies from the normal development process for new buildings in that:

- The importance of the initial financial appraisal and technical evaluation is increased.

- Finely tuned judgements must be made in short time scales and with limited information.

- A variety of parties may be involved in the development process each with different objectives.

The problem with vacant inner city industrial stock is that it is of marginal value. Its reuse relies on marginal solutions, where the latitude for uncertainty is reduced.

The process is not a simple sequence but a cyclical process in which the project team should give initial consideration to the following key issues:

- Where is the building located?
Accessibility for staff, visitors and goods.

- What is the building like?
Condition of structure, services and fabric.

- What could the building be used for?
Internal space planning for alternative uses.

- What are the constraints on re-use?
Planning and statutory requirements.

- What work needs to be undertaken?
Rehabilitation or conversion.

- How viable is reuse?
Economic appraisal of options.

Each question should be addressed in greater and greater detail as the opportunities for reuse become more viable with each step of the development process.

1.02 Actions in the process

Figure 1 identifies the key stages in the development process (based on the RIBA's *Plan of Work*) from project inception to post-contract, and highlights the level of participation to be expected from the private, public and voluntary sections at each phase.

Projects initiated by the public sector often rely on private sector participation, while projects initiated privately may need support from central and local government to make them viable. Building reuse projects may unite public, private and voluntary group interests, brought together by common goals of maintaining a well loved landmark, improving the environment, and rejuvenating the local economy. St Mary's, Rotherhithe, which only a few years ago was a run-down part of docklands in the London Borough of Southwark, is an exciting example of how an area can be brought to life by a mixture of initiatives by the local authority, private developers, voluntary groups, and private individuals.

2.00 The development checklist

The checklist which follows sets down the points to be considered at each stage, with cross references to the relevant section and chapter in the book.

The format was derived from experience of converting redundant industrial buildings for multiple lettings to small firms. The sequence of actions and information is equally valid for other uses, such as community centres, and new buildings which are being designed to be subdivided for use by small firms.

The development check list *(Figure 1)*

A PROJECT INCEPTION

B FEASIBILITY

PARTICIPANT: PRIVATE SECTOR

PRIVATE DEVELOPER

FINANCIAL INSTITUTIONS

TRADE ASSOCIATIONS

ESTATE AGENTS

DEVELOPMENT PROCESS

PRIVATE DEVELOPER

BUILDING OWNER

PUBLIC AUTHORITY

NON PROFIT ORGANISATION

BUILDING LOOKING FOR NEW USES:
Owned
Option to buy
Interest

USERS LOOKING FOR BUILDING

MARKET EVALUATION
FINANCIAL VIABILITY

LOCAL AREA SURVEY
INITIAL FEASIBILITY STUDIES
SIFT AVAILABLE BUILDINGS

SELECT OPTIONS FOR IN DEPTH TESTING

FINANCIAL APPRAISAL
POTENTIAL & EFFECTIVE DEMAND

SITE & LOCATIONAL EVALUATION:
Character of neighbourhood
Access for people & cars
Access for goods

LEGAL & PLANNING CHECKS:
Allowable uses
Means of escape & fire protection
Ownership & length of lease

STRUCTURAL & PHYSICAL EVALUATION:
Condition of structure, fabric, finishes, services
Specification & cost of building work

SPACE PLANNING
EVALUATION OF ALTERNATIVE USES

STRATEGY FOR IMPEMENTATION:
Typing of development organisation
Sources of funding
Phasing

PARTICIPANT: PUBLIC / VOLUNTARY SECTOR

FUND STUDIES

STAFF SUPPORT

PREPARE MARKET INFORMATION

STATUTORY AUTHORITIES

PLANNING DEPARTMENT

INDUSTRIAL DEVELOPMENT OFFICER

NEIGHBOURHOOD GROUPS

C/D OUTLINE PROPOSALS / SCHEME DESIGN   IMPLEMENTATION — SUPERVISION   L/M POST CONTRACT

FINANCIAL INSTITUTIONS

PRIVATE BUSINESS

PROFESSIONAL ADVICE   ⎞ ACTION RESOURCE   ESTATE AGENTS
                            ⎟ CENTRE (ARC)
PROVISION OF MATERIALS   ⎬ LONDON ENTERPRISE   LAWYER
                            ⎟ AGENCY
COMMERCIAL BANKS (BRIDGING LOANS)   ACCOUNTANT

ESTATE AGENTS

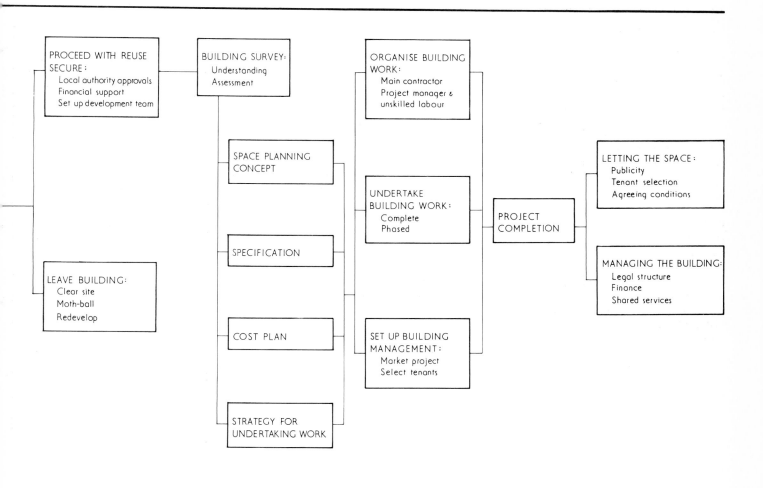

GRANTS & LOANS

INCENTIVES

LOCAL AUTHORITY COVENANTS

INFRASTRUCTURE & SITE IMPROVEMENTS

PROMOTION

JOB CREATION LABOUR

PROFESSIONAL INPUTS

INDUSTRIAL DEVELOPMENT
OFFICE (finding tenants)

FEDERATION OF WORKING COMMUNITIES

ASSOCIATION OF USERS

STAFF TRAINING

MANAGEMENT ADVISE

MARKETING OUTLETS

3.00 Alternative starting points

3.01 Building looking for users
Various clients may be found:
Local amenity groups, conservation groups or building preservation trusts.
Building owners wishing to provide a return on their asset.
Local authority concerned to forestall further deterioration of the fabric and blighting of the neighbourhood.

3.02 Users looking for buildings
Groups of small firms having difficulty in finding accommodation or individual business looking for space.

Users who decide to group together to convert a large building into small units.

An organisation working on behalf of a specific group of users.

A developer with a particular type of tenant in mind, or looking for suitable space to subdivide for small firms.

A local authority which wants to help small firms and provide employment, remove a cause of dereliction and decay, or increase income from rates.

Local employment action groups who wish to retain industry in the area.

3.03 Local authorities taking stock
Wishing to:
Decide on development policy
Initiate environmental improvement schemes
Promote the area.

4.00 Assessing the opportunities

4.01 Local area survey

Purpose
Assess economic activity of area
Define effective and potential demand
Propose local planning initiatives, and degree of intervention required by local authority.

Information sources
Building inspector will give reliable insight into condition of building
Borough library, historical archives
Community groups
Local chamber of commerce
Kelly's street directory and GPO
Yellow pages, to define network of present businesses
Observation, word of mouth.

4.02 Initial feasibility study

Purpose
Take stock of opportunities
Grade strategies for development
Sift buildings for further study.

Inputs
External viewing and ordnance survey map

Agents' particulars and planning history
2/3 hours professional time required

Shortlist buildings
Define spatial and locational requirements of user, type of tenancy organisation
Available buildings and their characteristics eg:
Space criteria – small or large
     medium, narrow or deep plan
     rise
     single or repetitive plan
     configuration
Structural form
Aspect
Site.

4.03 Select options to test
Which to reject
Which to test
Which to leave to market forces.

Factors affecting choice:
Characteristics of building
Local planning objectives
Uses attractive to local community
Demand
Neighbourhood character
Transportation.

5.00 Financial appraisal

5.01 Preliminary examination

Purpose
Examine marginal buildings to test impact of varying:
Mix of uses
Specification

Development approach
Length of lease.

Input
Architect/quantity surveyor to test whether to:
Refurbish industrial use on the cheap
Refurbish mixed use
Redevelop.

5.02   Detailed appraisal
Decide on potential users and likely rents.
List all the items of building work required.
Establish the elementary costs by deciding on the condition of the building and the level of conversion work required for the use proposed.
Work out financial feasibility by establishing annual equivalent cost per unit lettable area for alteration works,

asking rent, legal fees on lease agency, project management/risk factor; compare this with anticipated rental.
Revise scheme where necessary (if market allows) by adjusting rentals, specification of building work, profit element or renegotiating landlord's asking rental.
Establish possible sources of finance from central government, local authority or private sector loans.

6.00   Detailed feasibility report

6.01   Select option to proceed
Decide on most appropriate use:
Employment (commercial or industrial)
Non employment (community, housing etc.)
Mixed (eg. residential and work).

Select use:
Canvass local opinion
Match shape of building to shape of proposed new use (size, degree of subdivision required, access)
Define market demand
Choose a use for which finances are available.

Choose a building:
Match the shape of the users
Availability
Ease of conversion
Minimum planning restrictions
Meet fire regulations and 'means of escape'
Accessibility.

6.02   Prepare detailed feasibility study
State objectives of scheme:
The case for conversion and reusing the building
The rentals to be achieved
The size of units to be provided
The type of tenants to be accommodated
The organisation of the management body and the common facilities to be provided
The timing of the project.

Space planning concept:
Defining separate tenancies
Allowing for expansion and change
Locations of common services and facilities
Provision of heating, gas, electricity, water
Zoning of office, production, storage and circulating areas.

Assessment of building work required:
The condition of structure, fabric, services, fittings and finishes
The building work required to make the building habitable or allow the tenant to finish his unit to his own specification after occupation, or provide units ready finished.

Review the planning and statutory requirements that will need to be met in different areas:
Is a change of use involved under the Town and Country Planning Act, 1971?
Into which purpose group or use class does the proposed development fall in terms of the building regulations?
Check compliance with the four principal areas of legislation (planning law; building regulations; Factories Act, Offices, Shops and Railway Premises Act).
Check compliance with wider range of legislation.
Check compliance with fire regulations, both statutory and insurance company rules.

Strategy for undertaking the conversion alternatives are:
Contractor and full professional services
Project manager, subcontractors, direct labour and partial professional services
Voluntary advice and labour.

Financial appraisal:
As detailed above, including estimates of running costs: rent, rates, insurance, heating, electricity and maintenance

Type of development organisation proposed:
Individual developer
Association of users etc
Building preservation trust with charitable status.

Timing of project:
Sources of funding and help
Cash flow
Phasing of leases to tenants
Future plans.

Proposal for undertaking work
The form of organisation should match the scale and complexity of the task in hand. The type of building, the sources of funding and the method of approach will vary with the different agents for development eg:
Property company
Local authority
Landlord
Locally based developers
Building preservation trusts
User association
Small firms.

RIBA STAGE OF WORK C/D: OUTLINE PROPOSALS/SCHEME DESIGN

7.00 Assessing the fabric

7.01 Understanding
Collect as much information as is available from people and library sources about the building fabric.
Evaluate advantages, problems and failures of the building type.

7.02 Assessment
Assess elements that have failed, discover causes and apply remedial treatment.
Select areas where testing and special measures will be needed.

Decide which elements will need upgrading for planning and statutory reasons.
Decide on general standards of repair and evaluate factors affecting them; relate to the life of the building.

7.03 Specification
Decide on the standard of specification for each element, decide on cost rating.
Carry out cost checks on selected building elements.
Draw up full specification and documents suitable for tender.
Break down building work according to priorities and quantities.

RIBA STAGE OF WORK C/D: OUTLINE PROPOSALS/SCHEME DESIGN

8.00 Assessing the structure

8.01 Survey of existing structure
Initial survey to obtain idea of overall condition, materials of construction and major defects. Information is available from two complementary sources – the structure itself and existing drawings and documentation.
A more detailed survey should:
Identify structural material and assess in situ strength
Record section dimension
Record material and thickness of applied finishes
Note signs of distress
Expose and record connections and bearings
Inspect foundations and subsoil
Ensure that adequate records are made.

8.02 Assessment of structure as it stands
Is the structure generally sound and stable? If not reuse for any purpose is unlikely to be feasible.
Are there any signs of continuing distress? If so, these must be diagnosed to establish the cause and remedial measures considered.
Are there signs of past distress? Their treatment must be considered.

8.03 Assessment of structure for new uses
Do the proposals and the implications of the building work that must be carried out jeopardise the integrity of the structure?
Eg. removing structural walls can affect the ability of the structure to withstand lateral loads.
Assess the ability of the structure to withstand increased loading implied by change of use.
Does the structure have adequate stiffness to function under severe conditions?
Does the structure possess adequate fire insulation for the proposed new use?

8.04 Specification of structural work
Check interpretation and assessment of the survey with the building control officer.
Establish realistic solutions in terms of the stability of the structure during building work, phasing, adequate working space, accessibility.
Consult specialist firms as necessary.
Provide adequate contingency for work that cannot be envisaged from survey.
Assess temporary structural work required.

RIBA STAGE OF WORK C/D: OUTLINE PROPOSALS/SCHEME DESIGN

9.00 Planning the space

9.01 Planning the site
Establish the degree of demolition, rehabilitation and new building work required, making provision for future expansion.
Establish the number and type of goods, deliveries and the amount of car parking space to be provided.
Establish strategy for providing access and parking space within the limitations of the particular site.
Establish site coverage consistent with proposed use.
Note probable influence of surrounding development.

9.02 Planning the building
Decide on the types of use to be accommodated in each building.
Decide on strategy for organising tenancies.
Test the subdivision capacity of the building.
From the types of access and degree of separation required to meet statutory requirements (direct or indirect access, open plan, self-contained, shared).
Decide on the allocation of common services and facilities, eg. common access, entrance areas, stairs, lifts, loading bays, delivery parking, corridors, washing facilities, first aid and doctors' rooms, canteens and creches.

RIBA STAGE OF WORK C/D: OUTLINE PROPOSALS/SCHEME DESIGN CONTINUED

9.03   Planning individual tenancies
Test the rental units against different user types.
Decide on the type of function and layout required: process type layout or product line layout (unit, batch).
Decide on future requirements, dependent on type of firm – satellite, specialist or marketeer, fast or slow growing.
Develop space requirements by computing production area requirements from an understanding of the operations involved, and adding support requirements.
Deciding on space type/module, (percentage of floor area) for different kinds of operation (work space, desk space assembly, storage, amenities etc.).

9.04   Servicing and equipping the unit
In connection with the fabric and structure assessment and different levels of planning.

Evaluate existing services (if any)
Availability of statutory undertakers' supplies together with any special needs and requirements collectively relating to users.

Assess environmental requirements
Access, noise, security, loading, lighting, heating, power, telephone, water services, waste disposal, any specialist services for both individual units (sharing), and the building collectively.
Decide on level of metering and control.
Select or anticipate particular machinery/equipment and the space related to it. Consider whether it could be shared between units.

For the building
Assess fire precautions and alarms, toilets, general servicing and clearing arrangements, security, safety/hazards, reception and special building services (eg. printing, secretarial, accounting etc).
Make reference in assessment and the selection of equipment and the services of how to get the work done.

RIBA STAGE OF WORK C/D: OUTLINE PROPOSALS/SCHEME DESIGN

10.00   Controlling the costs

10.1   Cost composition and sensitivity
An elemental cost analysis should be prepared by a qualified cost consultant. When planning the space and specifying the building work an understanding of the composition and sensitivity of the costs is important. The key to successful rehabilitation/conversion projects lies in determining whether the worst features of a building are particularly cost sensitive in the overall proposal.

10.02   Elemental cost analysis
Works associated with the structural condition of the building/fabric.
Works in order to comply with the current standards of health and safety and fire precautions.
Works in connection with the client's requirements.

RIBA STAGE OF WORK K: SUPERVISION

11.00   Project management

11.0   The variables
Size of project
Condition of the fabric
Quality of the end result
Type of tenure
Amount of user involvement in the decision-making process
Amount of work being left to the end user
Methods of funding.

11.02   Level of professional services
Full professional service
Partial service
Client/building team
Do-it-yourself.

11.03   Organising the building work
Select contractor and establish:
Sufficient experience
Adequate resources
Rates to negotiate extra works
A balanced price
Daywork rates.
Select voluntary or unskilled labour and provide the following:
Adequate drawings/calculations for planning, building control, environmental health and fire authorities
Adequate insurance for third parties, neighbouring property, works and materials
Project manager
Realistic assessment of administrative overheads
Realistic estimate of building costs
Adequate site supervision.

12.00   Building management

12.01   Deciding on the legal structure
Private limited company
Public limited company
Company limited by guarantee
Common ownership
Building preservation trust
Charity
Association of occupants
Consider personal liability, voting powers, tax situation and the objectives of the enterprise.

12.02   Finding and selecting tenants
Ensure compatibility
Have a mix of firms
Ensure a base of well established firms to cover risk
Get bank and trade references to establish credit-worthiness
Avoid the temptation to accept all-comers
Remember the nursery function of such an enterprise.

12.03   Day-to-day management
Financial outgoings
Rent
Rates
Maintenance
Adaptation
Administration of shared services.

Firm control and monitoring of finances is vital:
Forecast future expenditures and prepare budgets
Allocate annual budget figure for each category of projected expenditure
Control may be by analysis built into accountancy system or approval of priced purchase orders against a periodic financial allocation
Penal surcharge established to ensure commitments are met.

12.04   Joint services
Shared services include
Reception
Printing
Meeting areas
Canteen
Book-keeping
Telephone switchboard and telex
Deliveries
Cleaning.

Factors affecting the scope and type of services that can be provided:
Mix of type of firms
Number of firms
Size of firms
Size of enterprise/building.

In considering shared services there must be an agreement over service charges, extent of benefits and the cost of specialist services.

7 Assessing the Development Potential

1.00 Alternative starting points

A project will only be successful if the right uses are matched to the available buildings and the development approach has been carefully thought out (figures 1, 2, 3). A project may begin with:

• A group of users looking for a building; or a professional who has been asked to find suitable space for a client or group of clients.

• A redundant building which requires an alternative use to arrest decay. In some instances the building may be one of architectural or historical interest, whose cause is taken up by a local conservation group. In other cases the building may be architecturally undistinguished, but in sound condition and its reuse advocated by a local action group to bring life and prosperity back into a locality.

• A local authority or major land owner taking stock of vacancy in an area, so as to formulate policy, and to earmark buildings requiring specific action.

2.00 The feasibility study process

Feasibility studies have a vital role to play in the development process in both the private and the public sector. For the private developer, group of users or building owner, the feasibility study process should:

Provide an understanding of the opportunities and realistic value of a site or building

Test the economic viability of alternative uses

Help decide on the feasibility of proceeding with a project.

For the local authority a quick method of assessing buildings should help the planning department:

Take stock of the characteristics and possible development outcome of empty buildings in an area.

The purpose of the local authority undertaking such a study is to:

Isolate common problems requiring policy change

Define realistic development control policy
Decide on whether to purchase or financially support specific buildings.

2.01 Main issues
The information which follows sets out the four main issues for consideration in testing the feasibility of a project, from its inception stage to the decision to proceed:

Picking the best building for a particular use
Finding the best use for a particular building
Taking stock of development options (local area survey and initial building assessment)
Undertaking an in-depth feasibility study.

3.00 Picking the best building for a particular use

In any locality there will usually be a range of possible buildings ranging from a small chapel or gatehouse with perhaps less than 100m^2 to a giant factory or warehouse with over 20,000m^2 of space. With such varied possibilities it is vital to pick the most promising ones by:

Establishing the potential users
Taking stock of the available buildings
Preparing a shortlist of the best buildings.

3.01 Establishing the potential users
Though it is not necessary to know precisely who each tenant is going to be, it is essential to have some idea of what kind of users are involved since they will vary in what they require and what they can afford. Often the best policy will be to go for a building that allows the widest range of choices and then carry out the work and tenant selection in a way which makes the most of the building.
Projects of this kind can be initiated by a number of types of organisations: See 'Users looking for buildings' (Development Checklist, chapter 6 section 3).

3.02 Taking stock of the available buildings
Which locality?
The next stage is to define the most suitable locality and to

51

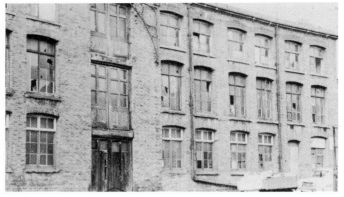

Figure 1   *Industrial building ripe for rehab and looking for a use.*

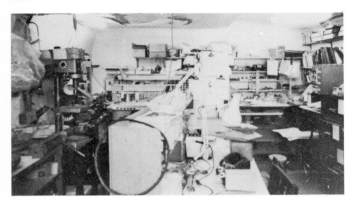

Figure 2   *Use looking for a suitable building*

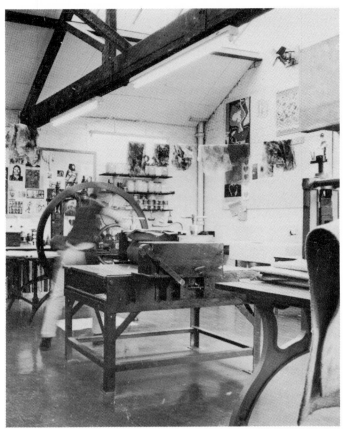

Figure 3   *Print workshop: needs matched to a building.*

carry out an inventory of what is on the market or might become available in that area. To allow a comparison of available opportunities, and an identification of most promising possibilities, empty buildings in the locality should be mapped. The physical or spatial characteristics of the available empty buildings should then be summarised in a format which allows rapid comparison (table 1).

Weighing up supply and demand
The economic viability of the scheme will depend on the relationship between supply and demand for premises. On the supply side, it is important to know the terms on which buildings will be available and the cost of converting them. The terms asked will depend on such factors as who owns the building, whether it was bought for redevelopment, what the attitudes of the planning authority are to redevelopment and how attractive the location is: clearly a building close to a main railway station in an area with many offices will be worth more as a development site than a similar building in a conservation area, or one where the local authority will not allow offices.

On the demand side, the main considerations are the numbers of potential tenants, their minimum requirements, what they can afford to pay and the suitability of the location in terms of accessibility for both goods and people. Thus a design studio may well require less in the way of floor space and services, such as gas and water, while at the same time being able to afford more in rent. However, such a firm may also be more choosy about its location, paying attention for example to the character of the area.

Information sources
● The local authority's estates department or industrial development officer may keep a list of properties available and a number of local authorities now publish a register giving basic details of buildings in both public and private ownership.

● Statutory undertakers' property departments (eg. British Rail Property Division).

● Local estate agents will keep fuller particulars. They can be identified both from the property register and from a street-by-street survey.

● The local planning authority may know about buildings that are about to be vacated, such as schools or hospitals, or those of historic value where an initiative may be welcomed.

● A street-by-street survey will help to indicate which buildings are vacant but not on the market. Buildings owned by the local or statutory authorites may be empty awaiting a planning decision. A direct approach with a proposal for a sensible alternative use may result in a short-life lease being granted.

3.03   Shortlisting the best buildings
A shortlist of the buildings with greatest development potential should be based on the following factors:

● Condition of the structure and fabric.

● Present planning use category. A change of use, or special planning requirements (such as being a listed building) may

Table I Comparison of three vacant buildings, North Southwark, London

Location			
Address	182 Union Street	50 Southwark Bridge Road	Green Walk
Accessibility: for goods	Poor, no distributor roads	Southwark Street and Bridge Road nearby	Quite good
for employees	Only Blackfriars Road buses	10 mins London Bridge, Borough	Buses only
Configuration			
Number of floors	7	7	6
Floor area (m²): per floor	440		
total	2640	3575	9620
Ceiling heights	5m in basement		
Frontage	40m	18m	
Depth	18m	37m	
Site coverage	Total, alley at rear	Temporary car park to rear	3 intercommunicating blocks
Internal structure	Open planned		
External fabric	Reasonable brickwork	Good brickwork	
Facilities			
Lifts	Two goods lifts to all floors	two 1t goods lifts, one passenger lift	
Staircases			
Hoists			
Loading doors	2 large, 2 small	2	
Yards		No private yard	Central yard
Car parking	7 spaces in alley	Probably	
General services	Heating, 3 phase electricity, sprinklers	Heating, sprinklers	
Lavatories			
Daylight	Good to rear of top floors	Some dark areas	
Fire escapes			
Floor loadings	Concrete floors		
Image	Solid building	Good looking frontage	Huge building
Valuation			
Age	Varying		
Previous use	Envelope manufacture	Warehouse	Warehouse
Present planning permission	Industrial GIA	GIA	Not zoned
Leasehold/Freehold	Lease until 1986	Short term lease	Lease
Rent/price	Rent review 1981		£47,500 pa (£495/m²)
Years	11 or shorter		10 years
Comments	Empty since 1974	Awaiting office permit	

Taking stock of empty buildings

Before a building can be selected for development a survey should be made of the stock of vacant buildings in the locality.

During the month of October 1977 the Urban and Economic Development Group (URBED) carried out a survey in North Southwark, London, which showed that there were 59 vacant industrial buildings and 130,000m² of floor space with a potential, if they were in use, of providing between 1600 and 5800 jobs. The survey showed that there was remarkably little space available for tiny firms (those employing 5 to 10 persons and requring under 450m²) and that 71 per cent of all the floor space was available in units of over 2250m².

Information on each of the empty buildings was collected within a standard format so that a short list could be drawn up of buildings suitable for conversion to multiple uses and more detailed feasibility studies undertaken.

have implications for the amount, type and standard of alteration work required.

● Site coverage. This will affect access, parking and external storage.

● Type of construction and services. The condition and distribution of wcs, number and location of staircases and the mode of construction will influence the choice of uses and the amount of work required to meet statutory requirements. Buildings with existing fireproof (concrete) floors – most twentieth-century buildings – are inherently cheaper to convert than those with timber floors and lightweight roof construction which lack insulation (eighteenth and nineteenth-century warehouses). Likewise factories are usually cheaper to convert than warehouses, because they often have goods lifts, lavatories, and correct floor to ceiling heights.

● Accessibility. Ease of movement of goods and people within the building, as well as the ease of access into the building.

● Configuration. The amount of space on each floor, degree of compartmentation, depth of space, number of floors, floor to ceiling heights and range of different spaces provided will influence types of use. Conversion work on a space of under 500m² can often be financed by a group of tenants, whereas a larger building may require more investment and hence institutional funding bringing more onerous conditions.

● Cost of the building. The length and terms of the ground lease or freehold and the rateable value will influence the rents and service charge which will be required to make the project viable.

● The locality. Frequency of public transport, proximity to major roads and the ease of parking in the neighbourhood will all affect the attraction of the locality. Uses that might be accommodated will depend on the traditional activities of the locality, the interests of the local community and proposed plans for the future.

● Availability of finance. A small building or one in good condition might be financed out of income from tenants, perhaps with a bank loan. However, most of the available space is in large buildings, and here the costs of conversion will usually require longer term finance, affecting the choice of building.

Table II Checklist for evaluating alternative buildings

Aspect evaluated	Assessment Good (3 star) ***	Average (2 star) **	Poor (1 star) *
Accessibility			
Goods	Near trunk road	Near primary distributor	Distant from both
Employees: Rail	0–5 mins walk to station	5–10 mins walk to station	10 mins + walk to station
Visitors: Bus	5 routes, 0–5 mins to stops	3 routes, 0–10 mins to stops	Anything other than categories on left
Car	On site or licenced parking @ 1 space per 1500 sq ft (140m^2) or better	On site, licensed or street parking @ less than 1 space per 1500 sq ft (140m^2)	Metered or no parking
Site†			
Site coverage	60% or less	60–90%	90% or more
Access	Maximum length vehicle to loading doors without need for 3-point turn	With need for 3-point turn	No access for maximum length vehicles
Building condition	Structurally sound	Internal work required	External work required
Building configuration†			
Number of floors	Single storey	2–4 floors	5 or more floors
Floor area per floor Total floorspace	50 000–150 000 sq ft (4650–14 000m^2)	10 000–50 000 sq ft (930–4650m^2)	Below 10 000, above 150 000 sq ft
Ceiling heights: ground	14–16ft (4.3–4.9m)	8–14 ft (2.4–4.3m)	Below 8 ft (2.4m)
upper floor(s)	10–14 ft (3.0–4.3m)	8–10 ft (2.4–3.0m)	Below 8 ft (2.4m)
Frontage			
Depth			
Internal structure	Columns	Non load-bearing partitions	Load bearing internal partitions
Aspect	Detached, 4-way aspect, windows all round	3-way aspect + windows	2-way aspect or less
Floor loadings	Concrete on steel supports	Cast iron or heavy timber	Light timber
Building specifications			
Health:			
Lavatories	1 per 25 workers @ 250 sq ft (24m^2) per worker or better	1 per 25 workers @ 250–750 sq ft (24–70m^2) per worker	Worse than 1 per 25 workers @ (70m^2) per worker
Fire:			
Means of escape	2 fire escapes to ground less than 60m apart	Single escape, everyone within 30m, or fireproof access with same plus rudimentary alternative	No fire escape and unfireproofed access
Combustibility	Concrete columns + floors or sprinkler system	Thick wood floors	Unprotected timber joists; cast iron columns
Services:			
Water and soil	To all floors	To building	None
Electricity	Three phase to all floors minimum 200 KVA	60–200 KVA	Below 60 KVA or to some floors only
Gas	Gas to all floors	Gas to building	None
Valuation			
Age	Under 50 years	Under 100 years	Over 100 years
Previous use	General purpose, large firm factory		Special use (eg brewery), warehouse
Tenure	Freehold or 99 year lease	25–99 year lease	Less than 25 year lease
Rent/price	Cheap (less than market price)	Market price	More than market price
Example: North Southwark, London (price £/m^2)	Freehold: less than £80 Leasehold: less than £75	£80–150 £7.50–20	£150+ £200+
Planning			
Present planning permission for:	General industry	Light industry	Office, commercial, housing
Planning zone	Industrial improvement area (eg Rochdale), conservation area, general employment area	Mixed development	Housing action area

* This table can be used as a checklist to weight the characteristics of different buildings, for example allocating three stars for good, two for average and one for poor (as Consumer Reports do, in selecting a 'best-buy'). † See tables on pages 25–26 for suggested classification criteria.

Rapid assessment
To help rapidly assess the buildings most likely to be suitable for conversion a quick method is proposed which awards critical aspects (see table II) of a building 'stars' for being good, average or poor. The criteria have been developed through experience on analysis of projects already completed.

4.00   Finding the best use for a particular building

The main steps are to:

Identify potential 'clients' (ie building owners whose premises are available for reuse)

Find suitable uses for the buildings thus identified.

4.01   Identify potential clients
Possible driving forces behind a project to reuse a particular building include:

● Firms who have moved to more efficient premises and have been unable to sell their old buildings.

● Firms who are looking for alternative uses for parts of their buildings.

● Owners of buildings of quality (either listed or in conservation areas) who are not allowed to demolish the property.

● Local authorities who have compulsorily purchased buildings for comprehensive redevelopment, but no longer have the finance for demolition and rebuilding, or who are looking for short life uses while planning objectives are reformulated.

● Statutory authorities who own buildings which are redundant due to changes in catchment areas (schools and hospital authorities) processes (gas and electricity boards) or transportation networks (British Rail or the harbour authorities).

● Building owners such as local authorities who are left with buildings made redundant due to changing social habits (eg. public bath houses) or misguided planning predictions (vacated and vandalised multi-storey car parks).

● Estate agents or property companies concerned to secure an early return from a redundant building when redevelopment is unlikely.

● Conservation groups who are concerned to retain a disused building of character or amenity groups who wish to bring the empty buildings in the area back into use, rather than let them decay and blight the neighbourhood.

● Individual enthusiasts.

4.02   Find suitable uses
The decision having been made to conserve a building, the choice of use will be a combination of imagination, careful planning and straightforward entrepreneurship. It is important to:

● Understand what grants or loans are available for conversion work on buildings in the area (chapter 8 section 5).

● Analyse what types of firms and services are already in the locality and their networks of interdependence. *Kelly's street directory* is a useful source of data, recording perhaps 90 per cent of small firms in an area. The classified telephone directory is perhaps the best source of all, though it requires considerable analysis and still does not provide the size of firm.

● Study the advertisements in the local paper – the market for very small units of accommodation which are too small to interest estate agents is normally transacted through the papers.

● Place an advertisement in the local paper to test the market. If the development is aimed at a specific industry or profession (eg designers) then advertising or editorial in the appropriate trade publication will produce feedback.

● Spread the word among the local business community that a project to provide small units of accommodation is being considered (eg through the local Chamber of Commerce or Rotary Club).

5.00   Taking stock of development options

5.01   Levels of approach
Professional time for undertaking feasibility studies is valuable and the number of vacant buildings available in an area may be high. The problem can be overcome by following a sequential approach which successfully narrows the number of buildings to be studied and selects the projects with most potential, the following procedure can be used:

Defining the context: the local area survey

Sorting the field: the initial building assessment

Testing the options: the financial viability study

Increasing confidence: the in-depth feasibility study.

the objectives, an amount of work and information collected at each stage (following the local area survey) are shown in three levels in table III, working on vacant buildings.

5.02   Local area surveys
The potential development options for a particular building are dependent on both the existing and future characteristics of the immediate area. The local area survey describes the characteristics and defines appropriate local authority responses for specific areas. The objective is to survey a definable locality so as to:

● Take stock of the characteristics of the vacant buildings (instant assessment).

● Assess the economic activity of an area and classify whether it is a) an improvement area where investment depends largely on the private sector, and the local authorities' roles in relaxing constraints and providing incentives, b) a development area where investment depends largely on the public sector taking direct action or changing the climate of opinion.

● Define effective and potential demand.

Table III Characteristics of three levels of feasibility study

	LEVEL 1	LEVEL 2	LEVEL 3
PURPOSE	Take stock of opportunities in an area Grade strategies for development Isolate common problems requiring policy change Sift buildings for further study	Define development control strategy Decide on future action Test sensitivity of alternative approaches Agree investment of resources	Confirm hypothesis Increase confidence
INPUT	External viewing and Ordnance Survey map Agent's particulars and planning history One hour of planner/architect	Access to building Discussion with agent/owner 2 man days valuer/QS + planner/architect	4 man weeks QS and architect Discussions with statutory authorities Accurate floor plans
INFORMATION COLLECTED	Factual information - size, shape, use, percentage vacancy, access Assessment of location, site, building, planning constraints	Alternative development proposals Element costs Consider 5 grades of specification Quantified comparison	Brief survey Sketch proposals Costing Programme of implementation
DECISIONS	Which to leave alone Which to test Which to leave to market forces	How far to change mix of uses Local authority inputs Neighbourhood investment	Choose method of approach Degree of investment

● Propose initiatives to be implemented by the local authority.

● Help define local development control policy.

A large amount of the data required will be available from statistics already compiled by the local authority. The information will cover:

● The amount and type of vacancy and estate agents' data on vacant premises.

● Potential and effective demand. There is little point in refurbishing buildings or initiating area improvement schemes if there is unlikely to be sufficient demand to make use of the extra space at rents that will make the investment profitable.

Demand for premises
Demand can come from three main sources:

Existing firms moving to find more appropriate or cheaper premises

Firms from elsewhere setting up branches

New firms starting up.

The level of demand will very much depend on existing patterns of activity, as similar businesses tend to cluster together. It will also depend on the state of the local and national economies. Finally, there may be local deficiencies, such as poor transport, that stop an area achieving its full potential.
Although it is impossible to forecast accurately the likely demand for workspace the following sequence of steps should help:

1 Check the experience of previous conversions:
Occupancy levels
Rental
Types of occupant.

2 Look at the market
Rent levels asked
Vacancy levels
Turnover by size band
Shortages experienced.

3 Analyse the local economies (preferably by property market area):
Occupied floor space
Employment break-down by industry (those that can use upper floors or prefer ground floor)
Employment trends
Size distribution of firms.

4 Assess the likelihood of building activity. Study the local authority or commercial schemes that are planned or under construction for new or converted space for small industrial units.

Local authority initiatives
The information collected (table IV) will indicate the state of the local economy and the degree of intervention required by the local authority. Table IV, section F suggests initiatives that may be taken by a local authority to help a stagnant or dying area. These initiatives can be categorised as:

● Changing the climate of opinion, by preparing planning briefs for selected buildings, promoting the area, or initiating environmental improvement schemes.

● Relaxing constraints, by speeding up the planning process, policies for mixed use, traffic management schemes.

● Providing incentives, through grants, loans etc., or moral support.

● Taking direct action, by undertaking area improvement or building conversion projects.

5.03 Initial building assessment

Many buildings may be vacant because they are no longer physically suited to the types of uses originally planned or are in poor condition. The first stage is to establish whether a building is suited to refurbishment (improvement for the same use), conversion (upgrading for alternative use), or should be redeveloped. Buildings worth bothering about are marginal cases, where with the right development approach reuse may be economically viable.

The initial assessment examines all the vacant buildings in the area with the objective of:

Understanding the physical characteristics of the building.

Deciding on the possible development outcomes.

Understanding why buildings are standing vacant: and so isolating common problems requiring policy change.

Sifting the buildings, to select those for further study.

To use resources most effectively, the initial assessment should rely on an external view of the building, backed up by ordnance survey map and local estate agents' particulars. Approximately one hour of an experienced architect's or planner's time is required for each building. The information collected covers accessibility, building configuration (size, shape, aspect and height), structure and condition. The first sieve groups buildings into three categories:

Good: leave to market forces
Marginal: test for development potential
Bad: leave for redevelopment.

Table V provides a worked example of an instant assessment sheet. However, without being able to enter the buildings, a great many decisions concerning condition, subdivision, quality of services, fire protection and means of escape are informed guesswork.

What such a survey can provide is:

● A coarse sieve separating the good from hopeless buildings so as to narrow the field of study.

● A comparative profile of the characteristics of the vacant building stock in local areas.

● A source of data to highlight the problems and physical characteristics of vacant buildings in local areas, to help formulate planning policy.

Table IV   Typical local area survey

A.	AREA PROFILE				
1.	LOCATION	Clerkenwell, London EC1			
2.	BOUNDARIES	Clerkenwell Rd	Goswell Rd	St John St	Compton St
3.	BOUNDARY ACTIVITIES	Retail, Horologists	Publishers, Printing	Retail, Offices	Retail, School, Refurnished block

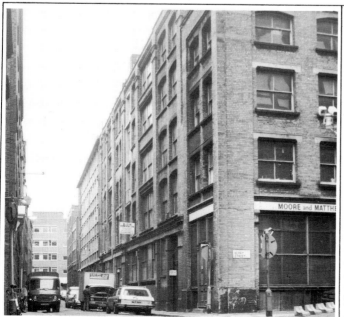

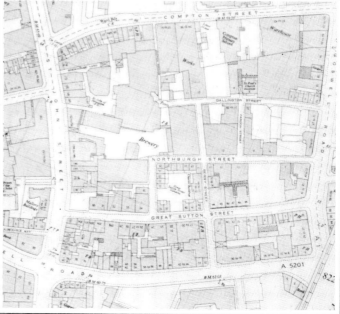

Table IV Typical local area survey—*continued*

		m²	per cent of total site area	per cent of total floor space
4. SITE AREA *		47,853	100	
5. GROUND FLOOR AREA		33,500	70	
6. HARD AREA*		14,350	30	
7. VACANCY*	Land	652	1	
	Buildings	24,792		16
8. PREDOMINANT USES* +	Industrial	42,734		29
	Office	25,745		17
	Commerce (storage)	37,532		26
	Residential	2,781		2
* 'Cluster' + Land Use Survey	Retail	3,826		3
	Others	10,397 +1		7

B.	AREA ASSESSMENT
9. DOMINANT EMPLOYERS	*Allied breweries, Small businessmen*
10. PREDOMINANT TYPES OF FIRMS	*Printers, Clockmakers, Small service firms, Publishers*

		+	o	–	
11. AREA UP-KEEP	Neat hoardings Well-maintained streets Painted buildings		✓		Broken fences Rough roads Broken pavements
12. BUILDING CONDITION	Maintained Recently vacated		✓		Broken windows Long empty, derelict Structural work needed
13. LOCAL SERVICES	Cafes, Pubs, Shops Busy streets Taxis	✓			No local services Deserted streets No taxis

C.	DEMAND	
14. PREDOMINANT SIZE OF VACANT UNITS	Size m²	Per cent of total
	0- 50	
	50-100	
	100-250	
	250-500	
	500+	
Vacancy level	Excessive (over 15%)	
	High (over 5%)	✓
	Low (below 5%)	

Table IV   Typical local area survey—*continued*

15. RENTALS £m²	Size	Storage	Industrial	Office
	< 250 m²			
	> 250 m²			

16. NEW DEVELOPMENT PLANNED OR UNDER CONSTRUCTION	Use	GFA (m²)	Rentals	Size of units	Per cent vacancy
17. MULTIPLE TENANCY BUILDINGS					
Compton St (rehab)					

			+	o	–	
18. EFFECTIVE DEMAND	Sold signs, building work, new growing firms, etc				✓	For sale signs, no building work, old established static firms
19. POTENTIAL DEMAND	Relevant firms near, easy access, support services		✓			No relevant firms near, Hard access, no service

D. ACCESSIBILITY			
20. GOODS VEHICLES	HGVs	MGVs	LGVs
	Narrow roads	*Fair*	*Fair*
21. UNLOADING (Predominant mode in area)	On street	Off street (lay-by or cul-de-sac)	Internal yard
	Generally	*No*	*No*
22. PUBLIC TRANSPORT	Bus	Tube	Train
	Good	*Barbican and Faringdon*	*No*
23. ON STREET PARKING	No restrictions	Restricted	Meters
			Predominantly
24. OFF STREET PARKING	Public	Covered	Open
		None	*None*
	Private	Covered	Open
		None	*Allied Breweries*

Table IV   Typical local area survey—*continued*

E. VACANT BUILDINGS (Summary of Vacant building survey)						
25. TOTAL FLOOR AREA (m^2)						
26. BUILDINGS	Size	Access	Config	Structure	Condition	Suggested outcome

6.00   Carrying out a feasibility study

6.01   Matching building and user

The assessment of the vacant buildings in the area will suggest a shortlist of possible buildings. From this shortlist the most likely building may be chosen for detailed analysis. A scheme can rapidly become uneconomic by trying to match the wrong use to the building or vice versa. The successful scheme will be the one that matches the building to uses and development options with a complimentary character so the minimum of adaptation is required.

To minimise time commitments and maximise on professional inputs the likely options should be tested by an economic appraisal before undertaking a detailed feasibility study.

6.02   Preliminary economic appraisal

This stage should aim to rapidly test the economic sensitivity of varying the mix of uses, level of specification, development approach, or method of funding. A format for undertaking economic appraisals, and the variables that may be adjusted to influence the economic viability of a scheme are described in chapter 8.

6.03   In-depth feasibility study

The purpose of an in-depth feasibility study is to:

● Confirm an hypothesis for a preferred development approach suggested at the preliminary economic appraisal stage.

● Decide the economics of a project, so as to be able to make a decision to proceed, and approach sources of funding for support.

● Increase confidence in the viability of the proposed development approach.

A detailed building feasibility study will require a major investment of experienced manpower if the results are to be of value. To arrive at an accurate assessment of the floor area available, the amount of building work required, and the need to insert new elements, the following information is required:

Accurate building dimensions
Outline survey of building condition
Checklist of statutory and planning requirements
Information on leases, and ownership.

Access to the building is essential, and the availability of accurate floor plans, constructional drawings, and a planning history file is assumed if the estimated four man weeks of input is to be met.

Table VI lists the information required, and useful sources of reference.

The in-depth feasibility study (table VII) should answer the following questions:

How viable is reuse?
What is the most suitable use?
How should the development be undertaken and funded?

The feasibility study provides the supporting evidence for a decision to be made to approach:

The building owner to negotiate a purchase or lease
Financial institutions for funding
Internal committees, and potential users for agreement on the proposed type of development.

The main steps to be included in the detailed feasibility report are shown in the development checklist (chapter 6, para. 6) under the following headings:

Statement of objectives of the scheme
Space planning concept
Assessment of building work required
Review of planning and statutory requirements
Strategy for undertaking the conversion
Financial appraisal
Type of development organisation proposed
Timing of project.

Table IV   Typical local area survey—*continued*

F. PROPOSED INITIATIVES	
Development control	
- Quick planning response for selected buildings	

(i) *Allow office conversion to encourage rehab. to high standard, mixed uses*
    (ii)
    (iii)
    (iv)	

- Preparation of planning briefs for selected buildings	

(i)
    (ii)
    (iii)
    (iv)	

- Policies for mixed use	
Selected areas Selected buildings	
Parking and Transport	
- Traffic management to improve movement	*Yes*
- Loading strips	

Lay-bys
    Service lanes
    Zoned parking and yellow lines
	
	Yes

- Car parking	
Reuse of wasteland for temporary park Reuse of surplus residential parking	*Yes*
- Improve public transport	
Environmental improvement	
- Wash and brush up (specify selected areas)	*Yes*
- Facelift (specify selected areas)	
- Landscaping	*Local park for lunchtime use (2,500 m^2)*
Vacant sites Streets	
Finance	
- Designate loans or grants for selected buildings	

(i) *No buildings of great architectural merit*
    (ii)
    (iii)
    (iv)	

- Purchase building or sites	

(i)
    (ii)
    (iii)	

Promotion	
- Space exchange	
- Planning shop	
- Training centre	

Table V Instant assessment survey sheet

VACANT BUILDING SURVEY

ADDRESS	230–240 STOKE NEWINGTON HIGH STREET, HACKNEY N.16
GROSS FLOOR AREA	3000 m²
PRESENT USE	VACANT PERCENTAGE VACANCY 100%
PREVIOUS USE	DEPARTMENT STORE

TENURE

	+		o		−	
Off street parking & delivery			✓			On street parking/narrow street
60 per cent site coverage					✓	100 per cent site coverage
Good site access					✓	No site access
5 min. tube and bus			✓			10 min bus
Goods lift/wide staircase			✓			No lifts/narrow staircase
Single-storeyed					✓	4 or more storeys
ACCESS						
Four-way aspect			✓			Single aspect
10–15 m deep	✓					20 m or more deep
Simple shape	✓					Complex shape
3.00 m Fl/FL (upper floor)	✓					3.60 m + FL/FL
CONFIGURATION			✓			
Frame	✓					Load bearing walls
Brick, concrete plasterboard	✓					Timber, cast iron, steel
STRUCTURE					✓	
CONDITION Good					✓	Bad

PROPOSED OUTCOME

1   Leave alone

2   Mothball or short term use (eg studio)

3   Clear for temporary use (eg parking)

4   Refurbish for industrial use

⑤   Clear and redevelop   LIGHT INDUSTRIAL/RESIDENTIAL/RETAIL

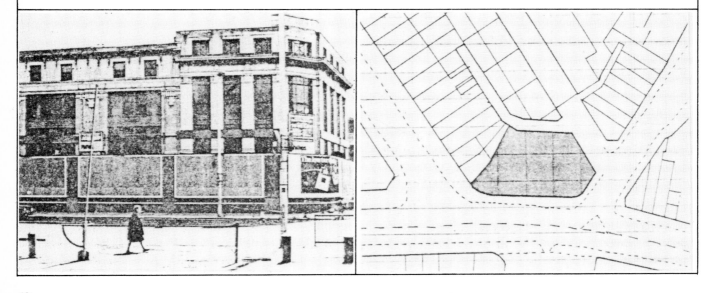

Table VI   Survey checklist for redundant buildings

Item to be checked	Information required	Source of information
1 Organisational factors		
1.01 Name of owner (including his intentions)		Estate agent; rate book
1.02 Name of estate agent		
1.03 Form of lease	Type: full repairing and insuring? Term/length/date of termination	Agent)there can be several) Space exchange agency
1.04 Assessment	Rateable value	Local authority
1.05 Rent/price	£ per annum (per month). Amount per sq ft (or m²)	Agent
1.05 Availability of space	Vacant or part possession Nature and number of tenants if applicable Form of management Rents, service charge	Agent
1.07 Previous uses	Names of organisations, type of manufacturing etc	Agents Local history archives/records
1.08 Age	Date of building/period	Local societies (history/archaeological)
1.09 Image	Dark, light, easily identifiable, typical of area etc	Inspection/maps
2 Site factors		
2.01 Location	Address	Agent (Post Office)
2.02 Accessibility	Employees/people: eg distance from transport (stations); number of buses passing Goods: eg narrowness of street, loading capabilities	Local maps; public transport information Site plan—1:2500 Ordnance Survey, street directory
2.03 Approach road	Width, construction	Site plan 1:2500 Ordnance Survey
2.04 Outside space (yard/garden)	Size for unloading, servicing parking (numbers)	street directory, or survey
2.05 Surrounding buildings	Uses, degree of enclosure to building under consideration	Local authority maps, and by inspection
2.06 Local community users	Types of use, frequency, length of time in use	As above
2.07 External influences	Noise, pollution, aircraft, roads, railways	Local authority, Dept of Environmental Health
3 Town planning		
3.01 Use classes	Town and Country (Use Classes) Order 1972 lays down 18 different classes. Existing limits of what could be proposed or would be approved	Local authority planning department
3.02 Local plan information	Zoning; General opportunities and constraints in neighbourhood; Major neighbouring uses existing and proposed; road proposals	Local authority planning department
3.03 Special orders	Existing or proposed; closing; clearance; demolition, repair; enforcement; Special control; compulsory purchase	Local authority
3.04 Notices	Preservation; purchase; dangerous structure	
3.05 Historic/listed building, ancient monument	Grade	Local authority; Department of Environment, Fortress House, Savile Row
3.06 Conservation area	Outstanding/ordinary; extent of area	Local authority or civic trust
3.07 Outstanding planning applications		Local authority
4 Building factors		
4.01 Configuration	Number of floors; ceiling heights; frontage; depth; space per floor m²; internal structure/compartments; external structure/enclosing elements; construction of floors and roof; daylight potential for floors	Survey; plans/elevations/sections. Local authorities, estate agents, archives
4.02 Facilities	Lifts (capacity, persons/goods); staircases (construction; hoists); loading doors; yards/ gardens; fire escapes; floor loading possibilities	Agents; inspection surveys
4.03 Services	Toilets; main drainage; water supply; electricity—phase, capacity; gas; (already existing/feasibility of supply); heating—method/type	Local authority Engineers Dept; Local; statutory authorities
5 Commercial viability		
5.01 Anticipated income/outgoings	Asking rent; rates; alteration works (estimate); fees—legal, architect, qs, agents, profit margin. Overall cost	

7.00   The decision to proceed

Even if the project looks viable there will still be much to do before work can begin.

Firstly, the present owner must be persuaded to take immediate steps to halt deterioration of the building if it is vacant. Once empty, a building will deteriorate rapidly, especially if it is located in an already blighted area.

Secondly, brochures for fund raising must be prepared and sources of finance for grant aid should be contacted. This period of the project will require boundless energy and co-ordination, making sure that the deadlines for grant submissions are met and organising the flow of money and resources so that when the team is ready to start on site, money is available to buy materials.

8.00   The role of the professionals

Unlike the new building project where its inception is planned, formalised, and funding is already set aside, the inception of a project to reuse an existing building is usually unplanned, informal and has limited funding. Many of the most successful projects to date (such as Clerkenwell Workshops London; or Trinity Arts Centre Birmingham) have been started by individuals with energy, ideas and perseverence.

Table VII   Contents and drawings for in-depth feasibility study

CONTENTS	EXHIBITS	FORMAT/SCALE
O.O SUMMARY AND CONCLUSIONS	STATISTICAL AND ECONOMIC APPRAISAL	TABLE
1.O WHERE IS THE BUILDING LOCATED?		
Location Main activities Change Demand Facilities Amenity	Location plan Site plan Summary of local area survey	Extract from street plan 1:1250 Table
2.O WHAT IS THE BUILDING LIKE?		
Description Access Ownership Configuration Structure and fabric Services Problems and opportunities	General view of site Space available Evaluation of existing building Summary of condition Evaluation of building	Photograph or axonometric Table Annotated plan Annotated plan Table
3.O WHAT COULD THE BUILDING BE USED FOR?		
Workspace Alternative uses	Options and areas yielded Preferred option Stacking plan of tenancies	Table Plan and section Plan
4.O WHAT ARE THE CONSTRAINTS ON RE-USE?		
Planning Fire Public health Energy Parking, access for goods and people		
5.O WHAT WORK NEEDS TO BE DONE?		
Summary of rehabilitation work Summary of conversion work		
6.O HOW VIABLE IS RE-USE?		
Assumptions Summary of building costs Net annual rental income Total development costs Capital value of completed development Financial appraisal	Elemental costs	Table

Table VII Contents and drawings for in-depth feasibility study—*continued*

CONTENTS	EXHIBITS	FORMAT/SCALE
7.O APPENDICES		

Background data
Sources of information
Specification of rehabilitation
  and conversion work
Analysis of total development
  costs		

Such projects have to rely on goodwill and voluntary advice until the viability of the project is assured. In the early stages the project may be too fragile to support the financial burden of a major input by professionals and any finance will be needed to make a start on building work.

The professionals may however, initiate projects (as at 5 Dryden Street and Barley Mow in London); become members of the steering committees; provide professional advice to clients wishing to undertake much of the work themselves; provide free advice through an organisation such as Action Research Centre; or act directly as an agent of the client body.

The advice required will range over a wide area and may include: finding a building; planning the space; assessing the construction and services; appraising economic viability; budgeting and cost control; advising on raising finance and finding cheap resources; organising the building work; managing the space; finding and vetting possible users.

In the early stages limited finances and the uncertain nature of the project require a flexibility of approach and a willingness to cover a wide range of subjects.

8 Assessing the Financial Viability

1.00 Introduction

1.01 Selecting suitable buildings
The success of a project depends on the choice of the most appropriate building. Unrecognised problems of poor access, structural defects, a need to meet statutory requirements or planning complications associated with a change of use, can rapidly turn a project into a financial disaster.

1.02 Need for feasibility study
There is little point in conserving and reusing old buildings if they are going to be uneconomic or more costly than building afresh (unless, of course, the environmental benefits exceed the extra costs). Conservation will only be substantially cheaper than redevelopment where a suitable building is chosen and appropriate uses are selected. Hence the arguments concerning re-use inevitably revolve around the economics of conversion.

1.03 Why schemes fail
The economic viability of a scheme depends mainly on four factors, discussed in section 2, the most fundamental being whether there are likely to be users requiring space in that area and willing to pay rentals high enough to exceed the cost of acquiring and adapting a building to both meet their needs and meet the requirements of the Building Regulations. Problems often arise because of a failure to do a proper assessment of the comparative economics of alternative schemes.

Feasibility study essential
The importance of undertaking a proper feasibility study cannot be over-estimated. The feasibility study makes it possible to bridge the gap between the idea and practicality, and links the needs of the ultimate user with the requirements of the financier.

Because of the cost in professional time of carrying out a feasibility study, it is important to concentrate only on the most promising conversion possibilities wherever there is a substantial choice of available buildings. We draw together, below, the major elements involved in carrying out such a feasibility study.

Table I provides a summary checklist of the steps to be taken in determining the viability of reuse.

2.00 The economics of conversion

There are many factors which determine whether re-use is economically feasible, the principal ones being:

Expected rental income
Likely development cost
Cost of acquiring a substantial leasehold or freehold interest in the site
Cost and availability of finance.

2.01 Assessing rental income
Information about prevailing rents and likely demand can be obtained from local estate agents, or the local industrial development officer.
Likely income rental depends on:

● Location.

● Types of new uses possible.

● Level of demand for accommodation (comprising both new firms that might set up or move into the area, and existing firms who want to expand or improve their premises).

● Rents that users can afford, and the likelihood of the space being occupied or the rent being paid all the time.

● Relative attractiveness of the area concerned (ie amenity of the surrounding neighbourhood, its accessibility, the degree of uncertainty, etc).

● The other sorts of property available in the area, and the terms on which they are available.

2.02 Estimating likely development costs
The critical factor affecting the feasibility of re-use tends to be the cost of redevelopment which will vary according to the building and location. Thus for an old warehouse in a dock area redevelopment costs are likely to represent well over 80 per cent of the total cost, whereas in a recently vacated factory in an attractive area, the acquisition costs of the site might exceed the cost of carrying out the building works.
Construction costs may be analysed in a number of ways.

Table I   A check-list of the sequence of steps to be taken in assessing the financial viability of conversion and re-use, at feasibility stage.

Step 1	Take stock of all the empty buildings in the area
1 . 1	Map the empty buildings
1 . 2	Summarise their characteristics

Step 2	Survey most attractive possibilities and compare with user requirements
2 . 1	Establish type of users
2 . 3	Survey appropriate buildings
2 . 3	Evaluate buildings against a checklist

Step 3	Establish feasibility of reuse
3 . 1	Decide on potential users and likely rents
3 . 2	Estimate the likely costs of development
3 . 3	Workout financial feasibility (see tables VII & VIII)
3 . 4	Revise scheme where necessary by adjusting rentals, specification of work to be undertaken , profit element, or re-negotiating the landlords asking rental

Step 4	Decide on the source of finance and the method of organising the project if the results are favourable
4 . 1	Establish possible sources of finance (see section 5)
4 . 2	Devise the appropriate organisational structure (see section 4)
4 . 3	Draw up a financial proposal

Table II   Summary of seven situations studied in Covent Garden

Description of new units to be provided	Description of existing buildings, divided into two categories in terms of repair work required	
	Category B★ Repairs to fabric Fire escapes and fireproofing New services	**Category C★** Non-structural partitions Overhauling services Upgrading finishes
Individual ground floor unit	Deep plan warehouse Cast iron columns and timber floors Open timber staircase	Ground floor shop with basement
Individual upper floor unit		Medium depth brick and concrete structure. Converted for floor use, additional fire escape required.
Co-operative or subleased Individual units	Medium depth warehouse Central lightwell Timber floors	Shallow depth brick and timber floor warehouse
Co-operative shared open plan space	Deep plan warehouse Steel frame and timber floors	Warehouse Concrete structure and floors

* For definition of categories see Levels of specification

Table III   Elementary conversion costs: analysis of seven feasibility studies undertaken in Covent Garden, London

Proposed new use of building	Category of building work required (see Levels of specification)			
	Costs given in £m^2 gross floor area			
	Category A	**Category B**	**Category C**	**Category D**
Office	£150–200	£100–150	£50–100	£20–50
Workshop studio	£130–175	£80–130	£40–80	£15–40
Average costs	£150–200	£100–150	£50–100	£20–50

The cost of building work varied between £40.00m^2 of GFA and £175.00m^2 GFA with an average cost of around £100.00 GFA.

Feasibility studies undertaken by Duffy Eley Giffone Worthington for the URBED Research Trust and described in *Accommodating small enterprises in Covent Garden*

Analysis by trades

One useful breakdown is into the trades involved, this affects how much work can be carried out by unskilled effort.

Analysis by user/legal requirements

A second way of looking at construction costs is to distinguish between those costs which must be incurred in meeting user requirements, and those necessitated in order to meet legal requirements, (e.g. the Building Regulations). This ratio will vary in accordance with type of user, and type of building. Table II summarises the type of building work required for seven conversions in London's Covent Garden area; and table III summarises the results of the feasibility studies which were undertaken: these showed that as soon as new fire escapes and services were required (as was the case with many of the units) costs increased steeply, sometimes by 100 per cent.

The precise cost of conversion work therefore depends on negotiations with statutory authorities. Approximately 30 per cent of the overall budget in the examples looked at was concerned with providing for fire protection, means of escape and sanitary accommodation (table IV).

Analysis by repair/conversion costs

A third way of looking at construction costs, and possibly the most useful, is to distinguish between repair and conversion work.

Repair can be defined as restoring a building so that it is in a good state for its original purpose. This is particularly hard to estimate as so much depends on the existing condition and what the users will tolerate. This is where experience really counts, unless a detailed schedule of delapidations is drawn up and costed by a qualified surveyor or builder, together with a structural survey where there are signs of structural faults.

However, there is evidence that costs are generally influenced by the length of time before the building is reused, and the level of security on the site. Thus a building recently vacated may only require £40–60/m^2 gross floor

Table IV Breakdown of Covent Garden conversion costs★, showing amount directly attributable to statutory requirements

	Costs necessitated by: statutory requirements Fire—means of escape Public health Other Cost £/m² GFA†	% of total	Other modernisations Alterations Decorations Electrics Heating, etc Cost £/m² GFA†	% of total	Total Cost £/m² GFA†
Medium depth warehouse, steel and timber floors	25	34	50	66	75
Warehouse, with steel frame and timber floors	30	24	105	76	135
Deep plan warehouse, steel and timber structure, open timber staircase	40	27	110	73	150
Ground floor shop with basement	28	28	72	72	100
Shallow depth brick and timber warehouse	27	26	78	74	105
Concrete framed warehouse	21	30	49	70	70
Medium depth brick and concrete warehouse (very good condition and minimum work required)	10	25	30	75	40

★ Costs current as at 3rd quarter 1983 but are exclusive of VAT and professional fees.
† Gross floor area.

area to be spent on carrying out a basic schedule of dilapidations. If the building is left for say three years or more its condition is likely to have deteriorated to such an extent due to vandalism, fire and the elements that the cost of making good basic defects could be as much as £200/m² gross floor area, which would obviously render any conversion scheme totally uneconomic.

Rehabilitation costs are likely to be higher where timber-floored buildings are involved. Labour costs are difficult to estimate as there are so many unknowns and builders normally include allowances for contingencies which tend to undermine the viability of a scheme.

In summary, the main factors determining the repair bill tend to be:

Age and quality of building and structure
Previous use and type of tenant
Period for which building has been empty
Character of neighbourhood and security against vandalism.

Conversion can be defined as adapting the building to a different use. Costs therefore will depend in part on how appropriate the building is already for the uses proposed. Though in practice the work overlaps with repair, it can be more readily estimated. The costs of conversion will be greatly affected by the specification of the building as it stands and the requirements of the new use proposed, possibly involving compliance with the various fire, health and building regulations.

The most expensive elements in the conversion costs are services, including gas, electricity, water etc (see table V). The fire regulations require staircases to be compartmented, cast iron columns to be encased and timber floors to be protected on the underside. The public health regulations require lavatory fittings in proportion to the anticipated

Table V Typical breakdown of conversion costs (light industrial option)

	High £	Medium £	Low £	Range* £	Average £ cost*	Average per cent
Structure-fabric	3.00	–	2.00	0–9.00	4.00	7
Internal sub-division	5.00	5.00	6.00	3.00–11.00	7.00	12
Services	35.00	25.00	13.00	9.00–48.00	29.00	49
Finishes	13.00	8.00	10.00	5.00–13.00	9.00	16
Contingencies	12.00	6.00	5.00	5.00–13.00	9.00	16
Total conversion cost £/m² lettable	68.00	44.00	36.00	22.00–94.00	58.00	100

workforce. These requirements will be easier to satisfy where a building was previously in industrial use.

Conversion costs, therefore, will principally depend on:

The original use and configuration of the building
The proposed new uses, and their implications in terms of structural alterations fire and health regulations
The degree of finish required, ranging from an empty serviced shell to a fully equipped unit
The level of specification required (see below).

Levels of specification

To arrive at conversion cost estimates for a scheme, buildings may be classified into five categories according to the levels of specification required:

A: involving major structural alterations, additions, new services etc.

B: general repairs to fabric, additional fire escapes, fireproofing and services

C: non-structural partitions, upgrading, finishes, overhauling services.

D: upgrading finishes only.

E: no work required at all.

As stated above, one lesson to emerge from the Covent Garden feasibility studies was that a major jump in conversion costs is encountered in moving from category C to category B. A redundant building requiring additional fire escapes and sanitary accommodation before it can be reused therefore needs particularly careful costing.

2.03   Cost of the site

The amount that is paid in order to acquire a freehold or substantial leasehold interest in a site should never exceed the difference between the capital value of the completed development, and the development costs. This difference is known as the residual site value.

As over-expenditure on a site can leave little finance for upgrading, great care should be taken to assess the proper value. Key determinants of site value, are:

Location of site (and hence the kinds of potential users)
Planning permission available
Owner and his expectations
Terms of any subleases
Capitalised income from computed development
Total development costs.

Table VI allows a broad-brush relationship to be established between the three key factors: development costs; rental income and residual site value (worked example in 3.02).

2.04   Securing the finance

The cost and availability of finance is most appropriately considered last, as it depends in part on the soundness of the scheme.

Cost and availability of finance will depend on:

Proposed uses and numbers of tenancies (the fewer the better)
Age of building (the newer the easier)
Configuration of building (single storey is most attractive)
The terms of tenure (freehold or long lease is best)
The organisation concerned (a previous track record may be essential)
The type of area and protected uses (which affect the availability of public loans and grants and the prospect of rental growth).

Table VI   Serviceability – analysis of economic viability

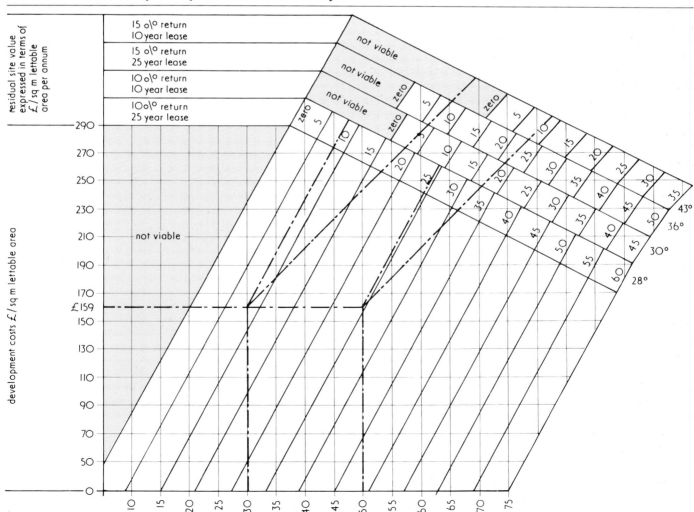

Table VII   Suggested format for organising and presenting a feasibility study (1)

1 SITE	Docklands				GROSS FLOOR AREA (GFA)	800 m²		
2 CONDITIONS	Category B (see paragraph 2.02)				NET LETTABLE FLOOR AREA	725 m²		

3 DESCRIPTION OF BUILDING

   Five-storey nineteenth-century warehouse
   Medium depth, with narrow width frontage and yard
   Natural light from three sides
   Brickwork structure, timber columns and floor joists

4 FLOOR	Existing use	GFA m²	Net m²	Landlord's asking rent £ m²	Proposed use	GFA m²	Net m²	Anticipated rent £ m²
Ground	Warehouse	160	145	15.00	Studio workshop	160	145	35.00
First	"	160	145	15.00	"	160	145	35.00
Second	"	160	145	14.00	"	160	145	32.50
Third	"	160	145	13.00	"	160	145	32.50
Fourth	"	160	145	13.00	"	160	145	30.00
Total		800	725	14.00 (ave)		800	725	33.00 (ave)

5 CONDITION OF FABRIC	BUILDING WORK REQUIRED
External elevation in reasonable condition Roof structurally sound Exposed floor and roof joists Stairs timber: open tread No evidence of serious dampness Surface water drainage only No heating No gas supply Electrics in bad condition	Works on site: clear out rubbish Floors: bring up to ½hr fire resistance Roof: overhaul existing coverings and flashings Stairs: strip out existing and provide 2 no. new Partitions/doors: form stair fire enclosures and wc cubicles Windows: unblock, overhaul, and replacement Services: new plumbing and sanitary equipment, kitchen services, lighting and power, gas supply, fire alarm Drainage: new soil drains required

6 CONDITIONS OF LEASE   11 years' full repairing and insuring

7 FINANCIAL VIABILITY AND RECOMMENDATIONS   (Feasibility study worked off-line: see table VIII)

   It will be evident that a fairly large capital investment will be required in order to convert the building into usable units. In the present market it is likely that the rent at £44.50 (over the ten-year lease - see table VIII) will prove to be too expensive for a small concern bearing in mind that rates and running costs must be added to the equation. Therefore either the initial asking rent must be renegotiated on more favourable terms, or the capital costs must be spread over a longer term (ie 25 years or more) in which case the rent will reduce to approximately £35.10 m² which will make it a more attractive proposition for a prospective tenant.

3.00   Testing financial viability

3.01   Financial viability calculations
Having set out the basic factors which influence the economic viability of conversion schemes, the next stage is to find a method of assimilating the basic information and testing the financial viability of a scheme – an essential step before embarking on a conversion project.

The method adopted here is that of calculating the 'annual equivalent cost' of the proposed conversion works. All the anticipated costs involved in the conversion and purchase of site are aggregated and expressed as an annual equivalent (capital sums are therefore amortised to an annual figure), and the resultant annual equivalent cost indicates what sort of annual rent will have to be recovered from prospective tenants to make the scheme viable.

Ways of raising finance are discussed in more detail in section 5.

Table VIII Suggested format for organising and presenting a feasibility study (2)

SITE Dockland EXISTING USE Warehouse PROPOSED USE Studio workshops GROSS FLOOR AREA 800 m^2 NET FLOOR AREA 725 m^2	ANNUAL EQUIVALENT COST Assuming interest rate at 12%		
	Expressed over a 10 years' lease (divide capital sum by 5.65)	Expressed over a 25 years' lease (divide capital sum by 7.84)	Expressed over a 50 years' lease (divide capital sum by 8.30)
1 ALTERATION WORKS Assuming 12% interest rate, say 1¼ year building contract, £ 78 200 x 1.253* 16% professional fees = £ 97 985 amortised . . .	£ $\frac{97.985}{5.65}$ £ 17 350	£ $\frac{97\ 985}{7.84}$ £ 12 500	£ $\frac{97\ 985}{8.30}$ £ 11 815
2 ASKING RENT 725 m^2 @ say £14.00 m^2 £ 10,000 Ignoring rent reviews and assuming a 10% reduction by negotiation: less 10% £ 1 000 NB Any additional premiums £ 9 000 etc should be amortised	£ 9 000	£ 9 000	£ 9 000
3 LEGAL FEES ON LEASE 5% of £ 9 000 Associated with obtaining £ 450 lease: amortised . . .	£ $\frac{450}{5.65}$ £ 80	£ $\frac{450}{7.84}$ £ 57	£ $\frac{450}{8.30}$ £ 54
4 AGENCY AND LEGAL FEES 10% of say £ 30 000 Letting agent' fees on = £ 3 000 first year's rent and associated legal fees: amortised . . .	£ $\frac{3\ 000}{5.65}$ £ 530	£ $\frac{3\ 000}{7.84}$ £ 380	£ $\frac{3\ 000}{8.30}$ £ 360
5 PROJECT MANAGEMENT/RISK FACTOR Allow say 20% of subtotal of items 1, 2, 3 and 4:	£ 26 960 x20% = £5 350	£ 21 937 x20% + £4 387	£ 21 229 x20% = £4 245
6 ANNUAL EQUIVALENT COST Add together items 1,2,3,4,5 Annual equivalent cost per m^2 of lettable area (divide a.e.c. by 725)	£ 32 310 £ $\frac{32\ 310}{725}$ = £44.50 m^2	£ 26 324 £ $\frac{26\ 324}{725}$ = £36.30 m^2	£ 25 474 £ $\frac{25\ 474}{725}$ = £35.10 m^2

Notes
In box 1 table VIII the factor 1.253 by which the building cost is multiplied is designed to take account of the cost of bridging finance and professional fees on the basic £78,200 building costs. See para 3.02 for further explanation.
In boxes 1, 3 and 4 of table VIII amortise' is the method whereby the repayment of a capital sum together with any interest that may accrue is expressed as an annual payment. The amortisation factors 5.65, 7.84 and 8.30 used in this exercise may be obtained from standard discounting/mortgage repayment tables.

In box 5, 'management/risk factor' includes an allowance for a working profit on the conversion scheme. Therefore this need not be calculated separately.

References

Property development feasibility tables 1982, obtainable from Building Economics Bureau, 5 Carlton Chambers, Station Road, Shortlands, Bromley, Kent, explains in detail the factors touched upon in the above calculations and provides a range of pro-formas to be used for the computations involved.

In developing and presenting a scheme in order to obtain finance, it is essential to organise the basic information in such a way that it is clearly understood. Tables VII and VIII show how a rapid financial appraisal may be undertaken.

Uses of tables VII and VIII
The purpose of these charts is to enable the designer to bring together the three major elements which underlie financial feasibility (cost of acquiring the redundant premises; cost of converting them to a new use, incorporating a profit element; and anticipated income).
This information is summarised on table VII together with

the conclusions drawn and the recommendation. Table VIII displays the calculations which have to be carried out to arrive at the 'cost' figure for acquiring and converting the premises (and which are best separated from table VII for the sake of clarity).

Step A fill in landlord's asking rent for existing redundant premises, on table VII, this figure will be known at the outset.

Step B fill in anticipated rent which is expected for premises, after conversion, on table VII.

Step C bring together all costs and fees on table VIII and convert any capital sums involved into annual equivalents (so that like can be compared with like, when relating estimated *cost* to anticipated annual *income*).

Step D having expressed the total of all costs involved as an annual equivalent cost; compare this with the anticipated rental income; and decide whether scheme is viable (box 7, table VII). If it is not, revise one or more of the inputs if market conditions allow, in order to bring the equation into balance.

Rental income may be increased by changing the mix of uses. One floor of offices, where previously it had been all light industrial, is likely to increase the return. Negotiate with the planning authority by showing how the scheme can be made financially viable by allowing a mix of uses (which incidentally may produce a better overall result for everyone).

Cost of acquiring the existing redundant building may be reappraised by renegotiating with the landlord.

Development costs may be reduced by changing the specification of the work done.
Table VI provides a quick method of trying different permutations of the three major factors to achieve a broadbrush indication of potential viability (more accurate calculations can only be carried out with the assistance of a development consultant).

3.02 Quick viability calculations
If, following the above calculations, the financial viability of the proposed scheme is in doubt (for instance, the required asking rent may be higher than prospective tenants are willing to pay for the quality of accommodation offered), then the scheme must be revised. The specification of conversion work may be altered, the landlord's asking rental may be negotiated, the profit element reduced, (see table VI). Below is a worked example:

Development cost
First, the building cost for the proposed rehab/conversion scheme must be estimated. This is assumed to be £78,200, ie £105.00/M² ($£9.76$/sq ft) of gross floor area. Two multiplying factors must now be applied to convert building costs/sq ft gross floor area (the form in which most quantity surveying consultants will present their figures) to development costs/sq ft lettable floor area.

● The first factor will adjust for professional fees, building contract period and interest charges (i.e. cost of finance). Its derivation is too complex to be explained here (consultants will be able to advise in detail). But as a rule of thumb this factor will normally fall between 1.20 (if professional and interest charges are at the low end of the range, and the contract period short) and 1.40 (if professional and interest charges are at the high end of the range, and the contract period longer).
If, for instance, professional fees are 10 per cent, interest charges 10 per cent pa and the contract period one year, the factor comes out at 1.16. If, at the other end of the scale, professional fees are 18 per cent, interest charges 15 per cent

pa and the contract period two years, then the factor comes out at 1.38.
For the present example, we will assume professional fees at 15 per cent, interest charges at 13 per cent pa and the building contract programme at 1½ years. The multiplication factor then works out at 1.273.

● The second factor will adjust from £/sq ft gross floor area to £/sq ft net floor area. Thus if the non-lettable area constitutes some 20 per cent of the gross, the factor will be 100 ÷ 80 = 1.25. We will assume non lettable area in this example to be 22 per cent of gross floor area: 100 ÷ 78 = 1.28.

● Applying the two multiplication factors to the building cost of £9.76/sq ft GFA, we therefore find:
£9.76 × 1.273 × 1.28 = £15.9/sq ft lettable floor area. Therefore the development costs for the proposed scheme in this example are £15.90/sq ft lettable floor area.

Estimated rent
This is the annual rent in £/sq ft lettable area that could reasonably be expected on the open market assuming a full repairing and insuring lease. It is assumed that these rents are exclusive of any service or running and maintenance charges that may obtain.
We assume that a survey of rentals in the same general location indicates that a rent of between £3 and £5/sq ft of lettable area can be expected.

Residual site value
If development costs are taken away from the capital value of the completed development, the 'residue' is the maximum amount that should be paid for the freehold or leasehold interest in the site.
The detailed calculations are beyond the scope of this study, and a development consultant's advice should be sought where necessary.
But for a broad-brush estimation of financial viability, plot the already calculated *development cost* on the vertical axis of table VI and the already estimated *rent* on the horizontal axis; and connect the point of intersection with the *site value* scales on the oblique scales.
For a development cost of £15.90, and a rental to the new occupants of £5/sq ft of lettable area per annum, it is seen that a 25 year lease at approx £2.45/sq ft payable to the existing landlord will yield a 10 per cent rate of return. For a 15 per cent return over 10 years, a site value of only £0.98 pa/sq ft lettable area could be afforded.
Had the anticipated rent been only £3/sq ft lettable area, then for a 15 per cent return over 10 years the scheme would be non-viable; but for a 10 per cent return over 25 years it would be viable provided the site value did not exceed about £0.80/sq ft lettable area per annum.

Note
In addition to the required rate of return described above, a further element has been built into table VI to cover overheads and profit on the initial capital expenditure. This additional margin has been taken at 20 per cent.

3.03 Undertaking an economic appraisal
Having set out the basic factors which influence the broad financial viability of conversion schemes, the economic feasibility of possible buildings for reuse can be tested.

Factors affecting the economic viability

The economic viability of a scheme depends on the balance between the cost of land, profit and overheads, building costs, and the income (rental asked) (see table IX). The most direct method of improving the economic viability is to reconsider the mix of uses. An assessment of over a hundred completed projects (by URBED) concluded that their viability depended on following an entrepreneurial or informal approach in contrast to the more usual institutional approach. The advantages of the approach are discussed in detail in section 4.

Table IX   Factors affecting the economic viability of conversion

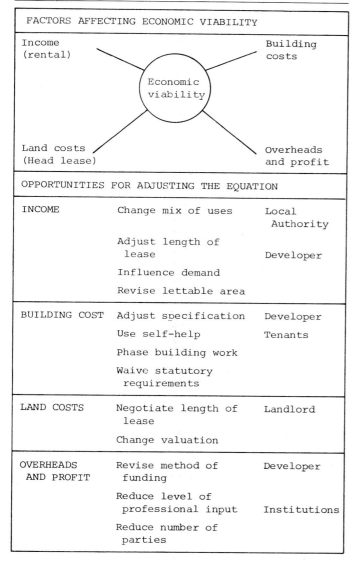

FACTORS AFFECTING ECONOMIC VIABILITY

Income (rental) — Economic viability — Building costs

Land costs (Head lease) — Overheads and profit

OPPORTUNITIES FOR ADJUSTING THE EQUATION

INCOME	Change mix of uses	Local Authority
	Adjust length of lease	Developer
	Influence demand	
	Revise lettable area	
BUILDING COST	Adjust specification	Developer
	Use self-help	Tenants
	Phase building work	
	Waive statutory requirements	
LAND COSTS	Negotiate length of lease	Landlord
	Change valuation	
OVERHEADS AND PROFIT	Revise method of funding	Developer
	Reduce level of professional input	Institutions
	Reduce number of parties	

Economic feasibility study

An economic feasibility study may be used by building owners or developers to decide on:

● The most viable mix of uses.

● A realistic site value or ground rent development approach.

For a local authority the economic approach may be used to:

● Agree development control policy for selected buildings by understanding the economic viability of different development options.

● Test the economic viability of existing planned uses.

● Provide development control officers with data on the economic viability of conversion or redevelopment.

● Assess the feasibility of direct local authority involvement with a specific building.

The prime objective of the economic appraisal is rapidly to appraise alternative strategies by testing alternative mixes of use and development approaches. Table X provides a typical worked example of an economic appraisal. Three options are assessed:

Refurbish for industrial use, 'on the cheap'
Refurbish for mixed use, limited professional input
Redevelop for office use, full professional service.

Taking into account the amount of building work required, the development approach, and the method of funding, a financial approach is drawn up for each option, and conclusions drawn. Table XI describes on a five point scale the levels of specifications and options available for implementation.

The success of a rapid economic appraisal is dependent on the experience of the professional inputs, and the range of both mixes of use and development approach considered.

It is assumed that an economic appraisal would take two man days each of an experienced valuer or quantity surveyor working with a planner/architect. The duo of a building economic expert and planning/building expert is seen as essential in coming to a balanced view in assessing the opportunities.

4.00   Setting up the appropriate organisation

4.01   The entrepreneurial approach

The economic viability of a project depends not only on the work to be done but also on the way that it is undertaken. In reusing old buildings, perhaps as much as 25 per cent of the total development costs can be saved by following an entrepreneurial or informal development approach, in contrast to the usual more conservative institutional style. The experience of a number of entrepreneurial developers who have converted old buildings suggest the costs can be reduced in a number of ways:

● By undertaking conversions which cater primarily for those small firms who want to keep their rents and other overheads as low as possible.

● By keeping expenditure on conversion to a minimum, leaving the occupant to decide whether he wants a higher standard of finish;

● By selecting an appropriate building and paying little for it, either because the prospects of redevelopment are low or because it is already owned by the developer;

● By cutting building costs and doing the minimum necessary to make the building sound and in compliance with legal requirements, with any item of expenditure being carefully assessed to see whether it will bring in extra rents;

Table X Economic appraisal sheet. Each option appraised against the five point scale of characteristics and specification shown in table XI

44–49 Gt Sutton St 13–17 Northburgh St		EXISTING	OPTION 1 *Refurbish Industrial use*	OPTION 2 *Refurbish Mixed uses: Industrial 30% Office 70%*	OPTION 3 *Redevelop Office uses*
ACCESS	Site coverage	85 per cent	85 per cent	75 per cent	100 per cent
	Goods vehicle access	One on-street point per 1000 m^2	Ditto	Internal courtyard	–
	Car parking	Off-site pay parking	Off-site	Off-site	Off-site
	Interior circulation	One goods lift per 1000 m^2 floor	Ditto	One goods lift per 500 m^2 floor	Four passenger lifts
	Number of floors	3–5	3–5	3–5	6
CONFIG.	Aspect	2 way	2 way	2 way	3 way
	Depth	15–20 m	15–20 m	15–20 m	20 m +
	FL/FL height	2.4–3.6 m	2.4–3.6 m	2.4–3.6 m	3 m
SPECIFICATION	Demolition		Demolish 10% building	Demolish 15% building	Demolish 100%
	Structure	Timber frame load-bearing brickwork	Ditto	Ditto	Reinforced concrete frame
	Fabric	Pointing; roof, windows need repair	Overhaul fabric	Overhaul fabric	Double glazing, brick infill
	Internal subdivision	80 per cent cellularised	Reduce cellularisation	40 per cent cellular offices	Open plan
	Finishes	Plaster defective and needs redecoration	Make good plaster. Redecorate	Carpet in office. Redecorate	Carpet. Suspended ceiling
	Services	Basic electrics. No heating	Adapt electrics No heating	Central heating. New electrics	Full air-conditioning
USAGE	Gross floor area	7000m^2	6500m^2	6050m^2	9300m^2
	Lettable floor area	5400m^2	5400m^2	5400m^2	7600m^2
	Size of units	10–200m^2	100–220m^2	–	1000m^2
TENURE	Freehold cost and finance amortised at 17% over 20 years = £ p.a. (1)				Freehold assume £1 M £170,000 p.a.
	Annual rental £ m^2 lettable floor area (1)		£58000 (£10.75 m^2)	£87000 (£16.00 m^2)	
	Development approach		Entrepreneurial do-it-yourself	Entrepreneurial Limited professional help	Institutional Full professional service

Table X   Economic appraisal sheet. Each option appriased against the five point scale of characteristics and specification shown in table XI—*continued*

44-49 Gt Sutton St 13-17 Northburgh St		EXISTING	OPTION 1 *Refurbish Industrial use*	OPTION 2 *Refurbish Mixed uses: Industrial 30% Office 70%*	OPTION 3 *Redevelop Office uses*
FINANCIAL APPRAISAL	Source of finance		*Self-finance through rents*	*Commercial mortgage*	*Institutional*
	Building costs		£350,000	£650,000	£4,000,000
	Professional fees (%)		£14,000 (4)	£65,000 (10)	£400,000 (10)
	Finance charges (%)		£20,000	£80,000 (15)	£570,000 (13)
	Overheads and profit (%)		£10,000 (supervise)	£80,000 (10)	£600,000 (13)
	Total development costs £		£394,000	£875,000	£5,570,000
	Costs amortised at 17% over 20 years = £ p.a. (2)		£71,000	£170,000	£950,000
	Total annual costs 1+2 ÷ LFA		£129,000	£257,000	£1,120,000
RENTALS	Industrial £ m^2 LFA (% of total)		£24 m^2 (100)	£18 m^2 (30)	
	Office £ m^2 LFA (% of total)			£60 m^2 (70)	£140 m^2 (100)

CONCLUSIONS	PREFERRED OPTION			✔	
	Development control policy	Change mix of use ✔	Change plot ratio	Review access, and parking requirements ✔	
	Local Authority intervention	Covenant	Grants	Act as developers	
	Local Authority support	Speed up planning process ✔	Provide management support	Publicity	

• By using small builders to carry out the work or direct sub-contractors with tight site management, or by using the occupants themselves;

• By keeping down overheads and using an informal approach with professionals used sparingly, e.g. to provide advice on overall viability;

• By phasing the work over a period of time, to minimise borrowings and to enable the space to be let gradually. In this way it can be adapted to occupants' requirements, and rent free periods may be given in return for occupants doing much of the work;

• By employing an on-site caretaker or manager in large buildings to sort out problems as they arise.
The entrepreneurial approach inevitably carries with it greater uncertainty and risk. Its success is dependent on the quality and commitment of the developer, a fact that is impossible to predict when undertaking a feasibility study.

5.00   Raising the finance

Once a viable scheme has been devised and an appropriate form of organisation chosen, it is necessary to find the finance. Any project that ties up resources has to find a way of financing the period before the money is returned either through rent or outright sale. There are three main possibilities:

Grants
Help in kind
Loans.

5.01   Grants
Unlike housing, there are no automatic grants for improving industrial buildings or meeting the regulations, though in some cases an element of public housing included in the industrial development, may reduce the total finance required. Government grants may be available when a building is of historic or architectural interest, where there are socially beneficial uses, and in certain other situations where new jobs will be created.

Grants for historic buildings
Where a historic building is involved, grants may be available for those that are 'listed' ancient monuments, or fall within outstanding conservation areas.

• Listed buildings are elegible for grants from local authorities, under the Local Authorities (Historic Buildings) Act 1962.

Table XI Description of building characteristics and specification

		1	2	3	4	5
ACCESS	Site coverage	40 per cent	40-60 per cent	60-80 per cent	80-99 per cent	100 per cent
	Goods vehicle access	One on-site delivery point per 1000 m^2	One off-site delivery point per 1000 m^2	One delivery point on cul-de-sac per 1000 m^2	One on-street delivery point per 1000 m^2	Nil
	Car parking	On site 1 per 6 persons	On site 1 per 6-12 persons	On site 1 per 12-24 persons	Off site on street	Off site pay parking
	Internal circulation	1 goods lift per 250 m^2 per floor	1 goods lift per 500 m^2 per floor	1 goods lift per 1000 m^2 per floor	1 pass. lift per 1000 m^2 per floor	No lifts
CONFIGURATION	Number of floors	Single floor		2-3 floors		4 or more
	Aspect	4 way aspect	3 way aspect	2 way corner aspect	2 way aspect	1 way aspect
	Depth	Under 15 m		15-20 m		Over 20 m
	FL/FL height (upper storeys)	2.4-3.6 m		3.6-4.2 m		4.8 m
SPECIFICATION	Structure	Concrete framed. Structurally sound. Adequate staircases		Exposed steel-work: some structural work required. Need to encase for fire		Exposed timber frame inadequate stairs, encase timber frame
	Fabric	Roof, brick-work, windows sound weathertight condition		Roof sound, minimum repointing, windows need overhauling		Roof leaks, brickwork spalling windows rotten
	Services	All mains services. Existing condition clean and sound		Mains services exist:overhaul internal services generally		No mains services-all new internal services required
	Internal subdivision	Open plan	0-15 per cent compartmented	15-25 per cent compartmented	25-40 per cent compartmented	40 per cent compartmented
IMPLEMENTATION	Internal finishes	Wall/ceiling plaster and floors cleaning and redecoration only		Some repairs to plasterwork, timber/concrete floors require attention, redecoration		All plaster 'shot'. Timber floors need replacement. Damp affects decorations
	Size of units	under 50 m^2	50-100 m^2	100-250 m^2	250-500 m^2	over 500 m^2
	Development approach	Institutional. Full professional service		Entrepreneurial, professional help		Entrepreneurial Do-it-yourself
	Source of finance	Institutional	Commercial mortgage	Bank loan	Self financing through rents	Personal investment

• Ancient monuments are designated by the Department of the Environment, who can offer grants towards the cost of renovating buildings that are of significance from an (industrial) archaeological viewpoint.

• Outstanding conservation areas are designated by the Secretary of State advised by the Historic Buildings Council, on the basis of an application for a specific building. If the area is classified as 'outstanding', grants are then available for the restoration of the fabric.

Grants are also available under Section 4 of the Historic Buildings and Ancient Monuments Act 1953, for the repair of buildings which are of outstanding historic or architectural interest. In certain cases 'town scheme' grants available from the DOE may contribute towards the cost of repairing buildings which inevitably may not be of outstanding interest but which are of particular value as part of a group. For repair work in conservation areas other than those accepted by the Secretary of State as outstanding under Section 10 of the 1972 Act, the Civic Trust administers a special government grant fund.

• Charitable foundations can contribute towards restoration schemes undertaken by building preservation trusts and amenity trusts. Two notable examples are the Pilgrim Trust and the Landmark Trust, which renovates old buildings as holiday homes. A number of charitable trusts have also been set up by private companies.

Grants for socially beneficial uses
Grants may also be secured according to the use to which the building is being put. In the case of workshops, there are a number of bodies who may contribute grants:

Crafts Advisory Committee (grants for artists/craftsmen)
Council for Small Industries (grants for workshops in the countryside and small towns)
Scottish and Welsh Development Agencies
Charitable foundations (workshops for the disadvantaged)
Department of Health and Social Security (sheltered workshops for the elderly, handicapped etc)
Home Office (help for ex-prisoners)
Department of Education and Science (school or college related workshops)
Urban Aid Programme (DOE funded community workshop facilities)
Manpower Services Commission (Special Opportunities Programme including training workshops for school leavers; special temporary employment programmes for adults, enterprise workshops).

Grants for employment creation
Certain bodies may be approached for financial assistance where projects involve an element of job creation:

English Industrial Estates (subsidiary of the Department of Industry)
Welsh and Scottish Development Agencies
Local authorities (under the Inner Urban Areas Act of 1978, grants are available in industrial improvement areas towards conversion projects where jobs will be created).

5.02 Help in kind
Help in kind means gifts of expertise, labour or materials. While these are not as flexible as cash, they are often easier to come by:

Expertise
A major problem for most projects when they are starting is obtaining good advice and professional help when there are no funds to pay for them. There are three main sources of help:

• Large companies are sometimes prepared to lend executives to socially beneficial projects, particularly when these can help career development of the person concerned.

• Retired managers or professionals may be interested in doing part-time work.

• Colleges can help through student projects. Students make up a great untapped body of enthusiasm and ability.

Labour
There are a number of ways of obtaining labour free or at a reduced cost including government funded programmes and voluntary schemes.

Government funded programmes for employing young people which might be tapped include:

MSC's Youth Training Scheme or Special Temporary Employment Programme
Training Opportunities Scheme (Government funded training programme for the building trade)
Community Industry (for the hard to employ)
Bulldog Enterprises (run by Home Office for probationers)
Community Service Orders (offenders sentenced by courts)

Voluntary schemes include:

Community Service Volunteers (where living accommodation and expenses must be found)
Conservation Corps
Friends of the Earth.

Advice on setting up voluntary projects can be obtained from the Community Projects Foundation, local Councils of Voluntary Service or the National Council of Social Service.

Materials
Companies may well donate materials where they would not give money, particularly if the company's name can be associated with a successful scheme. However, it may be better to order materials through a sympathetic firm that already obtains quantity discounts. The same applies to hiring or borrowing equipment. It is worth remembering that VAT is not charged on new works, but applies to maintenance work.
As renovation often requires the use of old materials, it can be worth coming to an arrangement with the local authority to recover materials from demolished buildings for reuse.

5.03 Loans

Short-term finance
There are several alternative sources of short-term finance.

• Clearing banks are generally reluctant to become involved in property development.

• Merchant banks tend to invest only in established companies.

• Finance for Industry is the largest source of finance for small companies. Set up by the Bank of England and the clearing banks, its property division invests in conversion schemes (A full list of banking finance is contained in the review by the London Chamber of Commerce and for the Bank of England).

• Financial institutions including pension funds and insurance companies invest over £1 billion a year, although most are interested only in 'prime' property. Smaller pension funds and property trusts are possibly better bets.

• Local authorities can offer mortgages and can tap finance from private financial institutions by offering some kind of guarantee or entering into a profit sharing arrangement.

• Architectural Heritage Fund loans, administered by the Civic Trust, provide capital to Building Preservation Trusts for renovations and resale schemes at low rates of interest.

Long-term finance

Financial institutions are normally reluctant to invest in conversion schemes because old buildings are seen as having relatively short lives. Workshops are also thought to involve lower rental growth, inadequate covenants and higher rent collection costs.

• Pension funds invest over £500 million a year in property. They differ in their investment policies, and some of the Union funds have begun to consider investing in situations that help economic development and may now be interested in industrial development. However, leases of at least 125 years need to be available, and the area should be one where rental growth can be expected. The smaller pension funds tend to be more interested in 'secondary' property than the big names.

• Insurance companies, investing over £600 million a year in property, like pension funds tend to be conservative, and follow established policies. However, in certain cases the social arguments could become compelling. If local authorities could be persuaded to act as intermediaries between the financial institution and the tenant, it may be possible for some proportion of insurance company investment to be directed specifically towards financing workshops.

• Landlords are the final source of long-term finance. The landlord may be prepared to invest in the building in return for higher rentals. Where an industrial company owns the building, the argument that investment will help create jobs and will improve the company image may be persuasive. A number of large companies such as the British Steel Corporation recently have begun to look at the scope for reusing buildings in their ownership to house small enterprises.

9 Assessing the Cost

1.00 Conversion versus rebuilding

1.01 The arguments for conversion
The stock economic arguments in favour of reusing redundant buildings are:

Cheaper building costs
No need for demolition
A shorter development period, so fewer finance charges.

These are examined below and are followed by a case study.

1.02 Building costs
On the face of it, the cost of converting a building ought to be lower than building a new one since many of the building elements are already constructed. However, as discussed in the previous chapter, costs depend on the condition of the building; the type of construction, particularly in industrial buildings; and the problem of the Building Regulations, especially those relating to fire.

1.03 Demolition costs
Conversion avoids demolition costs, but, on the other hand, it has sometimes cost almost as much to clean the rubbish out of a converted building as it would have done to knock it down. Demolition should not normally be a sufficiently expensive operation with older buildings to sway the economics one way or the other (except in the case of reinforced concrete-framed buildings, and basements).

1.04 Development period
The length of the development period has a direct bearing on the interest charges associated with site costs. As table 1 shows, new redevelopment work has much longer delays in the pre-contract design stage; and even where there is no change of use, planning permission will inevitably take longer by comparison with conservation. Taken together with the longer building period, this means an average overall increase in time from start to finish of about a third.

This difference in time will, however, again depend on the standard of building to be converted. If major elements (such as the roof) are in a bad state, it might take almost as long to repair or replace them as to demolish the whole building and rebuild. The nature of the firms engaged in alterations and improvements, coupled with hidden faults emerging, frequently lead to contract periods being greatly extended.

1.05 Finance charges
The importance of a longer development period depends partly on the prevailing interest rate. When the rate was around 12 per cent per annum, the shorter development period associated with conservation work was not so significant. With a rate of interest of 15 per cent or more per annum, the difference is much more important. The situation is, of course, highly volatile.

2.00 Case study

2.01 Introduction
To test these arguments a survey was made of a redundant warehouse in South London, and a scheme drawn up to convert it into studio workshops. The total budget for conversion was calculated, and compared with that of a notional purpose built new development.

2.02 Building costs
Table II gives an element-by-element comparison between the conservation scheme and the redevelopment alternative. The basis of the estimated costs is listed, together with explanations of the difference in costs of the two schemes.
The warehouse to be converted was chosen primarily because it was in reasonably good condition. Even so, the cost of conversion to studios and workshops comes to about 77 per cent of the cost of a new building. Just one major element found to be in bad state would result in the *difference* between the cost of conversion and the cost of redevelopment becoming insignificant.

2.03 Development period and finance charges
In the development budgets in table II the finance charges on the site costs were taken over 61 weeks for conversion, and 79 weeks for redevelopment. With an interest rate of 15 per cent per annum this amounted to a difference of just

Table I Development period comparison between conversion scheme and redevelopment scheme. These figures apply only to the particular scheme investigated in this case study (see paragraph 2.01) and should not be used as generalisations.

COMPARISON OF DEVELOPMENT PERIODS		
ITEM	CONVERSION SCHEME TIME IN WEEKS	REDEVELOP-MENT SCHEME TIME IN WEEKS
Purchase site	-	-
Draw up scheme	5	10
Obtain planning consent	8	12
Demolition	-	5
Building works	40	48
Sell (if applicable) complete building	8	4
TOTAL PERIOD	61	79

Table II Development budget comparison between conversion scheme and redevelopment scheme. The higher the prevailing interest rate, the greater the advantage of a short development period (and therefore, probably the 'conversion' alternative).

COMPARISON OF TOTAL DEVELOPMENT BUDGETS		
ITEM	CONVERSION SCHEME £	REDEVELOP-MENT SCHEME £
Purchase existing warehouse (includes legal fees)	35,000	35,000
Finance charges on site cost at say 15% p.a. for 61 weeks (conversion); 79 weeks (new work)	6,159	7,977
Demolition costs		15,000
Building costs	128,150	165,400
Fees - architect, QS, engineer at 16% for conversion 10% for new work	20,504	16,540
Bridging finance on building cost and fees at 15% p.a. (taken over HALF contract period, to approximate actual monthly cash flow) 48 weeks (conversion) 57 weeks (redevelopment)	10,291	16,191
Agency and legal fees (normally 10% of first year's rent) say	5,000	6,100
	205,104	262,208
Profit and risk: 20% (conversion scheme) 16.66% (redevpt scheme)	40,896	43,892
TOTAL BUDGET £	246,000	306,100

under £2,000 – about 3 per cent of the total difference between the costs of conversion and new redevelopment. Similarly, today's high interest rate has increased the significance of bridging finance in the argument for conservation. In table III the interest on cost of conversion work and fees (£148,654) was taken at 15 per cent p.a. over *half* the building contract and disposal period of 48 weeks (a rule of thumb commonly adopted to approximate monthly cash-flow). In the new work the same interest rate was taken on the building cost and fees (£196,940) over *half* a 57–week building and disposal period. The resulting interest charges were nearly £6,000 in favour of conversion – almost 10 per cent of the difference in the total development budgets.

2.04 Fees

Professional fee scales are higher in conversion because of the nature of the works undertaken. Therefore 16 per cent was taken on the conversion building costs and 10 per cent was taken on the new work building costs (table II). Estate agency fees on the new work will usually be slightly higher than on the converted properties as the fees are calculated as a percentage of the selling price and the property would normally have a higher value.

2.05 Profit and risk

There is a large risk element in conversion work. Although most defects in the building are obvious, and can be picked up on the initial survey, others – sometimes crippling – only come to light during the works. Whether the risk is contractually with the employer or the contractor, it has a habit of ending up in the employer's lap. This, coupled with the fact that new work is patently more substantial, means that con-

version work requires a greater profit margin. Hence the higher percentage (20 per cent instead of 16⅔ per cent) to cover profit and risk for the conversion work.

As can be seen from table II there is a difference between the two development budgets, in favour of conversion of some £60,100 when the total figures are compared; or £64,100 prior to any adjustment for professional fees. It will be seen that in this instance the total additional budget for building anew is a mere 25 per cent more than the cost of conversion.

Table III   Element-by-element building cost comparison between rehabilitation/conversion scheme and new development. In the conversion scheme, costs are broken down into rehabilitation (repairs and maintenance), and conversion

ELEMENT	REHABILITATION/CONVERSION NEW WORK	Rehab £/m² GFA	Conv £/m² GFA	New £/m² GFA	REMARKS
WORKS ON SITE	R/C: Clean out rubbish	2.30			Demolition of existing building for redevelopment is included elsewhere in budget
WORK BELOW LOWEST FLOOR FINISH	R/C: Nil NEW: Strip foundations, cavity wall of commons, lead-cored damp-proof course, hardcore, and 150 mm oversite concrete			10.00	Condition of surveyed warehouse was reasonable: no need for shoring and underpinning or new ground floor slab
UPPER FLOORS INC. FLOOR AND CEILING FINISHES	R/C: Clean floorboards, fill in depressions, sand down, new skirting, flameproof hardboard, 3 mm thermoplastic tiles. Board and 2 coats plaster to ceiling NEW: Reinforced concrete floor and beams, 50 mm screed, 3 mm thermoplastic tiles, skirting. Render and set to soffit of concrete floor	7.40	18.40	38.70	Existing floor had to be fireproofed, even so, reinforced concrete floor is still more expensive
ROOF	R/C: Overhaul existing slated roof. Take down coping, clean, re-bed and point NEW: Reinforced concrete roof and beams, screed laid to falls, 3 coats asphalt, 225 mm parapet wall in facings with precast concrete coping	9.90	1.60	23.00	Existing warehouse roof was fairly sound But others in the same area were much worse and would have been expensive
STAIRCASE	R/C: Strip out existing. Provide softwood staircase including fireproofing NEW: Reinforced concrete staircase, steel balustrading	4.90		2.60	Because of existing design the warehouse needed two staircases. These were timber because of the existing floor construction
EXTERNAL WALLS (INC. INTERNAL PLASTER)	R/C: Repair cracks, replaster and repoint as necessary NEW: 265 mm cavity – outer skin fair faced brickwork, inner skin blockwork. Flush pointing. Render and set internally	10.20		25.00	Again, the external walls were in reasonable condition: no major cracks
WINDOWS	R/C: Re-open blocked window openings, overhaul existing windows and sills. Provide and fix new metal windows, reglaze NEW: Provide and fix softwood casement windows including glazing. Precast concrete sills, softwood internal window boards	8.20		5.60	Most of the original windows had been blocked up. These had to be opened to comply with regulated natural light levels
DOORS (INTERNAL AND EXTERNAL)	R/C: Overhaul existing doors. Provide and fix ½hr fire-resistant doors and frames including ironmongery NEW: Panelled external doors. One panel glazed softwood, flush doors to ½hr fire resistance including frames and ironmongery	2.10	4.30	5.10	
INTERNAL LOAD-BEARING WALLS AND PARTITIONS (INC. PLASTER)	R/C: 75 mm stud partition, 9-5 mm plasterboard, scrim joints and set NEW: 225 mm commons partition, render and set, 75 mm stud partitions, 9-5 mm plasterboard, scrim joints and set		6.70	17.60	Load-bearing wall in to carry the reinforced concrete suspended floor

Table III Element-by-element building cost comparison between rehabilitation/conversion scheme and new development. In the conversion scheme, costs are broken down into rehabilitation (repairs and maintenance), and conversion

ELEMENT	REHABILITATION/CONVERSION NEW WORK	Rehab £/m² GFA	Conv £/m² GFA	New £/m² GFA	REMARKS
CEILING FINISH	R/C and NEW: See upper floors and roofs				
DECORATIONS	R/C: 2 coats emulsion to walls and ceilings; burn-off and prepare existing wood surfaces, knot, prime, stop and 2 coats oil paint	10.20	3.40		Note the additional expense in preparing existing surface
	NEW: 2 coats emulsion to walls and ceilings; knot, prime stop and 2 coats oil paint to wood surfaces			12.60	
FITTINGS	R/C: Wall, floor, sink units, worktops		2.60		
	NEW: Wall, floor, sink units, worktops			2.60	
PLUMBING AND RAINWATER INSTALLATION	R/C: Low level wc, lavatory basins, hot and cold water services, soil and ventpipes	1.80	7.00		
	NEW: Low level wc, lavatory basins, hot and cold water services, soil and ventpipes			8.00	
HEATING INSTALLATION	R/C: Electric unit heaters		4.00		
	NEW: Electric unit heaters			4.00	
GAS INSTALLATION	R/C: Install gas service	2.50			
	NEW: Install gas service			2.50	
ELECTRICAL INSTALLATION	R/C: Strip out where necessary, rewire and extend existing lighting and power installation including fittings	21.30			Note the additional expense of stripping out existing services
	NEW: New light, power installation inc fittings			18.00	
SPECIAL INSTALLATION	R/C: Attendance on Telecoms, fire alarm, hoses etc.		4.90		
	NEW: Attendance on Telecoms, fire alarm, hoses, etc.			5.00	
DRAINAGE EXTERNAL WORKS	R/C: Modify and extend existing drainage installation, including connection to main sewer. Take up and renew pavings where necessary		8.50		Existing drainage system accomodates surface water drainage only
	NEW: New drainage installation. Provide and fix new fence and pavings			4.00	
CONTINGENCIES	R/C: Design and contract contingencies	8.00	6.00		Included as a percentage (10%) of the total cost
	NEW: Design and contract contingencies			18.70	
PRELIMINARIES	R/C: Foreman, increased costs, insurance, water, power, scaffolding, hoarding, etc	8.90	6.90		Preliminaries higher in new work as they are largely related to the contract period and the value of the work
	NEW: Foreman, increased costs, insurance, water, power, scaffolding, hoarding, etc			19.00	

R/C: Total cost per m² of gross floor area: £ 97.70 74.30

     £ 172.00 x 745 m²
                                          74.30

              = £ 128,150   £172.00

NEW: Total cost per m² of gross floor area: £ 222.00

     £ 222.00 x 745 m²

              = £ 165,400

Table III   Element-by-element building cost comparison bewtween rehabilitation/conversion scheme and new development. In the conversion scheme, costs are broken down into rehabilitation (reparis and maintenance), and conversion—*continued*

NOTE:

The costs are current as at the third quarter of 1983 for a fixed price contract

The costs are exclusive of VAT. Approximately 60% of the works to the existing building will be taxed. New works are zero rated

The costs are exclusive of professional fees

Gross floor area (GFA) = 745 m^2

2.06   Conclusions

In conclusion, therefore: in this particular example conversion is more economical than redevelopment, but, owing to the large number of unknown factors in conversion it would be extremely foolish to make this a generalisation. In any particular instance two other factors should also be considered, i.e. categories of specification and amount of usable floor space.

Category of specification

Five main categories are suggested as a measure of the amount of building work required (see chapter 8, para 2.02).

The building under consideration in table II falls into category B (general repairs to fabric, additional fire escapes, fireproofing, and services). Analysis of the costs shows that the ratio between 'repair' (that is, restoring the building to a good state for its original purpose) and 'conversion' (that is, converting the restored building for its new purpose) is in the order of 55:45 per cent. Had the building been in category A (major structural alterations, additions, new services), this ratio could have been in the order of 65:35 per cent, and the cost of conserving the existing building and converting it for the new use could therefore be as much as building anew.

Amount of usable floor space

When changing a building from one use to another it is unlikely that the best possible use will be made of the existing space because of the layout of the original building. Therefore, even with two buildings of the same gross floor area, it is likely that the new building, because of the more efficient design, will have a higher percentage of usable floor space than the old.

3.00   Cost in use: capital and running costs

3.01   The importance of life costs

To compare two developments by analysis of their total development budgets is to take a slightly blinkered view of the overall situation. Developments should not be examined solely on their initial capital costs. An important component in the building cost equation is the cost of running and maintaining the building. The summation of these costs over the life of the building can be over three times the initial expenditure. Any decision which substantially reduces these running costs can be a decision well made.

3.02   Case study

To illustrate cost-in-use appraisal techniques we have analysed typical capital, running and maintenance costs for two different building types – an office and a workshop – and have further subdivided these into new and converted buildings.

3.03   Running costs

Table IV compares the likely running costs for the four buildings, incorporating the maintenance and repair of the fabric and services and all the energy costs. (Note: no allowance has been made for air-conditioning to the office buildings; if this were present the running costs would be significantly higher). It should be noted that these are *typical* running costs for the types of buildings illustrated based on personal experience with particular buildings and should, therefore, only be used as a guide.

3.04   Rates

Rates will, of course, vary widely around the country. If the buildings were in the inner area of a major provincial City the rates might be as in table V.

3.05   Capital costs

Table VI gives typical total budget costs for studio workshops and we have included these in the table together with typical office building costs calculated on a similar basis:

The annual equivalent of the capital cost is given in the right hand column: the mortgage cost of 100% funding of the project, including profit and risk.

The total life cycle costs of the buildings can, therefore, be expressed in the terms shown in tables IV to VII.

The figures show clearly the significance of the 'non-building' portion of annual premises costs relative to the total life-cycle costs; the significance is less the shorter the period over which the capital costs are amortised and, of course, rents work out a lot higher than mortgage repayments. Obviously rate-free periods such as those now available in the new Enterprise Zones do have an important effect on the budget.

3.06   Taxes

However, it is important to have regard to the effects of current fiscal legislation before drawing economic conclusions from these examples. The most relevant forms of taxation are:

Table IV   Typical annual running and maintenance costs of different types of buildings

	OFFICES		WORKSHOPS		REMARKS Costs as at third quarter 1983
	NEW £/m² GFA p.a.	CON-VERSION £/m² GFA p.a.	NEW £/m² GFA p.a.	CON-VERSION £/m² GFA p.a.	
MAINTENANCE OF FABRIC Replacement and redecoration both internally and externally	7.00	18.50	5.25	12.75	REDECORATION: External every 3 years Internal every 5 years Lower quality materials associated with low budget conversion lead to constant or frequent replacement. Prestige function of workshops not so vital as in offices: standard of decoration can be low
CLEANING COSTS Includes cleaning windows and all routine daily and internal cleaning	5.75	5.75	6.50	6.50	Dirt and dust generated more in workshop conditions, while a high standard of cleanliness may still need to be maintained
M & E RUNNING COSTS Energy and water costs	4.50	5.25	4.00	4.50	Services designed at same time as building for new development lead to a more efficient layout and design. Current legislation means that insulation values of new and converted buildings will be similar. Work carried out in workshops will not be as sedatory, and heat generated by machines will lead to lower heating costs. Also, statutory heating levels are lower for industrial than for office buildings
LAMP CLEANING AND CHANGING	1.00	1.00	1.00	1.00	
PLANT EQUIPMENT AND MAINTENANCE	9.50	9.50	10.25	10.25	Services are usually renewed complete, even in low budget conversions. If this were not the case then the figure would be considerably higher. Additional ventilation may be required in the workshop
£	27.75	40.00	27.00	35.00	

Table V   Typical rates for major provincial city

BUILDING TYPE	RATES £/m² GFA
New office development	45.00
Office conversion	36.00
New workshop development	34.00
Workshop conversion (Figures as at third quarter 1983)	27.00

Table VI   Annual equivalent costs of total capital budget

BUILDING TYPE	TOTAL CAPITAL BUDGET £/m² GFA	ANNUAL EQUIVALENT OF TOTAL CAPITAL BUDGET £/m² GFA Mortgage interest 15% Term: 7 yrs 15 yrs
New office development	620.00	149.22 106.11
Office conversion	400.00	96.47 68.60
New workshop development	325.00	78.44 55.78
Workshop conversion (Figures as at third quarter 1983)	260.00	62.06 44.14

Table VII   Total life cycle costs per square metre GFA at 3rd quarter 1983

BUILDING TYPE	MORTGAGE TERM Years	ANNUAL EQUIVALENT OF CAPITAL COSTS £	RUNNING AND MAINTENANCE COSTS £	RATES £	ANNUAL TOTAL LIFE CYCLE COSTS £ Mortgage 7 yrs	15 yrs
New office development	7	149.22	27.75	45.00	221.97	
	15	106.11				178.86
Office conversion	7	96.47	40.00	36.00	172.47	
	15	68.60				144.60
New workshop development	7	78.44	27.00	34.00	139.44	
	15	55.78				116.78
Workshop conversion	7	62.06	35.00	27.00	124.06	
	15	44.14				106.14

1   Development Land Tax

Development Land Tax is payable on part of the expected development value, and as such would have the effect of increasing the capital cost of the development. However, the tax is not paid on the first £100,000 of a development value if there has not been a change in use. Consequently, it is quite possible, especially in smaller developments (like most conversion schemes) that the effect of this tax would be negligible. No development land tax is payable in the Enterprise Zones for appropriate projects.

2   Corporation Tax

Apart from a few exceptions (e.g. research buildings) only the interest part of capital costs on buildings are subject to any corporation tax relief. However, the costs associated with the normal day-to-day running of a business-rent (if applicable), rates, heating, lighting, maintenance, moveable items etc., are subject to tax relief.

Therefore, a cheap material with a high maintenance cost could end up being more economical than expensive higher quality material once tax advantages are accounted for. Although, it must be noted here that the material might only be more economical from a maintenance point of view; other factors such as disruption of staff and work processes by constant/frequent maintenance progress should also be accounted for.

Note, however, that in the Enterprise Zones 100% of the capital cost of appropriate projects may be claimed against corporation tax in the first year.

4.00   Rehabilitation and conversion costs

4.01   Principal factors influencing construction costs

There are three principal factors influencing the overall cost of work to redundant buildings.

Rehabilitation

1 The structural condition of the building/fabric in the first instance (architects' and engineers' requirements)

2 The amount of work required to bring the building into line with current health and safety standards (fire officer/ district surveyor and public health requirements)

Conversion

3 The extent and standard of the conversion/planning proposals (client requirements)

4.02   Cost sensitive elements in the building estimate

The key to any successful rehabilitation/conversion project lies not in assiduously avoiding the problem buildings but rather in determining whether the worst features of these buildings are particularly cost sensitive in the overall proposal. Clearly, the involvement of an experienced cost consultant is vital at the early stages of decision making.

These are some of the more cost sensitive elements.

Work below lowest floor

Renewing the ground floor will have a far greater significance in a single-storey than a multi-storey building.

Upper floors

This element will always be particularly cost sensitive and care should be taken in assessing the amount of remedial work that will be required.

Roof

As with the floor slab this will have far greater significance in a single-storey building. Particular care should be taken in assessing the amount of damage that may have been caused to the roof structure due to the ingress of water.

Stairs

Will not have a significant effect on the overall equation if they are in the correct locations with regard to 'direct' and 'travel' distances. Be particularly wary if you have to form new openings in reinforced concrete floors.

External walls

Vertical elements of buildings such as walls/wall finishes etc are not only affected by the area of the building but also by the storey height and the wall to floor ratio. The wall to floor ratio is the mathematical relationship between the gross area of the external walls and the gross floor area of the building, i.e.

$$\frac{\text{Gross area of external walls}}{\text{Gross floor area of the building}} = \text{wall to floor ratio}$$

Thus a square-shaped building has a more economical plan form and a lower wall to floor ratio than a rectangular building. To summarise, if the storey height and the wall to floor ratio is low, then the element will not be as cost sensitive as a building with a high storey height and high wall to floor ratio.

Windows
Not normally cost sensitive unless there is a high wall/floor ratio and a profusion of expensive defective windows.

Internal partitions/doors
Defective studwork and associated plaster will clearly not present any problem if the proposal is to gut the interior of the building and vice-versa.

Ceiling plaster
Will only be cost sensitive if there is excessive damage and all the ceilings need to be replaced; relative, that is, to the cost of replacing other more expensive items.

Wall plaster/Decorations
See the notes on wall to floor ratios.
Seems unlikely to be a major determinant in taking a building as any scheme is bound to call for new decorations.

Services
May be a cost sensitive element especially if no mains services exist. Bringing in new incoming mains and mains drainage can be an expensive exercise especially if the building is in a remote country area.

Preliminaries
Must be considered in the initial appraisal especially if there are likely to be problems of access (inner city site), obtaining labour (inaccessibility), deliveries and storage of materials, protection of the public (hoarding, gantries) etc.

4.03   Other factors to be considered in the overall cost equation

Professional fees
The overall fee percentage will vary depending on the complexity of the project and the need to involve specialist consultants. For budgetary purposes full professional fees would normally be between 17 per cent and 22 per cent on a contract value of £100,000 as follows.
Architect 10 per cent to 12 per cent, cost consultant 4 per cent to 5 per cent, building services consultants (whose fees are taken as a percentage of the overall value of the services element) 2 per cent to 3 per cent, and the structural engineer, whose fees are taken as a percentage of the structural element or alternatively on a time basis, 1 per cent to 2 per cent.

Value added tax
In accordance with the provisions of the 1972 Finance Act works of a repair or maintenance nature are standard rated,

currently at 15 per cent, while new works or alteration works are zero rated. Although some anomalies do exist (eg renewing a defective window is subject to VAT, whereas enlarging the same opening by 25 mm and then renewing the window is classified as alteration works and therefore zero rated), the system is normally quite easy to follow. VAT is generally ignored by most consultants and treated as nothing more than a minor irritant and, indeed, if your client is registered for VAT then he will be fully entitled to recover any amounts expended and then it merely becomes a book transaction.

The problem arises, however, when your client is not registered and then it becomes a direct charge on the contract and must be taken into account in the initial appraisal. On rehabilitation/conversion works some 60 per cent of the works may be subject to VAT and on a £100,000 contract this would add a further £9000 to the overall cost of the project.

Regional variations
It is very difficult to determine accurately regional variations in tender price levels. They tend to fluctuate very much on a local level and in particular may be affected by such factors as:

1 location of material suppliers
2 availability of skilled and unskilled labour
3 current workload of firms in the immediate area (eg Aberdeen and the oil industry)
Availability of Government grants in the area (ie interest free loans to develop industrial estates in new development areas would be more attractive to building firms than rehab). In order to give some rule of thumb of regional variations in tender price levels we have grouped the main geographic regions into the four bands, listed below.

Table VIII   Regional variations in tender prices

Region	Index
Northern Ireland Northern East Anglia South West West Midlands East Midlands	85
Wales North West Yorkshire and Humberside	90
South East Scotland	100
London	120

Tender procedures
Methods of contractor selection, detail of tender documents and length of tendering period all have some effect on the overall level of costs.

Limited competitive tendering normally results in the most competitive price but if time is critical the contract could be negotiated or let on one of the cost-plus types of contract. Any benefit that may accrue from the reduction in the start-completion dates must be weighed against the additional premium that normally accompanies these types of contract. Similarly the detail of the tender documents may have a beneficial or an adverse effect. Some contractors prefer pricing bills of quantities; other less sophisticated contractors are frightened by the welter of detail and prefer to price on specification and drawings.

Finally, if the tendering period is too short, the contractor will have had insufficient time to get quotations from his various subcontractors and may overprice a particular item of work in order to cover himself.

Cost control

We cannot over-emphasise the critical importance of obtaining strategic cost control from the initial inception of the scheme. Such control would span elemental cost planning, the method of contractor selection, tendering procedures and contract arrangements together with continuous monitoring of possible changes in the cost structure and detailed financial reporting.

It is extremely unlikely that any initial estimates given by a qualified cost consultant would hold good in the absence of any of the above facets of the cost control function.

4.04   Elemental analysis

Basis of costs

The costs are current as at the third quarter of 1983 for a fixed price contract in the South East with a contract value in the region of £100,000 to £140,000: see tables IX, X and XI.

The costs are exclusive of professional fees and VAT.

It should be appreciated that it is not the intention to produce a detailed pricing guide for rehabilitation and conversion works, but merely to indicate the relative costs of typical items of work that are normally encountered in this type of building operation, and to indicate the costs of alternative specifications where appropriate. The figures should not be used in isolation and cannot be considered as a suitable alternative for the expert advice of a qualified cost consultant.

The range factor is given to indicate how the cost of each of these items may vary depending on the relative quantities involved – eg new concrete floor, unit cost of £30/m^2 of actual area. If there is a larger area involved, then apply the low factor of $0.80 \times £30 = £24/m^2$. If there is a smaller area involved, then apply the 'high' factor of $1.25 \times £30/m^2 = £37.50$ (possibly the area of a rear extension or the like). The costs have also been segregated into four separate work categories, namely works associated with:

a the structural condition of the building/fabric
b complying with current standards of health and safety
c complying with client's requirements
d contingencies and preliminaries.

Future trends

The building industry has been so savagely mauled in past years by repeated cutbacks in Government spending and a marked slowdown in development activity in the private sector, that given a sudden upsurge in commissions it will quickly become over-stretched and at a far earlier point this time than it did in 1973.

How will this affect the cost of rehab? Well, the pointers are very clear. Figure 1 indicates the changes in tender levels and building costs since the end of the development boom. It will be seen that whereas the general cost of building (ie labour and materials increases) has risen by some 233 per cent the actual cost of works to the client has risen by only 140 per cent; a direct result of reduced profit margins etc, with too many contractors chasing too few jobs.

The effects on the overall level of costs, therefore, are likely to be dramatic, tender levels will rise substantially as the gap between the respective indices closes and the first sector to suffer will be rehab or 'dirty work' as it is known in the industry.

Table IX   Works associated with the structural condition of the building/fabric

	UNIT COST	RANGE (FACTOR		REMARKS
		LOW	HIGH	

WORKS ON SITE
 	
Clear away existing rubbish
  Cost per skip (in £)
  Hire   30.00
  Labour (10 hrs at £3.50/hr)   35.00
                                 ――――
                                 65.00
	£65.00/each			Average skip 6m^3 for bulky items

WORKS BELOW LOWEST FLOOR LEVEL Underpinning existing foundations 1 m wide x 2 m deep in 1 m stages	£320.00/m	0.76	1.20	Should leave at least two weeks before commencing adjacent stage
Cut and insert new slate dpc in 1 b wall (225 mm)	£21.00/m			
Silicone injection dpc in 225 mm wall (excluding plaster)	£15.00/m			Maximum effective injection 350 mm
Strip out existing defective timber floor, reduce level dig, hardcore, 150 mm concrete and three coats bituminous waterproof compound and 50 mm cement and sand screed	£30.00/m^2	0.80	1.25	Check levels to be made up or reduced under old timber floors

Table IX Works associated with the structural condition of the building/fabric continued

	UNIT COST	RANGE (FACTOR)		REMARKS
		LOW	HIGH	
WORKS BELOW LOWEST FLOOR LEVEL (CONTINUED)				Check heights of sleeper walls under old floors
Strip out existing timber floor, insert new sleeper walls (750 mm) and provide and fix new 175 x 50 mm joists at 400 mm centres with 25 mm tongued and grooved boarding	£36.00/m^2	0.85	1.25	
150 mm hardcore bed	£ 1.70/m^2	0.83	1.25	
150 mm sulphate resisting concrete bed	£ 7.50/m^2	0.82	1.18	
3 coats bituminous waterproofing compound	£ 3.90/m^2	0.70	1.10	
65 mm cement/sand screed	£ 4.20/m^2	0.92	1.20	
UPPER FLOORS				
Take out and renew defective floor joists (175 x 50 mm)	£ 4.90/m^2			
Take up existing floor, piece in where defective and relay boards	£ 5.60/m^2	0.85	1.10	20 % renewing
Take up defective boarding, clear away and renew with 25 mm tongued and grooved boarding	£15.50/m^2	0.85	1.10	Plain edge 10% cheaper
ROOF (PITCHED)				
Prepare and apply two coats bitumen based sealer	£ 7.00/m^2	0.80	1.10	Limited life
Strip existing covering and provide and fix new felt, battens and new Redland concrete tiles	£12.50/m^2	0.95	1.05	
Ditto secondhand Welsh slates	£14.00/m^2	0.80	1.10	Currently in great demand in rehab sector
Ditto new Welsh slates	£28.00/m^2	0.85	1.15	
Take up and renew defective zinc valley gutter and boarding (1100 mm girth)	£50.00/m	0.85	1.15	Check any evidence of staining internally
Renew zinc stepped flashings (225 mm girth)	£11.50/m	0.94	1.15	
Renew cement and sand fillet	£ 2.00/m	0.86	1.16	
Take out and renew defective rafter 150 x 50 mm	£ 5.50/m			Excludes any temporary support
Ditto defective purlin 150 x 75 mm	£ 9.00/m			Ditto
ROOF (FLAT)				
Take up existing covering and renew with three layer felt and chippings	£11.00/m^2	0.87	1.12	
Ditto two layer asphalt on felt underlay	£12.50/m^2	0.85	1.15	
Ditto new zinc sheet on felt underlay	£25.00/m^2	0.83	1.10	
Take up and renew defective roof boarding (25 mm featheredged)	£12.00/m^2	0.88	1.12	Normally defective if covering holed
150 mm three layer felt upstand including tucking into brickwork joint	£ 4.20/m	0.82	1.10	
150 mm asphalt skirting	£ 7.00/m	0.90	1.10	
RAINWATER				
Take off and renew 225 x 19 mm softwood fascia	£ 4.20/m			
Ditto fascia and 300 mm asbestos cement soffit board on bearers	£11.00/m			
Take off and renew half round cast iron gutter and brackets	£ 9.75/m			Add 30% for fittings
Ditto pvc gutter and brackets	£ 5.50/m			Ditto
Renew defective cast iron downpipe 75 mm in diameter	£11.00/m			Ditto
Ditto pvc	£ 6.25/m			Ditto

Table IX Works associated with the structural condition of the building/fabric continued

	UNIT COST	RANGE (FACTOR)		REMARKS
		LOW	HIGH	
STAIRCASE				
Renew 1 no defective tread and riser (750 mm wide)	£19.50/each			
Renew defective baluster 1200 mm	£ 5.60/each			
Take off and renew 75 x 50 mm rounded softwood handrail on and including brackets	£14.00/m			
EXTERNAL WALLS				
Raking out existing joints and repointing	£ 5.60/m²	0.85	1.25	Depends on condition of existing mortar
Cut out defective facing brickwork and rebuild, including all cutting, toothing and bonding, to existing	£50.00/m²			
Take down and rebuild 225 mm parapet wall faced both sides	£42.00/m²			
New brick on edge coping	£ 7.00/m			
New precast concrete coping to 225 mm wall	£11.00/m			
Cut out fractures in existing brickwork and stitch in (450 mm wide in 225 mm wall) facings one side	£21.00/m			Excludes making good plaster. NOTE: No allowance for scaffolding in above rates
WINDOWS				
Overhaul existing double hung sash window	£55.00/each			New cords, weights etc
Provide and fix new sash and glazing to double hung sash window	£55.00/m²			Includes decoration
Cut out defective timber sill and renew	£22.25/m			
Cut out existing stone sub-sill and renew in concrete	£28.00/m			
Hack out existing and reglaze in 4 mm clear sheet glass	£13.00/m²			
Ditto and reglaze in 6 mm georgian wire polished plate glass	£25.00/m²			
WALLS AND CEILINGS				
Hack off existing plaster and apply three coats waterproof rendering	£ 8.90/m²	0.92	1.08	
Hack off existing plaster, apply two coats bituminous waterproof compound and fix Gyproc dry lining on metal firrings	£12.50/m²	0.94	1.22	
Hack off existing plaster, dub out as necessary and render and set including jointing new to existing to brickwork	£ 7.50/m²	0.90	1.14	
Ditto to stud partitions	£ 8.50/m²	0.92	1.08	
Ditto ceilings	£ 9.75/m²	0.85	1.07	
Hack off and re-render plinth externally	£ 7.00/m²			
Hack off and renew stucco work externally including forming new profiles	£ 9.75/m²	0.92	1.28	

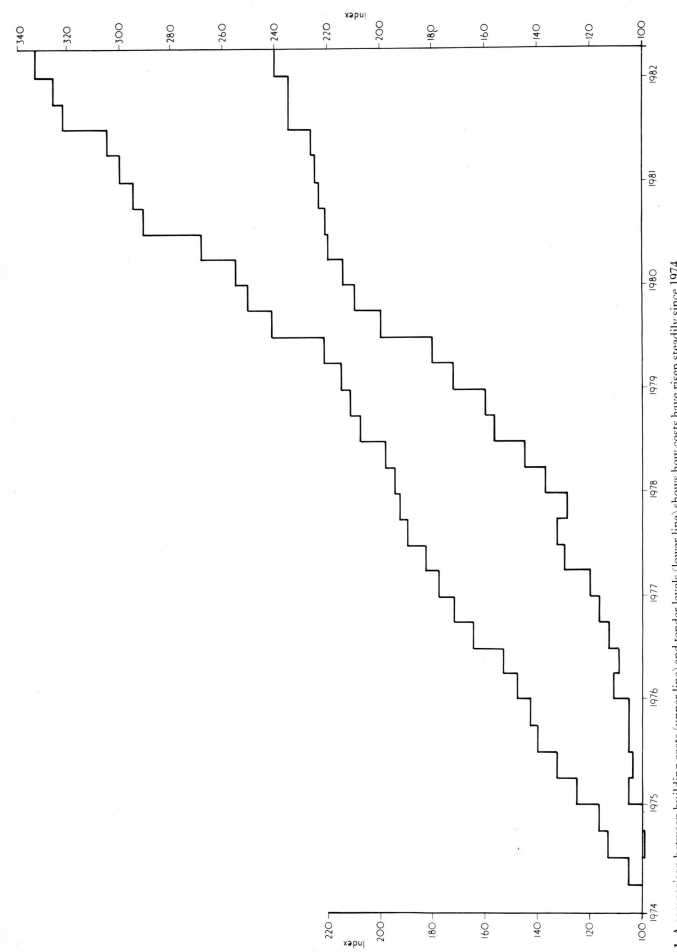

1 A comparison between building costs (upper line) and tender levels (lower line) shows how costs have risen steadily since 1974. Tender levels have not risen correspondingly. Indications are that contractors will be increasingly reluctant to allow this situation to continue.

Table X   Works in order to comply with current standards of health and safety

	UNIT COST	RANGE (FACTOR)		REMARKS
		LOW	HIGH	
FIRE PROTECTION/MEANS OF ESCAPE				
Provide all temporary supports, needles etc and form standard door opening in 225 mm brick wall including new lintel and making good all areas disturbed	£140/each			Excludes cost of new door and frame
Ditto 337 mm wall	£175/each			Ditto
Provide and fix new one hour stud partition with two layers of 12 mm plasterboard both sides, skim coat, timber skirting and two coats emulsion	£ 34.00/m^2	0.83	1.10	
Provide and fix two skins of plasterboard skim coat and two coats emulsion to exposed timber joists	£ 11.00/m^2	0.88	1.06	Affords 1 hour fire resistance
New half-hour fire door and frame with glazed viewing panel and all ironmongery and decorations	£200/each			Ironmongery pc £35.00 supply only
Ditto, pair of doors, with ironmongery and decorations	£360/each			Ditto, £60.00 supply only
Provide and fix new stairs in existing openings, 3 m storey height in two flights and one half landing. Alternative specifications:				
Timber, including asbestos cement to soffit, decorations, handrail and vinyl covering	£1000/lift			
Reinforced concrete with grano finish and metal handrail	£1500/lift			
External steel staircase, including decorations and all associated builder's work in connection	£1750/lift			
Encase cast iron column/beam in asbestos cement on framing 1200 mm girth	£35.00/m	0.90	1.30	
Ditto sprayed asbestos cement compound	£25.00/m	0.88	1.20	
THERMAL INSULATION				
Form new access hatch to existing roof space	£55/each			
75 mm fibreglass quilt insulation	£ 4.00/m^2	0.85	1.05	
PUBLIC HEALTH/SANITARY				
White glazed wc suite complete including cold water supply (excludes soil pipe)	£200/each			Assumes at least 4 no wc units in building
Lavatory basin complete including hot and cold water supply and wastes	£340/each			Includes 1½ gall electric hot water heater
100 mm diameter pvc soil stack including all fittings	£ 25.00/m			
SERVICES				
Mechanical ventilation plus pipework to wcs	£200/toilet			Assume 3 m run to outside wall
CO_2 fire extinguishers	£ 70.00/each			Two gallon type
150 mm salt-glazed stoneware drain including all excavation and haunching (assume invert approx 1000 mm)	£ 28.00/m	0.90	1.20	
Form new manhole externally 600 x 600 mm, invert 1500 mm	£250/each			
Ditto internally, with double seal double cover invert 1500 mm	£350/each			Double seal cover very expensive

Table XI   Work in connection with client's requirements

	UNIT COST	RANGE (FACTOR)		REMARKS
		LOW	HIGH	
INTERNAL DIVISIONS/ACCESS				
Provide and fix 100 mm blockwork partition, plastered both sides with timber skirting and two coats emulsion	£ 22.00/m²	0.85	1.12	
Ditto 150 mm thick	£ 25.00/m²	0.85	1.12	
Ditto stud partition, one layer of plasterboard both sides, skim coat, timber skirting, two coats emulsion	£ 26.00/m²	0.89	1.05	It may be necessary to strengthen existing joists under
New plywood faced flush door and frame, ironmongery and decoration	£150/each	0.90	1.18	Ironmongery pc £20, supply only
Ditto sapele-faced self-closing flush door, ironmongery and decoration	£200/each	0.93	1.20	Ironmongery pc £50, supply only
FLOOR FINISHES				
Punch down nails, remove tacks etc, fill nail holes etc on existing floor and machine sand surface and two coats polyurethane	£ 7.00/m²	0.90	1.25	
Prepare concrete and lay 300 x 300 mm pvc tiles, 3 mm thick fixed with adhesive	£ 9.00/m²	0.95	1.15	
Ditto on 3.2 mm hardboard fixed to timber floors	£ 11.00/m²	0.95	1.15	
Prepare subfloor and lay foam underlay and carpet pc £ 8.00 supply only	£ 12.50/m²	0.94	1.05	Carpet only pc £ 8.00/m²
Prepare subfloor and lay 152 x 152 x 22 mm quarry tiles to level base	£ 22.00/m²	0.94	1.10	Screed elsewhere
100 mm pvc skirting fixed with adhesive	£ 2.50/m	0.92	1.10	
150 x 19 mm plain softwood including decorations	£ 4.00/m	0.85	1.15	
152 x 22 mm quarry tile skirting with rounded top edge, coved bottom edge	£ 7.00/m	0.90	1.15	Add 20% for angles etc
WALL FINISHES				
Prepare existing surfaces and apply 152 x 152 x 6 mm white glazed ceramic tiles fixed with adhesive	£ 20.00/m²	0.92	1.15	Labour add 20%
CEILING FINISHES				
Provide and fix new suspended ceiling on Z section metal suspension system, fixed to structural soffit, (600 mm suspension, 600 x 600 tile module)	£ 17.00/m²	0.95	1.25	Profile tiles pc £ 8.00/m² supply only
DECORATIONS (EXISTING WORKS)				
Prepare and supply two coats emulsion to surfaces of blockwork walls	£ 2.70/m²	0.94	1.05	15% cheaper to plaster walls
Ditto to concrete ceilings	£ 3.00/m²	0.90	1.10	20% cheaper to plaster ceilings
Prepare and supply one undercoat and two gloss finishing coats to timber surfaces over 300 mm girth internally	£ 6.00/m²	0.95	1.10	Add 15% for external works
Ditto to windows medium panes	£ 7.50/m²	0.95	1.10	Ditto
Prepare and apply one undercoat and two gloss finishing coats to timber skirting 200 mm girth	£ 2.40/m	0.90	1.10	
NOTE: Add 50% to the above items for burning off existing paintwork				
DECORATIONS (NEW WORK)				
Prepare and apply two coats emulsion to plastered surface walls	£ 2.00/m²	0.80	1.05	
Ditto ceiling	£ 2.50/m²	0.85	1.10	

Table XI   Work in connection with client's requirements—*continued*

	UNIT COST	RANGE (FACTOR)		REMARKS
		LOW	HIGH	
DECORATIONS (NEW WORK) (CONTINUED) Prepare, knot, stop, prime and one undercoat and two gloss finishing coats to timber surfaces over 100 mm girth	£ 4.75/m^2	0.95	1.10	
Ditto to windows, medium panes	£ 6.00/m^2	0.90	1.15	
Ditto new skirting, 300 mm girth	£ 2.00/m	0.90	1.10	
SERVICES				
Electrical (includes all mains costs on consumer side only)				
Lighting circuits wired in pvc insulated cable installed in cavities and roof space, protected where buried by light gauge conduit	£ 30.00/point			Excludes light fittings
Ditto but in MICC	£ 55.00/point			Ditto
Ditto but in screwed welded conduit	£ 60.00/point			Ditto
Twin 13 amp power circuits in pvc insulated cable on a ring main protected where buried by light gauge conduit	£ 35.00/point			
Ditto but in MICC	£ 65.00/point			
Ditto in screwed welded conduit	£ 70.00/point			
NOTE: The above costs exclude builder's work in connection. As a rule of thumb add 10-15%				

HEATING VENTILATING, AIR-CONDITIONING

Will vary enormously depending on the degree of environmental comfort/control required and the industrial processes (if any) the system may be required to accommodate

At a very basic level a 3 kW fan heater including wiring may cost £ 150 each installed, whereas a fully air-conditioned space may cost between £100-140/m^2 of gross floor area depending on the area served

CONTINGENCIES AND PRELIMINARIES

Having established a basic order of cost from the rates contained in this chapter, consideration should then be given to the specific amounts to be included in the initial cost plan to allow for designand construction contingencies and main contractor's preliminaries

CONTINGENCIES

As a general rule of thumb allow 10% at the initial feasibility stage for design and construction contingencies

PRELIMINARIES

Contractors' preliminaries normally contain those site and ancillary costs that may be common to many of the building elements but which cannot easily be incorporated elsewhere in the overall tender analysis (ie site foreman, water, power, scaffolding, which will afford access for roof works, works to external walls and decoration works, etc)
    The cost of the preliminaries element will fluctuate according to site location, access, time of year the contract is undertaken etc. The following are some of the more important items to consider when assessing the likely cost of the preliminaries element:

1) Site supervision. On a small contract the foreman may well spend some of his time 'on the tools' in which case only include that percentage of his time that is non-productive in the preliminaries (ie 20-week contract: foreman at £ 300/week spends 60% of his time supervising; therefore non-productive time = 20 x 300 x 60% = £ 3600).

2) Provision of messroom, toilets, office accomodation, storage for plant and materials. Could be a problem on a confined inner-city site with offices having to be built over footpaths, etc

3) Insurances (personal and property). May involve a higher premium if the site is in a built-up area

4) Temporary telephones, power and water. Again, may be a problem on a remote country site

5) Overtime and weeke d working. Must be included in the rates or considered in the preliminaries. An important consideration if the contract programme is particularly tight

6) Security patrols, watchman. Vandals may be a problem, especially in run-down city areas

Table XI Work in connection with client's requirements—*continued*

7) Scaffolding, fans, staging

8) Hoarding could be an expensive exercise, especially on a large exposed site

9) Access and unloading of materials. May necessitate cranage of some nature, and/or weekend working if a built-up inner city area

10) Increased cost of labour and materials. On a fixed price contract increases are normally taken as an across-the-board increase on the specification/bill rates, or alternatively are allowed for in the preliminaries.

Proposed labour increases are particularly difficult to assess and are dependent to a large degree on the success or otherwise of successive governments in controlling the overall level of wage increases.

Materials on smaller rehab contracts are currently increasing at a rate of some 2% a month but this will obviously be affected by any favourable purchasing arrangements that the contractor may have with respective suppliers

There is therefore no general rule of thumb for assessing the overall preliminaries element. It may be as low as 4% on a multi-million pound contract, or as high as 20% on a small rehab contract. On the £ 100,000-£ 140,000 contract under consideration , given normal site conditions, etc, the percentage allowance would normally be about 8%-9% of the total contract value

Table I   (Chapter 10) Sequential approach to checking statutory compliance and financial viability

TENTATIVELY MATCH POTENTIAL USERS WITH AVAILABLE BUILDINGS

Identify possible users
Identify possible buildings
Tentatively match potential users with most suitable
of available buildings

CHECK FINANCIAL VIABILITY

See chapter 8
Estimate anticipated rental income from new use
Estimate the approximate costs of acquiring and developing the site
Estimate cost and availability of the scheme

CHECK STATUTORY COMPLIANCE

See this chapter
Check whether 'change of use' is involved
Carry out a general check against 4 principal Acts (table III)
Carry out a general check against the wider range of legislation (table IV)
Discuss fire protection requirements in particular, with statutory authorities and insurance companies

PRODUCE OUTLINE DESIGN

See chapter 13
Develop site layout, taking into account access, delivery, parking and future expansion requirements
Develop tenancy strategy and outline design for building shell
Develop outline plan for fitting out of individual tenancies

CHECK FINANCIAL VIABILITY
Repeat the checks already carried out at the feasibility stage above, but at a level of increased precision, based on more detailed design information

CHECK STATUTORY COMPLIANCE
Carry out a detailed check against 4 principal Acts (tables V and VI)
Carry out a detailed check against fire safety requirements, both legislative and insurance company rules (see this chapter)

PROCEED TO MORE DETAILED DESIGN STAGES,IN ACCORDANCE WITH LATER CHAPTERS

10 Meeting Statutory Requirements

1.00 Introduction

This chapter covers the problems of meeting statutory requirements and regulations under Acts of Parliament for two main areas:

Planning and the use of the building
Safety from fire.

Obtaining approvals for the conversion of industrial structures is particularly complex, because the previous planning history of the building can be as significant a factor as the intended use.

Fire requirements, which have been defined in various Acts, are now administered together under the Fire Precautions Act 1971, but insurance companies have their own, independent rules and procedures, through the code of the Fire Offices Committee. Fire safety is one of the most difficult areas for a conversion project to surmount: compartmentation requirements, upgrading of the structure and fabric, and provision of escape stairs can easily make an attractive seeming project economically impossible.

2.00 Complexity of legal framework

To the uninitiated, the number of Acts which may influence an inner city conversion project and the number of authorities who may need to be approached for approval, may seem daunting. It is clear that legislation is changing rapidly at present and requires careful checking. A methodical approach will, however, help the designer steer a relatively smooth course through these complexities.

There are a limited number of key provisions which apply widely and with which those involved in rehabilitation work need to be thoroughly conversant. Once this framework is understood, it will usually be found that only two or three Acts are encountered on any particular conversion project, and only on rare occasions will there be a need to meet the whole range of authorities.

The principal pieces of legislation to be checked are:

The Town and Country Planning Act 1971, and other planning controls in force
Building Regulations 1976

The Factories Act 1961
The Offices, Shops and Railway Premises Act 1963.

3.00 Sequential approach

Working together, the designer and developer should take a sequential approach to the design process, as shown in table I (facing page), this will bring them into contact with the controlling legislation in a logical progression.

4.00 Legal checks at feasibility stage

4.01 Introduction
The purpose at feasibility stage is to provide the client with an appraisal and recommendation which will enable him to decide whether the envisaged project is viable and should be carried out. This precedes the outline design. Table II shows the scope of legal checks to be carried out at this stage.

4.02 Use classification
One particular factor is fundamental to all conversion work in the industrial sector: 'the use classification of the previous occupancy'. Only when a change in the classification is proposed (eg shop, class I, to light industrial, class III) does the full weight of contemporary design standards apply to a building conversion.

Use classes abbreviated from the Town and Country Planning Act 1971 are:— 1:Shops, II:Offices, III:Light industrial, IV:General industrial, V–IX:Special industrial groups A–E, X:Wholesale warehouses, XI XII XIV:Residential institutions, XIII:Religious, XV:Health, XVI:Display galleries, XVII:Theatres, XVIII:Sports facilities.

To upgrade and convert a whole structure at one time will often be well beyond the financial resources of a developing agency, especially if conversion work is to be financed out of income from the earlier tenancies. To work within the constraints of existing planning use classifications will then be the only way to proceed, converting to new uses at a later date.

Table II Legal checks at feasibility stage

```
STEP 1

Is a change of use involved under the Town and
Country Planning Act 1971? See para 4.02
```

```
STEP 2

Into which purpose group or use class does the
proposed occupancy fall, in terms of the
Building Regulations? See tables VII and VIII
```

```
STEP 3
Check compliance with the four principal areas
of legislation which may apply: Planning Law,
Building Regulations, Factories Act, Offices,
Shops and Railway Premises Act. See table III
```

```
STEP 4

Check compliance with wider range of more
general legislation. See table IV
```

```
STEP 5

Check compliance with Fire Regulations, both
statutory, and insurance company rules. See
tables IX, X and XI
```

```
STEP 6

Proceed to more detailed design stages
```

4.03 Fire protection

Fire safety requirements are also of quite fundamental importance: the assessed risks and the required safeguards, as laid down both by statutory authorities and insurance companies, could easily spell the difference between financial viability and non-viability. The Building Regulations 1976 list and describe eight different purpose groups (table VIII). These have a critical effect on the fire compartmentation, structural fire protection and means of escape requirements which may be applied to a redundant building. They therefore need to be very clearly established at feasibility stage.

The London Building (Constructional) By-Laws define use in a different way. Their categories are given in table VII.
Note: at the time of writing, proposals have been made for extending the Building Regulations to London.

4.04 The principal four Acts

The principal checks to be carried out at feasibility stage, in relation to the four Acts most commonly encountered, are listed in table III. The Fire Precautions Act, sections 13 and 14, restricts the power of the fire authority to impose further requirements in the case of a building which already complies with the Building Regulations, so conflict between different requirements should be avoidable. Further simplifications are proposed in the Housing and Building Control Bill, before Parliament at the time of writing.

4.05 The full range of relevant legislation

In addition to the four main Acts, there is a wide range of legislation which may be relevant and table IV provides a checklist of the titles, the principal provisions, and the authorities responsible for enforcement. It is clearly the architect's task to co-ordinate the relevant approvals, particularly in so far as he can relate decisions to a realistic timetable.

5.00 Legal checks at outline proposals and scheme design stages

5.01 Introduction

Having taken the key strategic decisions, which are part of the feasibility study process and which determine whether or not the proposed conversion is going to be viable, the designer can now resolve more detailed problems as part of the outline proposals and scheme design stages.

5.02 The principal four Acts

Following the first set of checks carried out at feasibility stage (table III), a second set of checks at design stage is outlined in table V. A third set of checks relating to the same four Acts, is outlined for the later implementation stage of the project in table VI.

5.03 Fire safety

As at the feasibility stage, fire safety requirements are complex, they are referred to in section 6 below.

6.00 Fire requirements

6.01 Identifying main problems

Designers need a series of simple signposts to the main problems which will be encountered in making older premises safe by modern standards. Further detail will then come through direct contact with the relevant legislation or fire officers. Problems of fire safety can be conveniently subdivided into four categories.

● Protection of the *building*. This is a question of meeting the structural fire protection requirements of the building regulations, by means of proper 'compartmentation' and acceptable forms of construction. *See paragraph 6.02.*

● Protection of the *occupants*, by means of adequate escape routes, alarm systems and firefighting equipment. *See paragraph 6.03.*

● Developing a *tenancy strategy* for the building under consideration, which will satisfy both the compartmentation requirements and the escape route requirements identified above. *See paragraph 6.04.*

● Protection of the *contents* of the building, in terms of insurance company requirements. *See paragraph 6.05.*

6.02 Structural fire protection

Purpose groups and compartment sizes
The first step is always to establish the shape and extent of the risk involved.

If the work is being undertaken in inner London (the former LCC area) national building regulations do not at present apply, but 'Use classes' derived from the London Building Acts. These are shown in table VII and detailed provisions are to be found in the relevant GLC publications (see references in Bibliography).

Table III   A programme for complying with the critical Acts (feasibility stage)

Planning law and related procedures	Building Regulations	Factories	Offices, Shops and Railway Premises
1 Established use and change of use It is vital to determine the established use of a particular property. Planning permission will only be required if the use is to be changed or the quantity of space in use increased. In a warehouse there may, for example, be some existing ancillary offices relating to clerical work which was carried out within the space and these rights might be carried over to form an office portion of the rehabilitated space provided they could still be shown to be ancillary to the main use. If a change is proposed, then this should be in conformity with the approved development plan for the area. If a new plan is under preparation and has not yet been confirmed then the previous plan, however old, remains in force. A planning authority may nevertheless designate a particular area for compulsory purchase at any time, if this becomes the only way of obtaining a desired change or the comprehensively organised redevelopment of an area with numerous non-conforming uses.	**1 Previous use, change of use and application of the regulations** The presumption in Part A of the regulations is that all buildings in constant use are allowed to remain in their present state until such time as *either* an alteration or extension to the fabric is undertaken *or* the use is changed, at which time the regulations will be applied to the new parts (and to the old if non-compliance would otherwise increase). If a building was originally built before any regulations existed (eg an eighteenth century mill) or was exempt from control when first erected (eg army barracks) then the extent of alteration required, if there is a change of use, may be considerable. Note that the use classes for building regulations are not the same as for town planning. Buildings which are to be used mainly for storage, mechanical plant or animals and where no one works permanently are exempt from the majority of regulations.	**1 Definition of a factory** The act defines a factory as a place where two or more people are employed in manual labour. This is deemed to include trades ancillary to theatre and cinema production, printing works and laundries as well as places where manufacturing and repair work takes place. A factory need not be the whole building, and a building can be divided into any number of individual factories.	**1 Applications** An office is a part of a building where the principal use is for office purposes. A shop is either where the principal use is for retail trade or a wholesaler where goods are kept for sale, or a place where the public delivers goods for repair.
2 Minor changes Certain minor alterations such as exterior painting, the erection of fences, installation of new plant and extensions of up to 20 per cent of cubic volume or 750 sq m floor area may be allowed without a planning application. A frequent cause of complaint in residential areas is the need for permission to do such things as sell home-grown vegetables or craft objects made in a back extension. Planning law is absolute on the incompatibility of uses but enforcement seems to depend on the scale of operation involved. If the floor area concerned does not exceed 235 sq metres, a change of use may be made without permission from warehousing to light industrial use.	**2 Structural fire protection** Covered by Part E. A critical factor determining the level of fire protection for the structure itself is the size of 'compartments'. Normally these are defined by solid floors and dividing walls. Access ways and ducts passing through these will require metal barriers or shutters which operate automatically in the case of fire, so limiting its spread but also constraining escape routes. For industrial (factory) uses, a critical change in fire protection (from one to two hours standard) applies where the cubic capacity of a compartment exceeds 8500m³ in the upper floors of buildings up to 28m high. All hoist ways must be protected. Basements are almost always subject to more stringent standards to such a degree that it may be uneconomic to open the basement at all if rents for this kind of space are low. The revised London Constructional Bylaws now require that *all* buildings have some minimum period of fire resistance.	**2 Overcrowding** The cubic space available for each worker must reach a minimum level 11.32m³ although space more than 4.26m from the floor does not count). In practice this could mean that activities which use floor area very intensively (such as clothing manufacture) may not be accommodated in buildings with a low floor-ceiling height (say below 2.4m).	**2 Overcrowding** The cubic space available for each worker in a building where the ceiling height is less than 3.05m must be at least 11.32m³.
	3 Construction of fire escapes Most existing buildings have some sort of fire escape system but if the building is an old multi-storey structure it is unlikely to meet modern requirements. Protected stairways should, for example, have a smoke outlet at roof level and should not, if possible, contain vertical pipes or ducts. External stairways should be well away from openings in external walls: rooftop escape systems are to be avoided other than for small units of space where no other alternative is economic.	**3 Means of access and escape*** Safe access must be possible to all workplaces. The Acts provides that gangways, ladders, openings in floors should have appropriate handrails. Safe escape in case of fire is also necessary: generally this means an alternative exit for every area where more than 10 people work and alternative exit stairways for upper floors. This also means that escape routes must be kept clear of obstructions and doors open out without a key. There are more stringent codes for places of special danger eg where paint is sprayed and where cellulose film is stored or processed. The London Fire Brigade's Code of Practice is a good guide.	**3 Means of escape*** Recommendations are set out in BS3 CP Chap IV pt 3. Properly constructed corridors and stairways are considered 'safe areas'. Access to a safe area may be through no more than one internal office. Single stair buildings are possible provided corridor lengths do not exceed 12m. Sizing of escape routes must take account of all the people likely to be in the building at one time.

continued on page 98

Table III   A programme for complying with the critical Acts (feasibility stage)—*continued*

Planning law and related procedures	Building Regulations	Factories	Offices, Shops and Railway Premises
4 Construction areas and historic buildings Local authorities have special control over alterations to Grade 1 and Grade 2 historic buildings, and control over demolition is extended to cover *all* buildings in a conservation area. Otherwise location in conservation areas can be helpful to developers as grants and loans for improvement may be available. The presumption of the legislation is that new work will be designed not as a separate entity but as part of the larger whole. Special consideration should be given to bulk, height, materials, colour and the vertical or horizontal emphasis of design. Some relaxation of zoning, density, plot ratio and daylighting controls may well be justified. To assist them in considering applications of this kind, it is suggested that local authorities should establish advisory committees: doubtless architects with special local knowledge will be invited to serve on these.	**4 Inclusion of domestic uses** Changing to and from domestic uses presents particular problems which are unlike those experienced in other cases. In changes *from* domestic use to industrial or office functions (eg a Georgian house to be converted to flatted workshops and studios) fireproof means of escape will be required where none were provided before. In changes *to domestic use* (eg where flats are to be incorporated in upper levels of a multi-storey warehouse) it will normally not be possible for the new residential functions to share means of escape with the other uses and the highest standards of structural fire separation between functions may be demanded. Certain detailed regulations covering ventilation, thermal and sound insulation also apply only to domestic uses and are not covered here.	**4 Ventilation** All work space must have fresh air ventilation (six air changes per hour is recommended). This may have to be provided mechanically where internal rooms are planned.	**4 Ventilation** All work space must have adequate ventilation but offices are considered more likely to be mechanically ventilated.
	5 Inclusion of public uses If the general public is to be admitted, say to a studio-theatre, or there is some training/educational function with its own spaces in the building, then the parts concerned will be treated separately from the remainder. As a general rule, the regulations for fire escape are more stringent, but those for protection of the structure less stringent than for factory spaces of similar size.	**5 Underground rooms** These are subject to special control if used for purposes other than storage. Permission may be refused on 'any hygienic ground' such as the likely entry of dust and dirt from the street.	**5 Sanitary conveniences** Pro rata for each sex (if more than five persons are employed): approximately five fittings per 100 employees.
		6 Sanitary accommodation Separate accommodation is required for each sex, the number of fittings depending on the expected number of employees (1:25 is normal). Lavatory areas must be separated from workplaces by a ventilated lobby.	**6 Lifts** These are covered by special regulations. Passenger lifts must be enclosed.
			7 Markets It is worth noting that covered markets are considered a special case. It is likely that requirements for sanitary accommodation would be less stringent and for escape routes more stringent than for a shop of similar size.

* Approval of means of escape from offices, shops and factories has been administered under the Fire Precautions Act since 1 January 1977. The new regulations broadly continue and bring together arrangements set out in the earlier Acts.

Table IV   A checklist of relevant legislation

Responsible authority	Responsible officers	Title	Principal provisions	Application to industrial conversions
HM Land Registry		Land Registration Acts 1925, 1966. Land Registration and Land Changes Act 1971.	Being progressively introduced over whole country, this legislation will eventually make registration of all land ownership compulsory. Currently covers most urban areas.	All changes in land ownership.
Countryside Commission for National Parks, elsewhere local authorities		Countryside Acts (Scotland 1967: England and Wales 1968) Wildlife and Countryside Act 1981.	Conservation of the countryside etc. Facilitate provision of recreational facilities on waterways and protect right of way.	Canalside buildings, rural projects.

Table IV   A checklist of relevant legislation

Responsible authority	Responsible officers	Title	Principal provisions	Application to industrial conversions
Department of Education and Science		Education Act 1944	Regulations covering amenity health and safety in school premises, special schools, training premises.	Training activities
Department of Employment	Health and Safety Executive (formerly Factory Inspectorate)	Celluloid and Cinematographic Film Act 1922	Safety in premises where film is stored.	Film processing.
		Factories Act 1961 Health and Safety at Work etc Act 1974	Covers health and safety of people employed in manual labour: density, temperature, ventilation, sanitary provisions, drainage, fire protection, lifts, access routes, etc. Specific regulations also issued covering particular industries	All industrial uses.
Department of Industry	Alkali Inspectorate	Alkali Act	Provides for registration of all alkali works and control of commissions.	Chemical industries.
Department of Industry		Industry Act 1972, 1975	Provides improvement grants for industrial buildings in development and intermediate areas. Currently under revision.	Industrial areas outside London and the West Midlands.
Department of Industry		Welsh Development Agency Act 1975 Scottish Development Agency Act 1975	Acts concerned with industrial development promotion in these areas.	
Department of the Environment and Department of Industry		Control of Office and Industrial Development Act 1965	Is intended to control the location of new office and industrial workspace; requires issue of ODPs and IDCs for developments of certain sizes in certain Regions, provisions currently suspended.	
Department of the Environment & Local Authority		Local Government, Planning & Land Act 1980	Act under which Land Registers are required. Has considerably increased Central Government powers, including establishment of Urban Development Corporations.	London & Liverpool Docklands, & other; also Enterprise Zones.
Department of the Environment		Explosives Act 1875, 1923	Licensing of explosive factories and magazines: criteria include site layout, construction details, etc.	Chemical Industries.
		Inner Urban Areas Act 1978	Empowers local authorities to grant-aid conversions in industrial improvement areas.	Urban projects.
County Councils	Engineers Dept	Restriction of Ribbon Development Act 1935	Controls means of vehicular access to very large structures and some public buildings.	Multi-storey industrial estates.
		Highways Act 1959, 1971	Control of access to buildings from highways, and obstruction of streets by projections from buildings.	Buildings without service yard.
		Petroleum (Consolidation) Act 1928	Ventilation of areas where petroleum products are stored and structural separation from other uses. Car parks included.	Vehicle storage.
Shared between County and District Councils but with certain matters subject to approval by Department of Environment	Planning Dept	Town and Country Planning Act 1971 Town and Country Planning (Amendment) Act 1972 Local Government Planning (Amendment) Act 1981	Provides for making of structure plans and local plans as well as for the control of land use and of the appearance of all development. Change of use is defined, procedures are laid down for appeals against decisions and for the holding of planning inquiries. Local authorities may carry out work to preserve unoccupied listed buildings. Appeal procedures for unauthorised works.	All changes of use. Listed buildings.
District Councils, but Department of Environment may override	Planning Dept	Civic Amenities Act 1967 Town and Country Amenities Act 1974	Principal legislation covering conservation and preservation of buildings and trees; also deals with disposal of vehicles and similar rubbish.	Conservation areas.
District Councils	Environmental Health Dept	Clean Air Acts 1956, 1968	Established smokeless zones and controls emission of black smoke, dust and grit. Covers design of new furnaces and allows for grants to aid conversion of old ones. Height of chimneys is controlled.	Noxious processes
		Noise Abatement Act 1960	Requires producers of a noise or vibration to use the best practical means to counteract nuisance to others.	Noisy processes and building sites
		Food and Drugs Act 1955	Regulations covering design and construction of premises where milk products are handled and food is stored or prepared.	Food and drink processing

Table IV   A checklist of relevant legislation

Responsible authority	Responsible officers	Title	Principal provisions	Application to industrial conversions
		Prevention of Damage by Pests Act 1949	Prevention of infestation by rodents of premises where food is manufactured or stored.	Food processing
	Environmental Health Dept and Fire Dept	Offices, Shops and Railway Premises Act 1963	Provisions for the health, safety and welfare of employees. Covers occupancy, temperature, ventilation, lighting, sanitation, means of escape, fire-fighting equipment. Includes control of common parts in multi-occupied buildings.	Office space
	Environmental Health Dept and Building Control Dept	Public Health Acts 1936, 1961 Public Health (Drainage of Premises) Act 1937	Covers access for refuse disposal etc but also the use of unsuitable materials in general and the demolition of dangerous or dilapidated buildings. Sewerage, sanitation and the disposal of trade effluents come under this legislation. This is the enabling Act under which the Building Regulations 1976 and the Building Standards (Scotland) 1971, 1973, are made.	All buildings
	Building Controls Dept	Health and Safety at Work etc Act 1974	Gives additional powers for the making of Building Regulations, which control size, strength and safety, fire protection, drainage, insulation, stairs, lifts, circulation routes etc of most buildings and specifies materials and methods to be used in many cases. Adds to or modifies safety precautions of various other Acts. Enabling legislation for further control including the possibility of approval by stages, type approval and type relaxations. May in future cover inner London area where currently London Building Acts apply.	All buildings outside inner London*
	Fire Depts and Building Control Dept	Fire Precautions Act 1971	Issue of fire certificates for factories, offices, shops, hotels and hostels. Will in future apply to other public buildings. Covers means of escape, fire-fighting equipment, alarm systems, occupancy levels and storage of inflammable materials.	All buildings outside inner London*
Justices, but some local authorities (eg the GLC) have adopted these powers		Licensing Act 1964	Structural requirements for licensing of premises where intoxicating drinks are to be consumed. Includes clubs.	Social areas
Greater London Council*	Architects Department (District Surveyors and Building Regulation Division)	London Building Acts 1930, 1935 (Amendment Act 1939) The Greater London Council (General Powers) Acts 1966, 1968 London Building (Constructional) By-Laws 1979	Provides for inner London the equivalent of the Public Health Acts and the Building Regulations. Differences of detail apply in particular to structural stability and to precautions in case of fire.	Inner London projects
New Town development corporations	Relevant depts	New Towns Acts 1959, 1965	Covers all activities of New Town development corporations; land acquisition, land disposal, planning finance, building experiments.	New Town projects

* Inner London Borough Councils have powers over public health, planning and housing (as do District Councils elsewhere). The Greater London Council has strategic responsibilities in planning (like a County Council) and also (unlike counties) in housing. Highways (normally a county matter) are divided between GLC and boroughs depending on the importance of the routes concerned. Reorganisational charges are being discussed at the time of going to press.

Table V   A programme for complying with the critical Acts (design stage)

Planning law and related procedures	Building Regulations	Factories	Offices, Shops and Railway Premises
1 Vehicular access The local planning authority is required to consider the traffic and transport implications of a development proposal. The same authority is usually also the highway authority and may wish to impose modern engineering standards when the opportunity arises. Inadequate accommodation for delivery vehicles, as well as for employees' car parking, is a frequent cause of refusal to grant permission for change of use.	**1 Structural stability** Covered by Part D. Calculations may be required for all elements including roof and foundations. Self-weight, imposed floor loading, dynamic loads, wind loads, and snow load are to be resisted. The regulations refer to BS3 CP Chap V where imposed loands are specified by use class (these classes being similar to but not identical with the purpose groups specified in Part E). Deemed to	**1 Lighting** Sufficient lighting must be maintained everywhere people work or move about. This may, however, be natural or artificial. Skylights may be shaded to reduce glare.	**1 Lighting** Provisions similar to those for Factories except that offices are considered more likely to have artificial illumination.

Table V A programme for complying with the critical Acts (design stage)—continued

Planning law and related procedures	Building Regulations	Factories	Offices, Shops and Railway Premises
	satisfy provisions are made for traditional brick and timber construction but should be checked locally before use. Similar provisions for the other common structural materials are made by reference to various engineering Codes of Practice. If the building is five or more storeys high, its structure must resist lateral dynamic forces, such as those caused by a gas explosion, as well as those normally catered for.		
2 Aesthetic control Planning authorities can be asked to grant permission in outline only, to begin with, and reserve approval of details to a later stage. Aspects which are frequently the subject of disagreement include new windows and door openings, type and colour of facing materials, location and design of advertising, hoardings, etc.	**2 Design of staircases** Since 1975 a revised Part H applies to all buildings. No more than 16 successive rises are permitted without a landing nor more than 36 without a change in direction. Headroom is controlled, tapering steps or radiused stairs subject to width constraints and handrail(s) required. External stairs exposed to the weather not permitted if they exceed 6m height.	**2 Heating** The Act does not lay down a minimum temperature (except where the work is sedentary) but states that a reasonable level of heating must be maintained in all workrooms. In many instances this service will be provided by the tenant or employer and not the developer or building manager.	**2 Heating** Minimum standard 16°C.
	3 Resistance to moisture Covered by Part C. This section calls for external walls to be weather resistant, for roofs to be weatherproof, and for precautions to be taken against rising damp. The definition of an 'excepted' building includes cases where compliance with the regulations would not increase protection to the health of employees.	**3 Insulation** Thermal Insulation Regulations are Part FF of the building regulations and took effect from 1 June 1979. Factories require a U-value of 0.7W m² deg C on walls and roofs, and offices a U-value of 0.6, but the regulation will not apply to unheated spaces or to areas of less than 30m².	**3 Insulation** Designers are now expected to give due consideration to energy conservation.
	4 Heat-producing appliances Part M covers prevention of the emission of smoke and the provision of adequate ventilation for solid fuel and gas fired heating units.	**4 Materials** Those used for roof insulation must have Class I (high) resistance to the surface spread of flame.	

Table VI A programme for complying with the critical Acts (implementation stage)

Planning law and related procedures	Building Regulations	Factories	Offices, Shops and Railway Premises
1 Enforcement Authority may serve an enforcement notice, which must include a time limit, and after failure to comply, a stop notice. Disregard is a criminal offence, but if notice is invalidated on appeal, compensation is payable.	**1 Materials** In Part B the use of any material in full accordance with the appropriate BSCP is considered adequate. Particular precautions are required with roofing felt with asbestos-cement or steel sheeting on external walls or on roofs, and with external plasterwork. Softwood timber used in certain areas of Surrey and Hampshire must be protected against the longhorn beetle.	**1 Fire alarms and fire-fighting equipment** Audible alarms are required. Booklets are published covering the provision of extinguishers and other fire-fighting equipment. All buildings must have adequate provision. Exits must be marked.	**1 Fire alarms and fire-fighting equipment** Provisions similar to those for Factories Act.
2 Statutory undertakings The local authority is statutory undertaker for connection to public sewers, disposal of trade effluent, refuse collection. The local highway authority is statutory undertaker for connection to highway drains. Water supply, gas supply and electricity supply are the responsibility of the relevant local area board; the water authority is responsible for drainage into rivers; there is no control over drainage into the sea. Telephone services are supplied by the Post Office. All these parties may need to know about and agree with the details of a development project.	**2 Construction** The builder is responsible for providing adequate structural stability *during* construction. In some cases this will be a considerable problem in itself.	**2 Clothing** Facilities will be required for storing outdoor clothing. In many cases the tenant will take care of this.	**2 Clothing** Provisions similar to those for Factories
		3 Personal services In certain circumstances factory doctors must be catered for, canteens provided and so on. Tenants will normally be aware of these requirements as they relate to a particular industry	**3 Personal services** Provisions similar to those for Factories.

101

Table VII   Use classes: London Building (Constructional) By-laws 1972

Class I As a warehouse or for trade or manufacture.
Class II For Offices and/or for dwelling purposes, or for a purpose not included in this table, except as a public building.
Class III Partly for offices or for other purposes under Class II, except for dwelling purposes, and partly as a warehouse or for trade or manufacture.
Class IV Partly for dwelling purposes and partly as a warehouse or for trade or manufacture.
Class V For housing high voltage power type electrical transformers and/or high voltage power type switchgear, or for a purpose involving a similar risk.
Class VI For housing or displaying a petrol driven vehicle.

Table VIII shows the purpose groups under the Building Regulations; and table IX the permitted compartment sizes for the three purpose groups most relevant to this series: offices, shops and factories.

Table X explains the periods of fire resistance required for purpose group VI and defines the elements of construction; and table XI gives forms of construction.

Special risks under the Factories Act

Particular uses may be classed as a special risk. It is worth considering early in the design process how many of these the building can contain and reserving the best-protected part of the structure for them. Where trades are classed as special risk and extra high hazard under the Factories Act, spaces containing them should be enclosed with fire-resisting construction. (Some special risk premises, factories, are still covered by the Factories Act directly).

An operative sprinkler system will usually be thought to reduce the risks; owners of a sprinkled building may be able to negotiate an increase in the permitted compartment size.

6.03   Means of escape

Alarms, fire fighting equipment and escape routes.
The second and distinctly separate step is to ensure the safety of occupants by installing a good alarm system, local fire-fighting equipment and adequate means of escape. Table XII illustrates the kind of consideration relevant at this stage.

6.04   A tenancy strategy

Typical tenancy arrangements
Table XII gives examples of the way compartmentation and fire escape requirements apply in a number of typical multi-tenanted industrial structures.

6.05   Fire insurance

FOC recommendations
Insurance companies have their own criteria for assessing the risks involved to property. Some of the differences in definition and the problems which they create are given in table XIII which is based on the recommendations of the Fire Offices Committee (which represents most of the major fire insurance companies in the UK).

7.00   References

References to statutory regulations and fire precautions are given in the Bibliography, pp 180–181.

Table VIII   Purpose groups under the Building Regulations 1976

Purpose group	Descriptive title	Detailed definition of use	Critical problems in the use of redundant buildings
I	Small residential	Private dwelling-house (not including a flat or maisonette).	Means of escape
II	Institutional	Hospital, home, school or other sleeping and living accommodation for the care of old people, for persons suffering from physical or mental disability or for children under the age of five.	Means of escape
III	Other residential	Accommodation for residential purposes other than those covered in I and II.	Means of escape
IV	Office	Office, or premises used for office purposes, meaning administration, clerical work (including writing, book-keeping, sorting papers, filing, typing, duplicating, machine calculation, drawing and editorial work, handling money, telephone and telegraph operation.	Means of escape, lavatory accommodation
V	Shop	Shop, or shop premises, meaning premises not a shop but used for the carrying on of retail trade (including sale to members of the public of food or drink; retail sales by auction, the business of lending books or periodicals and the business of a barber or hairdresser) and premises to which members of the public are invited to deliver goods for repair or themselves carry out repairs.	Fire compartmentation
VI	Factory	Factory within the meaning of the word in the Factories Act 1961 (Section 175) (but not including slaughterhouses).	Fire compartmentation
VII	Other places of assembly	Places whether public or private, used for the attendance of persons for or in connection with their social, recreational, educational, business or other activities, and not within groups I to VI.	Means of escape
VIII	Storage and general	Places for storage, deposit or parking of goods and materials (including vehicles), and any other premises not within groups I to VII.	Structural fire protection

Table IX   Structural fire protection under the building regulations: Purpose groups IV to VI and compartment sizes.

Purpose group	General comments	Floor area restrictions	Cubic capacity limits
IV Offices	As for groups V and VI below.	No limitation as to compartment size.	
V Shops	No height limitation on single-storey buildings. In buildings over 28m high, floors over 9m above ground to be compartment floors.	Floors immediately over basement exceeding 100m² to be compartments. No compartment may be over 2000m².	No compartment to have cubic capacity over 7000m³. If with sprinklers, 14 000m³ possible.
VI Factories (see also table X)	No height limitation on single-storey buildings. In buildings over 28m high, floors over 9m above ground to be compartment floors.	In buildings over 28m high compartment size limited to 2000m².	In buildings under 28m high, capacity must not exceed 28 000m³. In buildings over 28m high capacity must not exceed 55 000m³.

Table X   Structural fire protection under the building regulations: periods of fire resistance for the structure of factory buildings (Purpose group VI).

Dimensional limits: Height (m)	Floor area (m²)	Volume (m³)	Minimum period of fire resistance (hours): Ground and upper floors	Basement
Single storey	2000		½ hour (d)	
Single storey	3000		1 hour (d)	
Single storey	No limit		2 hours (d)	
7.5 (a)	250	No limit	0 hours (d)	1 hour (c)
7.5	No limit	1700	½ hour (d)	1 hour
15	No limit	4250	1 hour (b) (d)	1 hour
28	No limit	8500	1 hour (d)	2 hours
28	No limit	28000	2 hours (d)	4 hours
over 28	2000	5500	2 hours (d)	4 hours

Definition of elements of structure

protected shaft — NOT members of roof only
any gallery
separating wall compartment wall
parts of structural frame
any loadbearing wall
floor
independent beams and columns
NOT lowest floor

(a) Applies to buildings, no compartments.
(b) Half an hour for secondary elements of non-compartment floor.
(c) Half an hour only required for basement less than 50m².
(d) Load-bearing external walls should normally be half an hour fire resistant, and separating walls one hour fire resistant.

Table XI   Structural fire protection under the building regulations: typical forms of construction which are deemed to satisfy the regulations

Form of construction★ Floors etc containing high alumina cement not permitted.	Thickness of construction required to achieve required period of fire resistance ½ hour	1 hour	2 hours	4 hours
Rc columns, no finish; see **1a**	150 mm	200 mm	300 mm	450mm
Solid encased stanchions, steel—sprayed asbestos; see **1b**	10 mm	20 mm	30 mm	70 mm
Hollow encased stanchions, steel – asbestos board; see **1c**	9 mm	12 mm	25 mm	—
Timber floors; see **1d**	Lined with 2 layers of plaster-board	Lined with mineral quilt plus asbestos board	—	—

★ See: BS 3590: 1970 for approved methods.

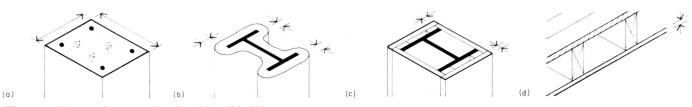

Figure 1 *Forms of construction listed in table XI*

Table XII Fire protection for typical tenancy arrangements

Configuration		Description	Compartmentation	Escape routes
Direct access	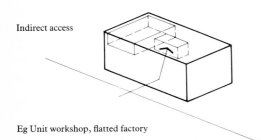 Eg Chambers, arcaded shops.	Units have a street (or yard) frontage, may receive visitors directly, extend vertically within the building and have their own stairs and/or lifts.	Each building contains a number of tenancies divided by fire-resisting walls. The standard of resistance is lower for the subdivisions than for the building as a whole.	Each tenant has his own fire resistant stairway but if: *either* the direct distance on a single floor exceeds 12m, *or* more than 10 people work on a single floor *or* there is an area of high fire risk then an alternative means of escape is required. This may not pass through another tenancy.
Indirect access	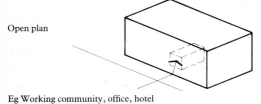 Eg Unit workshop, flatted factory	Units are reached through internal stairs or corridors which form an intermediate space common to a number of users.	Each tenant is separated from adjacent tenants by a fire-resisting wall and a fire-resisting floor. Groups of tenancies form compartments which are divided from each other by walls and/or floors to a higher standard of fire resistance.	Each individual tenant has a door onto the shared fire resistant escape corridor which leads to a fire resistant stairway, a second means of escape being needed in conditions similar to that described above. Where the corridor passes through a compartment wall this opening is protected by a fire shutter. Where there is only one fire exit, tenancy doors should be self-closing.
Open plan	 Eg Working community, office, hotel	Units as such do not exist but tenants take space within a large envelope having a single front door.	Each open area is a compartment (subject to its being within the permitted volume for the most dangerous use class concerned) surrounded by fire-resistant walls and floors to the highest applicable standard.	Each compartment has direct access to two or more fire-resistant stairways. If a stairway serves more than one compartment it may be necessary to protect the relevant doorways with a fire shutter.

Table XIII Insurance requirements: recommendations of the Fire Offices Committee

Aspect	Recommendation for Grade I construction (may qualify for a premium reduction)	Recommendation for Grade 2 construction (will not normally incur any additional rate)	Comment
Cubic capacity	Buildings occupied for trade, manufacturing or warehouse purposes should be subdivided into compartments not greater than 7000m³.	As for Grade I.	This is about one-quarter the capacity allowed under the building regulations for structures less than 29m high and is a serious constraint outside London.
Walls	External walls and internal load-bearing walls should be of non-combustible materials. Fire resistance 2 hours. At upper levels there should be an unbroken solid panel 1m high around the perimeter.	As for Grade I. Fire resistance ½ hour.	Building regulations use concept of unprotected area to limit size of windows. Results could differ.
Roofs	To be constructed of non-combustible materials although concrete decks may be covered with insulation and a waterproof membrane. Beams and trusses to 2 hour fire resistance. Rooflights may not exceed 25 per cent of plan area. No rooflight to be greater than 5m², space between at least 1.8m.	As for Grade I. Aluminium not permitted as a structural element. As for Grade I.	Building regulations do not consider roofs elements of structure: they may be unprotected. The codes conflict.
Floors	To be fire-break floors (similar to 2 hour fire resistance). Openings protected as if for a fire-break floor.	Materials to be non-combustible. Aluminium not permitted as a structural material. Openings to be surrounded with ½ hour fire resistance enclosures.	Note that timber joists are not covered by these provisions.
Finishes	Ceilings and linings to be of non-combustible materials.	As for Grade I.	This raises difficulties with regard to use of timber.

Note: Fire Offices requirements are being reviewed to relate them more closely to Building Regulations. Date review is to be completed not certain.

11 Investigating the Fabric and Structure

1.00 Introduction

This chapter covers the approach needed to investigate the fabric and structure of a building, once the economic feasibility and suitable uses have been established. It proposes a pattern of work and contrasts the various design approaches necessary for the different building types which may be encountered. The chapter also includes sources of information and methods of surveying buildings. The assessment of the structure and fabric drawn from the survey is discussed in chapter 12. It is necessary to recognise the distinction between the building fabric and structure. The structure is that part of the building which is load-bearing and is essential to its stability, while the fabric includes not only the structure, but also the covering, additional building components, and the applied surfaces.

2.00 Characteristics of the fabric

Some forms of construction do not lend themselves to simple analysis. There is often:

A great variation of building materials even within the same building type
A mixture of construction types within the same complex
A variety of unit sizes within a single example.

Tables I and II compare fabric properties and their attendant problems in relation to spatial and construction types. The tables are developed from chapter 3, where different types of redundant buildings were tabulated with possible new uses. (See chapter 3, table II). Figures 1–8 demonstrate some of the building types whose original use has ceased and which are suitable for conversion to new uses.

3.00 Problems with the fabric

3.01 Lack of maintenance

Problems concerning the fabric of redundant buildings are generally due to age, limited building technology and variable standards, compounded by a lack of maintenance, (table III). Buildings which are not regularly inspected and maintained can easily reach a stage where they cannot eco-

nomically be repaired. Old buildings often utilise timber in places which are easily overlooked; concealed timber or steel/iron members are vulnerable to rot or rust (failures and treatments are examined in the next chapter). By contrast, the specification of structure and materials is often a higher standard than can be afforded today, possessing greater tolerance to allow changing performance requirements, with the result that additional loading can often be borne without elaborate alterations. It is unlikely that complete restoration of the fabric will be necessary. The more modest techniques of repair (rectifying defects) and upgrading elements to a serviceable use will be sufficient, (figure 9).

3.02 Listed buildings

Most of the buildings studied in this book are not listed by the DoE as being of outstanding architectural interest. However, there is a growing number of structures of industrial archaeological interest which have received grants as either ancient monuments, historic buildings or for being within conservation areas. The possibility of obtaining such a grant should be pursued if the building in question qualifies. However, it is important to check which building elements qualify for improvement or any other grants which may now be available.

Buildings may need special techniques for the preservation of the fabric. Information on repair and conservation of old buildings has become a growth industry, with symposia, publications and research increasing steadily. Most of it is directed at a high quality of craftsmanship and a greater appreciation of the archaeological value of the original material. This attention to technique has tended to obscure the other simpler aspect of conservation, which is concerned with the best reuse of the building stock, as an economic resource.

4.00 Establishing a pattern of work

4.01 Organisation

Having focussed on a building suitable for reuse it is important to conduct a detailed examination of the fabric to assess its potential for space planning and statutory requirements.

Table I Relation of fabrics' properties to building types – Range of small & large space types

Space types Loadbearing	Variations	Structure Loadbearing and internal columns	Fabric Characteristics	Disadvantages	Failures
Small single gate house	farm building(s)	Not applicable	Internal finish often good standard.	Small spaces, difficult to provide large openings for expansion.	Minimal compared with others.
Large single church hall	meeting hall	barn	Internal finish usually good standard for social buildings.	Large space difficult to heat. Roof access difficult for maintenance.	Large roof prone to problems.
Small repetitive House	garages	interwar factory	Short spans no structural problem.	Spaces, if enclosed by loadbearing elements, create a restriction on interconnection. Domestic staircases and floor loading often inadequate.	Valley guttering and rainwater disposal.
Large repetitive warehouse	railway arches	textile mill	Internal finish usually basic. Can have long spans.	Warehouses and industrial buildings have minimum insulation and no ceiling. Viaducts have windows at ends only.	Differential settlement of foundations.
Small and large town hall	school	church	Possible clerestory or roof lighting. Internal finish usually good quality.	Mix of constructional types. Variety of building materials.	Differential settlement. Complex roof guttering. Redundant or expansion services.

Table I shows a classification by spatial types (see chapter 3 table II) and relates these to fabric properties. The buildings have different forms of structural system.
Table II lists type of construction by material and the related fabric problems. The most common types are nineteenth-century two-storey masonry box, twentieth-century single-storey, early twentieth-century multi-storey, and concrete frame with solid floor.

The organisation of the work on the fabric of the building may be done by a designer, architect or surveyor or by the owner or project leader instructing the builder directly. The different ways of undertaking the work are covered in detail in chapter 15 on project management.

4.02 Design approach to the fabric

The designer must be aware of the ways in which the physical fabric of the building developed in response to the aesthetic and social needs of a previous generation. This is a different situation from that of designing a new building, and can offer stimulating opportunities in design because of the constraints although it will call for a more modest design attitude. Existing buildings need careful investigation and analysis before a design can be finalised. Designers need to be wary of making alterations which affect the performance characteristics of the fabric. The most successful physical conversions have taken place where the designer involved with the change has thoroughly understood how and why the original building was made, before the new uses are decided.

The process of surveying and specifying the work for the fabric of a building can be divided into three interlinked stages: assessment, understanding, and specification, (table V). These stages can occur concurrently.

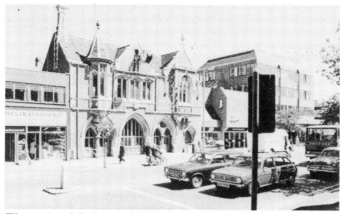

Figure 1   *Administrative changes leave civic buildings redundant.*

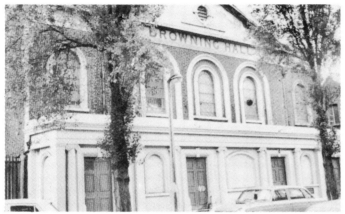

Figure 2   *Mission and public halls provide large clear spans.*

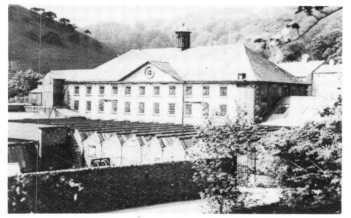

Figure 3   *A building of aesthetic merits makes additional demands.*

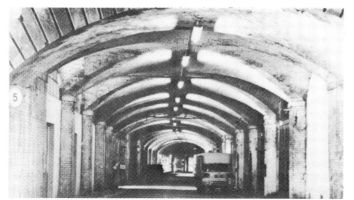

Figure 4   *Railway arches useful for less 'desirable' industry.*

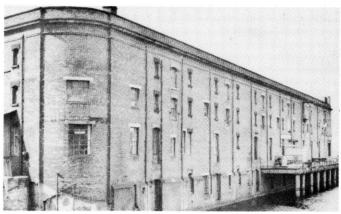

Figure 5   *Inner city canals are lined with sound vacant structures.*

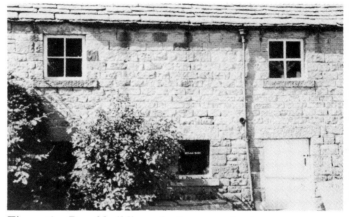

Figure 6   *Rural buildings also become redundant.*

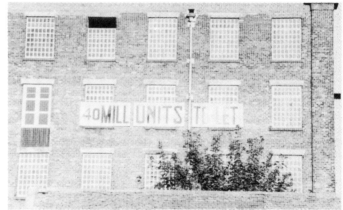

Figure 7   *Mills; large vacant floor areas in decline.*

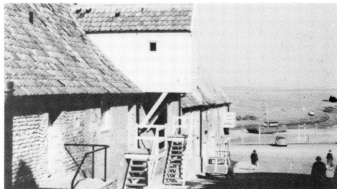

Figure 8   *Rural storage buildings; some compete with domestic market.*

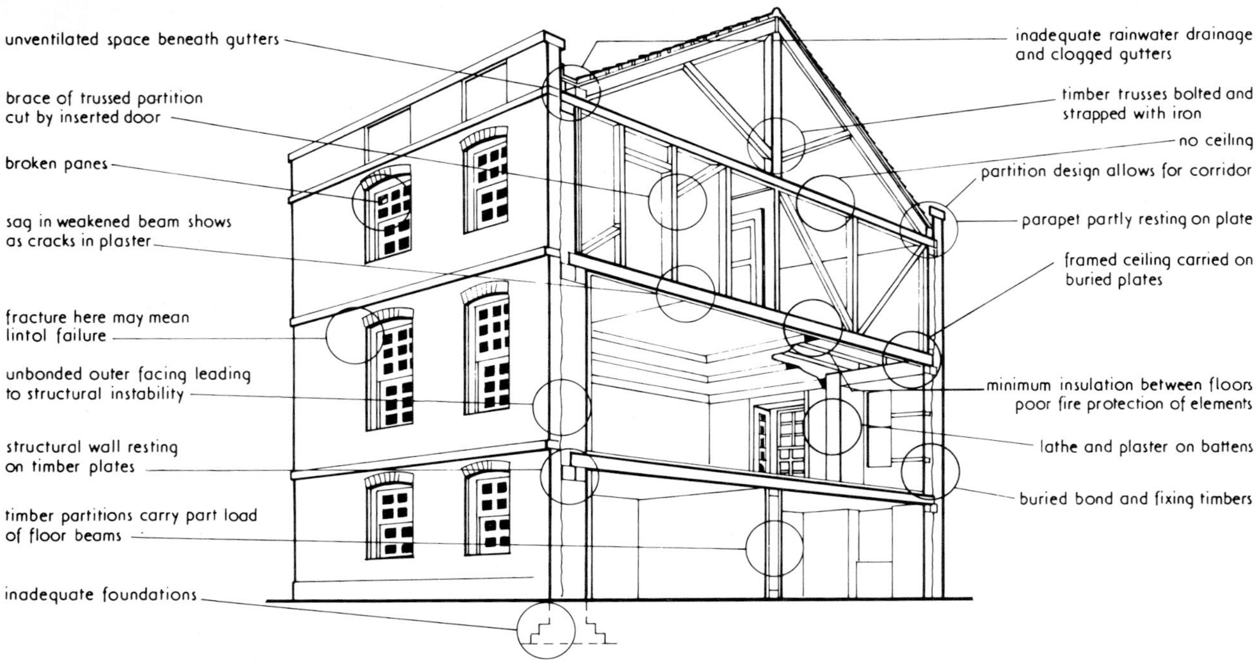
unventilated space beneath gutters
brace of trussed partition cut by inserted door
broken panes
sag in weakened beam shows as cracks in plaster
fracture here may mean lintol failure
unbonded outer facing leading to structural instability
structural wall resting on timber plates
timber partitions carry part load of floor beams
inadequate foundations
inadequate rainwater drainage and clogged gutters
timber trusses bolted and strapped with iron
no ceiling
partition design allows for corridor
parapet partly resting on plate
framed ceiling carried on buried plates
minimum insulation between floors
poor fire protection of elements
lathe and plaster on battens
buried bond and fixing timbers

Figure 9 *In any building there are certain danger spots where faults may develop as a result of the decay or failure of incorporated timber. Other problems stem from shortcomings in construction.*

Table II Material construction types and related fabric

Construction type	Fabric problem
Brick and timber or all timber	Combustibility, wet and dry rot and insect infestation.
Brick and cast iron.	Low fire resistance of elements, partial removal may be difficult.
Brick or stone and concrete.	Filler joint in concrete floors, difficulty of pronouncing on safety for new loadings. Corrosion problems with some concrete.
Steel frame and reinforced concrete.	Less likely to need structural alteration.

Also some structures may need the introduction of new floors where none were provided for the previous industrial use (eg breweries and maltings).

Table III Common fabric problems

Common problems	Resulting features
Lack of maintenance and failure to regularly inspect structure.	Blocked gutters Broken window panes Missing roof tiles Neglect of timber members leading to rot Neglect of steel/iron members leading to rust
Structural instability	Bulging walls Cracking Inadequate foundations
Fire hazard, poor fire protection of elements	Non-existent ceilings, especially in warehouses No protection to columns or floors
Poor standard of insulation	No insulation in roof, eg because of use as storage
Inadequate rain water drainage	Valley and parapet gutter failure Complex roof planes Missing downpipes
Insanitary disposal of wastes	Inadequate drainage system in size and capacity
Outdated or non-existent services	Electrical wiring outdated Boiler, rusting, poorly maintained

Step 1 Understanding

Collect as much available information from people and library sources about the building fabric

Survey the building, develop an hypothesis concerning the strategy of repair and upgrading, complete structural survey

Evaluate advantages, problems and failures of the building type

↓

Step 2 Assessment

Select areas where testing and special measures will be needed

Assess elements that have failed, discover causes, and apply remedial treatment

Assess structure as it stands and for new uses

Decide on which elements will need upgrading for planning and statutory reasons

Decide on general standards of repair and evaluate factors affecting them, relate to the life of the building

↓

Step 3 Specification

Decide on the standard of specification for each element

Carry out cost checks on selected building elements

Draw up full specification and documents suitable for tender

Break down building work according to priorities and quantities

Table IV *Steps to be taken in considering the fabric of the building.*

5.00 Collecting information

There are two methods, which when used together can reveal valuable information.

● Indirect method, where information is gathered from varied sources such as individuals involved with the building, (eg the caretaker) and from documentation (see sources below).

● Direct method, entailing a thorough physical examination of the structure and fabric, the product of which is a measured drawing survey, a structural appraisal and a written appraisal of the building elements and their dilapidations.

The purpose of collecting information is to understand completely the building construction and its materials, the existing structural principles and the existing services. It is important to assess the defects that are on the surface and check for hidden potential problems (damp, rot etc). In assessing the qualities of the fabric the following check list provides the basic categories to be investigated.

● Existing facilities: lifts, staircases, loading doors, fire escapes, floor loading possibilities.

● Existing building configuration: number of floors, ceiling heights, frontage, depth and construction of floors and roofs etc.

● Existing services: lavatories, mains drainage, water supply, electrical and gas services etc.

6.00 Sources of information

6.01 Documents and drawings

The survival and location of available records is often a matter of chance, especially for the more modest industrial buildings on which this study concentrates. A lot of time can be spent in apparently fruitless searching, and it will be a matter for the designer's own judgment to decide when to call a halt. The following list is not exhaustive, but does illustrate the variety of sources that may yield useful documentation.

● The present building owner and his agents (surveyor, solicitor, etc. It may be possible to identify and approach previous owners.

● The local building control authority. In inner London this would be both the district surveyor and the GLC Building Regulations Division, Middlesex House, 20 Vauxhall Bridge Road, London SW1. Elsewhere it would be the local building inspector or building control officer, etc. Policy on retention of records will vary according to the authority. It is unlikely that records will exist of the construction of buildings earlier than the year of the authority's establishment, but more recent alterations may be documented. Local health departments often hold good plans recording drainage information.

● Insurance plans. These were maintained for the commercial and industrial areas of most cities and towns, including London, at a scale of 40 ft. to 1 in. or similar. The best known are Goad's plans. They indicate materials of construction, use at time of survey, and some other structural information. Plans were periodically updated by the issue of revision slips. A full set is held at the British Library map room.

● Local libraries and record offices. These may contain old directories of the area (from which earlier owners and change of use can be determined, and perhaps also a tentative date for construction), as well as other information and further sources (local histories, large scale Ordnance Survey maps, industrial archaeological surveys and reports, etc).

● Specialist libraries and drawing collections. Libraries, museums and societies which may be able to offer information on historic buildings include the Royal Institute of British Architects; the Royal Institute of Chartered Surveyors; Victorian Society; Georgian Group; V&A Museum; local historic buildings societies; local conservation groups; and local authorities.

● The original, and later, architects and engineers. These can often be traced from one or other of the above sources, although this is obviously less likely to be the case for the many humbler buildings. Most practices retain their original drawings or microfilm copies, and some – especially consulting engineers – have their origins in the nineteenth century. The RIBA Drawings Collection and the Institution of Civil Engineers' library should also be approached particularly if the designer was well-known.

● Architectural and engineering periodicals. Once a construction date is known with reasonable accuracy, a search through periodicals such as *The Builder, The British Architect, Proceedings of the Institution of Civil Engineers* etc, may well turn up a surprisingly informative account of the then newly-erected building.

● Archives. The historical Manuscripts Commission publish lists of sources known to the National Register of Archives, Quality House, Quality Court, Chancery Lane, London WC2. The most useful are those on sources of business and sources of architectural history and the fine and applied arts; the latter is cross-indexed by location and designer.

● The Geological Survey maps and memoirs. These are essential sources for information on ground conditions and should be consulted to gain a broad picture of the underlying ground on the site. The local authority may also be able to supply information, and may point out site investigations carried out on adjacent sites. The reports of these investigations will indicate the local conditions likely to obtain, but this may be sufficient to rule out the need for trial holes to be dug.

● Public authority buildings. If dealing with a building now or once in the possession of a nationalised industry or public authority, it will usually be most productive to approach the appropriate body in the first instance. Examples:

Type of building	Appropriate authority
Canal buildings	British Waterways Board
Railway buildings	Public Record Office (for British Transport historical records), and the regional civil engineer; London Transport etc.
London dockside buildings	Port of London Authority
Colliery buildings	National Coal Board
Steelworks	British Steel Corporation

7.00 Surveys

7.01 Introduction
The survey stage is concerned not merely with looking at a building, but is a painstaking observation of its present form and construction, its historical derivations and implications for the future. It is important to watch for subtle distinctions in the use of local building materials, eg particular attitudes to bonding in brickwork or the influences of the other (local) industrial activities – for instance, the connection between shipbuilding and timber roof carpentry techniques. It is important that the survey is not done too fast and that the general context in which the building was built is established. The date of construction of the building must be established because it will tell the designer what to expect of the building construction and will reflect the influence of any planning by-laws. The passing of building legislation dictated different standards of construction for each building type. The designer surveyor must gain experience by looking at many buildings, learning about older building techniques and materials and assessing how they have withstood outside forces and change.

7.02 Types of survey
Surveys will need to take place at different periods of time during the project. Each successive survey is a more detailed development of part of the previous work.

• Feasibility survey. The initial survey will be based on a first look at the building to see if it is feasible for use. Factors affecting this are:

The overall impression of the condition
Materials of construction
Major defects.

The time available may be limited, but must be sufficient to identify any significant problems which could affect a decision to proceed further. Those making this initial survey should therefore be experienced in this type of work.
Evidence obtained from the sources above (para. 6) could now be of value in identifying what information should be sought on site.

• Full survey. The second survey, which will be a development of the initial survey, will need to be very thorough, and a checklist/schedule is shown in table V. The material and the condition of each element will need to be checked. This will itemise the elements that need to be tested and identify those that require specific treatments for repair and maintenance.
Having undertaken the initial survey, the designer must consider what the structural survey on-site is required to achieve and must also test its scope and detail. The help of a structural engineer will probably be required.
It would be appropriate to consult the local building control authority at this stage, to establish what structural information it will be required in considering the submission for building regulations approval.
A drawn survey will have to be completed, unless existing plans are available which can be used as a basis.
A photographic record is invaluable for:

Saving time, recording details of faults, serving as an *aide-mémoire*. It is very easy to miss things while surveying. Comparing with sketched elevations for interiors and details Consultations with authorities, amplifying applications Subsequent disagreements about faults.

• Detailed survey. A detailed survey of specific parts may be required later during the design period of the conversion work, so that production drawings can be prepared.

Table V Survey checklist: site factors

Element	Item to check : drawing eventually at 1:1250, 1:500, 1:200
External works:	
Boundaries	Defined in relation to the building line General orientation, aspect Position of benchmark (if any)
Ground surface	Level or sloping
Walls, fences and gates	Material/type Condition Heights Direction of swing of gates
Steps, ramps and paved areas	Material/type, condition
Natural features	Tree type, shrubs, creepers Condition, heights, spread etc
Ground condition	Liability to flooding – height above sea level (from maps), streams, evidence (marsh roads), water table Liability to subsidance (mining or other) – evidence (uneven ground, cracking) Liability to erosion (coastal)
Adjoining properties and outbuildings	Material/type Condition, construction/general form Proximity of undesirable features
Drainage:	
Manholes/inspection chambers	Type, size, direction of flow of pipes Invert level, cover level Adequacy of fall, condition
Drains, gulleys, vent shafts	Testing for water tightness by hydraulic, smoke, or pneumatic methods Material type and size
S and vps, wastepipes	Condition Adequacy (may be necessary to excavate)
Cess pools, septic tanks, soakaways, wells, (if present)	Understand drainage pattern and ultimate disposal system
Services:	
For all services	Main supply and position Material, adequacy, condition Protection
In addition: Water, rising main	Storage Stopcock and drain cock
Hot and cold water (if present)	Control Insulating material for hot water Degree of protection from frost
Electricity	Control and meter position Lighting and socket outlets – conduit runs, age etc
Gas	Control and meter position
Heating	Boiler, radiators – position, storage, capacity Fuel – gas, oil, solid fuel Pipe condition Supplementary provision/electric immersion
Telephone	Location of supply and outlet

Table VI   Survey checklist: building factors

Element	Item to check: drawing eventually at 1:100, 1.50
Roof exterior:	
Pitched, flat or mixed	Construction – hipped or gable, shape and slope, complexities, eg dormers
	Main finish, hips, ridge, verge
Eaves	Construction – parapet, exposed rafters, bargeboard projection
Gutters and rainwater pipes	Materials, size
	Condition, adequacy
	Fixing, discharge points
	Rib, valley and parapet gutters
	Is the rainwater system complete?
	Check elevations
Flashings	Chimneys, party walls, abutments, pipes traversing, gutters
Roof interior	Construction – main beams or trusses, rafters, spacing and size
Ceiling	Ceiling joist size and spacing (if different)
	Material and thickness
	Boarded areas
	Condition of timbers, infestations
Flues in roof space	Rain penetration
Party or gable walls	Back of stacks
	Torching (if applicable)
Insulation	Material, capacity
Storage cistern	Insulation, support, age, condition, cover, presence of valves (if any)
Pipework	Material, conditions, insulation, functions (supply, downfeed, overflows)
Walls:	
External finish/material	Materials
	Condition
	Thickness (insulation value)
	Pointing, condition
	Decoration
	Structural system in general (mass frame or mixed)
	If stone or brick – bonding, coursing method, rubble infill, reinforcement?
Elevations	Rainwater pipes
	Particular features – balconies, bay windows, dressings, overflows
Air bricks/grilles, ventilators	Type, size, adequacy, obstructions, connected to ducts? Disused?
Foundations	Plinth
	Subsoil, type, settlement
	Defects; cracking, bulging, patches, staining
Damp course	Material (slate, engineering brick, bituminous)
	Relative positive to ground level
	Obstructions, malfunctioning, continuity
	Rising damp
	Pointing, condition
Windows	Type and size
	Material, finish
	Glazing, beads or putty conditions
	Subframe
	Lintel, arch
	Sill threshold
	Position in rebate, flashings
	How fixed?
	Direction of swing of opening
Doors	As for windows, plus – additional fan light, single, double
Floors:	
Timber floor	Construction, joist size and direction
	Stability, deflection
	Finish, surface condition (square edged or tongued and grooved boarding)
	Infestation, damage, defects (likely points under windows, corners, near walls)
	Access traps

Table VI   Survey checklist: building factors

Element	Item to check: drawing eventually at 1:100, 1.50
Floors continued	
Stairs, timber concrete or steel	Construction sizes, tread and riser (pitch)
	Soffit, open or sealed
	Threads and riser, finish, nosing condition
	String, well apron, balustrade/railing
	Stability
	Deflection (movement relative to walls)
Concrete floor	Construction, screed thickness
	Position of downstand beams
	Ceiling finish and thickness (if appropriate)
	Damage
	Finish
Internal walls and ceilings:	
Recesses, projections	Are projections closed chimney breasts?
	Do they occur on other floors?
Plaster	Ceiling, walls, condition, thickness, ornamentation/roses/centres
	Is it alive? Loosely pinned to back of structure or only stuck to wallpaper?)
Finishes and trim	Woodwork condition (architraves, etc)
	Decorative repair and standard
	Are architraves, cornices complete
	Special decorations

The degree of detail in the survey and analysis of different elements will be related to the nature of the final specification, The specification itself is dependent on the proposed activity intended for the building, the length of lease and consideration of the factors listed in the next chapter. In order to avoid unnecessary examination of some parts, as well as to ensure adequate attention to others, the correct level of effort is best learnt from practical examples.

7.03   Basic information
It will be necessary to establish factual information early or prior to conducting any physical survey. The following paragraphs list the information and equipment required.

Summary of information
Age: date built, date of major alterations, etc, period style
Image: easily identifiable, typical of area etc
Plot: dimensions, boundaries
Access: pedestrian, vehicular (see below)
Building accommodation: space available in covered/partially enclosed, number of floors
General remarks
Address: name of street, including number of adjoining properties. (Useful for permissions and negotiations)

Access factors
Permission: from estate agents, present owner, future occupier
Occupancy: occupied or empty, period of occupation, people and goods
Keys: availability and location
Special instructions: necessary or required
Legal position: freehold, leasehold, restrictive covenants

7.04   Equipment to be taken
While it may appear obvious to list the equipment required for a survey, the surveyor may frequently be involved in deeper, more exhaustive investigations than normal. More

cutting away, and hence tools, will be essential to complete the work unless a contractor is on hand, but this can be time-consuming and expensive and should only be contemplated for major structural searches.

● Measuring: long tape, short tape, folding rule/rod.

● Tools (essential): spirit level (pocket type), dumpy level, pocket knife or probe.

● Tools (optional): binoculars, simple pocket compass, bolster, club hammer, length of galvanised tube, calipers, thickness measurer, profile measuring device.

● Equipment: ladder (folding) camera (Polaroid can be useful), torch, metal mirror, survey board, moisture meter.

● Clothes: overall/dungarees, head protection, waterproof protection, pockets to coats, stout shoes.

8.00 Structural survey

8.01 Carrying out the survey
The work can be broken down into four stages:

Survey of existing structure
Assessment of structure as it stands
Assessment of structure for new use
Specification of structural work.

In practice two or more of these stages may occur simultaneously, due to programme requirements. The assessment and specification are considered in detail in the next chapter.
The structural survey will usually be undertaken as part of the general survey of the building, from which the position of all elements and their overall size will be known. To establish size and details of the structural components, it will normally be necessary to remove finishes at selected points. The extent of this work will depend on the available documentary information and the degree of 'standardisation' in the choice of structural components. It will also depend on the designer's judgment based on a general inspection of the building and its visible structural defects. Traditional buildings in masonry and timber can generally be surveyed using the principles applicable to house surveys. (See Housing Rehab Handbook, Architectural Press 1980). Construction in metal and reinforced concrete may call for advice from a structural engineer. The following paragraphs are intended to assist the designer by pointing out matters on which the structural survey should concentrate, recognising that not all may be relevant for any particular project. Commonsense and experience should be used in defining the nature and scale of the survey.

Identify structural material and assess in situ strength
This may require sampling. Timber species can be identified by TRADA or the Forest Products Research Laboratory if necessary. Bricks and mortar may be removed from suitable lightly stressed areas to be crushed and analysed separately by a material testing laboratory. Concrete can be cored and reinforcement can be sampled from a lightly loaded area for tensile testing. Iron or steel members can usually be identified by eye, but if necessary these too can be carefully sampled for analysis and strength tests.

Record section dimensions
Concrete slabs and walls can be drilled through to establish thickness more accurately than by working back from storey-height and floor-to-floor dimensions. Rolled iron and steel sections should have web and flange thicknesses recorded in the course of the survey.

Record material and thickness of applied finishes
This is necessary in assessing existing load on structure, unless finishes are to be stripped off and replaced.

Note signs of distress
For example, sagging floors and roofs; bulging or out-of-plumb walls; cracking – record pattern of cracks and measure width at several points along each crack; distortion of members; movements at joints.
Cracks in structures require careful consideration – are they static or on the move, recent or old, evidence of significant distress or relief of relatively minor effects? It may be desirable to install 'tell-tales' across suspect cracks to establish whether movement is continuing. These should preferably be steel studs whose distance can be monitored by a strain gauge, rather than glass strips which – once cracked – cannot yield quantitative information. Readings should be taken over as long a period as possible, as diurnal temperature and dampness effects, and seasonal moisture movements in the ground, may be misinterpreted as significant evidence of further structural movement.

Expose and record connections and bearings
This can be the most 'troublesome' aspect in terms of justification for strength under new loading or structural behaviour. Spot-checks of joist, slab and beam bearings should be made especially where signs of movement are visible (eg out-of-plumb walls and spalled finishes under bearings).
Inaccessible connections in reinforced concrete and concrete-cased steelwork may have to be exposed or X-rayed, but both operations can be hazardous and expensive. Uncased connections in metal-framed structures should be sketched and measured, noting plate thicknesses, bolt/rivet/weld sizes etc.

Inspect foundations and subsoil
For shallow foundations, trial holes should suffice. If deep foundations are suspected (more probable in large old buildings of recent construction) every effort should be made to locate available documentation. Foundation material, size and condition should be noted; bearing strata should be inspected, probed and, perhaps, sampled.
A thorough site investigation involving deep boreholes may be unavoidable but this is expensive. Trial holes should be backfilled quickly after inspection, be adequately timbered while open and should not be located at 'sensitive' points where their excavation could cause damaging ground movement.

Ensure that adequate records are made
Full-time attendance may be necessary to guarantee that all relevant information is recorded as the investigation proceeds. Photographs are extremely valuable in this work. Site sketches should be clear and legibly annotated.

12 Assessing and Specifying the Building Work

1.00 Relation to the total plan of work

The process of assessing the building work can start at the same time as the full survey and continue, with special studies (laboratory tests) as appropriate, into the detailed design production and specification stages. The relation of this stage to the overall plan of work can be seen in tables I and II.

2.00 Assessment of building work

In assessing the building work the designer will need to:

• Assess the fabric for defects and apply the necessary remedial treatments (section 3).

• Assess the structure, both as it is and for new uses, (sections 4 and 5).

• Decide on the standard of repair/restoration (section 6):
Apply the 'planning principles' to the fabric
Check the regulations in relation to the proposed planning solution
Evaluate the building's use of energy
Check the watertightness of the fabric, drainage etc
Finalise the external covering/envelope, considering three aspects:

1 appearance – walls, roof, (new) openings etc
2 external factors – view, daylight, sunlight, etc
3 cleaning and maintenance – both during refurbishment and for the future.

Table I   Relation of work on the building fabric to the plan of work (RIBA)

Stage	Purpose and decisions	General tasks to be done	Particular work related to fabric
AB inception and feasibility.	To prepare general outline of requirements and plan future action. To provide the client with an appraisal and recommendations to determine how the project can proceed.	Client's briefing Consider requirements Carry out user studies Site conditions	Initial walk round the building 'Survey checklist'. Chapter 11. Prepare rough list of building work required. Establish cost related to standard of conversion required.
CD outline proposals scheme design.	To determine layout design and construction, outline specification and costs for approvals.	Develop tasks above in greater detail.	Thorough survey of building. Provide list of dilapidations. Testing the building. Carry out special surveys (damp, timber treatment).
EFG detail design and production information (and bills of quantities).	To obtain final decision on every matter related to design specification construction and cost. To prepare production information and arrangements for tendering.	Prepare elemental list of building work related to drawings and specifications complete cost checking.	Detailed survey of parts of building as necessary. Complete purchase of building and/or agreement of lease to allow contractor's possession.
GHJ tender action and project planning.	To enable contractor to submit a price and programme of work.	Follow code of procedure for selective tendering or alternatives.	Meet contractor(s) on site to explain work.
K site operations.	To follow plans through to practical completion of building.	Check work done and record progress in relation to programme. Review communications, organisation, information, labour position, materials supply, sub contractors etc.	Regular site meetings and visits.
LM completion and feedback.	To hand over for occupation. Analyse management construction and performance.	Remedy defects, settle the final account. Study building in use.	Final inspections.

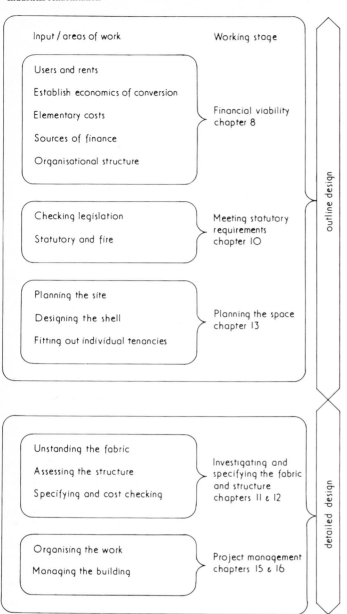

<table>
<thead>
<tr><th>Input / areas of work</th><th>Working stage</th></tr>
</thead>
</table>

Input / areas of work	Working stage
Users and rents Establish economics of conversion Elementary costs Sources of finance Organisational structure	Financial viability chapter 8
Checking legislation Statutory and fire	Meeting statutory requirements chapter 10
Planning the site Designing the shell Fitting out individual tenancies	Planning the space chapter 13
Unstanding the fabric Assessing the structure Specifying and cost checking	Investigating and specifying the fabric and structure chapters 11 & 12
Organising the work Managing the building	Project management chapters 15 & 16

outline design

detailed design

• Finalise the internal scheme in relation to performance requirements of the activities, to include:

1 Thermal insulation
2 Sound insulation
3 Ventilation
4 Accommodation for services
5 Fire resistance/security
6 Durability, maintenance, appearance
7 Cost plan check.

3.00 Assessing building defects and remedial treatment

3.01 Guide to building defects

The guide is set out in checklist form (table III) and is based broadly on the same information as the survey checklist in chapter 11. It is important to draw up a list of diagnoses and cures while actually touring the building. The remedial treatments indicated will help rationalise a priority list of steps to be taken immediately for occupation and safety and steps which can be delayed until funds and time permit.

In general, defects arise from:

Inadequate original design or poor supervision of building work
Bad workmanship
Application of forces that the building cannot stand
Effects of biological agents (fungi, insects)
Changes in temperature
Incompatibility of adjacent materials.

Table II *(left) Relation of work inputs to the end products of design. It will be necessary to sketch over lightly each of the inputs to the working stages before completing the outline design stage for one project. As the design is being worked up to a detailed stage a second check will be required.*

Table III   Guide to building defects and treatments

1 Roofs

1.1 Pitched – tiled and slated. Two sets of defects – structure and covering

Element	Defects	Reasons	Comment and remedial treatment
Ridge and hips	Rot in ridge timbers Rot in hip rafters Slipping hip tiles	Missing or defective pointing Missing hip irons Defective lead rolls Fungal and insect attack:	Rebedding, recovering, replacements required
Covering	Missing slates, loose tiles Breaking, splitting of tiles Uneven course of areas of tiles Humps over party walls, bowed ridge	Tired or rusting nailing Torching (lime mortar and horsehair) failure, holds acidic rain water Frost action Chemical attach (polluted air) Impact of workmans' boots and ladders Defective battens and rusting nails due to damp Deflection of rafters or battens not set properly over wall Long term overloading Fungal/beetle attack Deterioration of timber ends	Replace single tiles in the vulnerable positions If area exceeds 5 per cent to 10 per cent recovering will be necessary Depending on seriousness of structural weakening, use suitable struts for rafters only NB Check load on structure if covering is changed

Table III   Guide to building defects and treatments—*continued*

1 Roofs—*continued*

Element	Defects	Reasons	Comment and remedial treatment
Eaves	Rot in fascia or soffit	Exposed edge defective Tilting fillet absent Lack of painting	Replacement, allowing spacers between fascia and wall
	Rot in barge board	Defective tilting Defective pointing Rot in battens Defective timber supply	Resetting as necessary
	Old cracks in external walls of building near eaves level	Roof spread due to overloading, introduction of heavier roof covering, under-design of weakening of structure	Dependent on severity: consider use of steel ties or replacment Additional support or reducing overload
Ceilings (suspended)	Dampness under truss	Any of the above Defective valleys or parapet gutters Defective tiles, slates or other roof covering Absence of sarking felt	As above

1.2 Flat – asphalt and built-up bituminous felt coverings

Element	Defects	Reasons	Comment and remedial treatment
Verges	Rotted fascia	Defective check or absence of proper drip to fascia Defective gutter Asphalt brittle or too thin	Replace fascia Thicker edge for asphalt
Upstand and abutments	Damp on ceiling junction below or on adjacent wall due to rain	Crack in finish material tucked into brick joint Defective flashing, or cavity tray Capillary attraction Insufficient upstand Ill-bonded laps	Careful retucking of edges into upstand and/or abutment Renew items, extend upstand and flashing
Surface and corners	Minor split Major split and other defects below	Thermal structural stress on old asphalt Differential movement	Relaying treatment and/or bituminous sealant Strip and incorporate movement joint
Outlets	Damp in structure ceiling below	Not dressed into flange of rainwater outlet	Renew outlet and covering or repair defect
Dampness on ceilings fixed or suspended NB also occurs for shallow pitched roofed buildings (factories) and for walls: 'cold bridging'	May or may not be associated with rainfall; if it is, damp patches will be localised	Usual cause is condensation due to water vapour passing through ceiling construction into structural part of roof known as 'interstitial condensation' Surface of roof finish becomes very cold, risk depends on humidity conditions of air in space below roof	Depends on construction, can include provision of efficient vapour barrier on surface of ceiling Fitting ventilation to air spaces Careful detailing required

1.3 General

Element	Defects	Reasons	Comment and remedial treatment
Parapets	Defective bricks and mortar, loose copings, damp on ceiling or wall below	If parapet is saturated, possible frost damage Rainwater bypassing ineffective dpc Open joints in coping (if present) Back gutter and/or outlet defective	Insert new dpc under coping, attention to careful detailing (eg throatings) Rebuild parapet
	Cracking of wall Part of parapet projects beyond wall	Movement – thermal and moisture	If dangerous or water penetrating, rebuild
Gutters and rainwater pipes	Dip in gutter or misaligned pipe Rust if cast iron, leaking joints Blockages	Insufficient support or broken parts Lack of paint/maintenance Lack of gratings	Replace and renew Clean and repair or replace Clear system, replace gratings
Party wall projecting above roof surface	Wet brickwork	Defective soaker, flashings, omission of dpc	Remedial measures and check detailing to protect the wall Improved ventilation: one option would be take down and roof over

All infestation problems see section 3.1

2 Walls

2.1 Bricks

Element	Defects	Reasons	Comment and remedial treatment
		Caused by overloading of foundations	Redistribute load more evenly
Foundations	Leaning, bowing and cracking of walls Check for later additional storeys or window and door openings	Differential settlement Subsidence and soil movement	Provided it has stopped, tie two foundation elements together in acceptable way Underpinning may be required Take care not to introduce new hard spots in foundations or new stresses Structural engineer's advice required

Table III   Guide to building defects and treatments—*continued*

2 Walls

2.1 Bricks continued

Element	Defects	Reasons	Comment and remedial treatment
Walls	Leaning and bulging which is more serious than cracking		If distortion is not too great, tie back wall internally by metal rods or straps Support externally with buttresses, so that their thrust acts against the inclination of the wall 25mm in normal storey height would not need attention Danger point for collapse: degree of inclination of full height of wall exceeds one-third of wall thickness at base
	Diagonal crack through brick joints Crack through bricks themselves Cracking Defined as Fine – 1.5mm width max Medium – 1.5mm to 10mm width Wide – above 10mm width	Consider nature of brick: if dense and non-porous, there may be a risk of water penetration through capillary action	Cut out and rebuild: 1 Fine cracks in dense non-porous brickwork where there is little likelihood of water penetration 2 Medium cracks in brickwork built in strong mortar where the crack follows the joint 3 Medium cracks which pass through the bricks 4 All wide cracks Rake out and fill: 1 Fine cracks in porous brickwork 2 Medium cracks in brickwork in soft lime mortar Materials: in remedial measures care should be taken to avoid using a mortar stronger than that existing
	Cracks in vaults	Usually dampness and poor maintenance	Clean out and repoint, removing any moisture retentive finishes (lime wash or distemper)

2.2 Elements related to brick walls

Element	Defects	Reasons	Comment and remedial treatment
Built in timber members eg timber joints, bearers, plates	Open to insect and fungal attack, easy to overload	Absence of treatment or maintenance Slenderness of sections	Removal of rotten timber, elimination of rot and insect attack: see timber treatment, section 5.1
Lintels, stud framing and board timbers	Open to insect and fungal attack, easy to overload	Absence of treatment or maintenance Slenderness of sections	Retain lateral support to wall by removing short lengths at a time and filling the cavities with brick and concrete
Built in iron and steel members (including wall ties)	Corrosion causing fracturing, distortion and loosening of brickwork	Metal unprotected, twisted and distored	Remove if possible and brick up openings If possible, clean ends of rust and protect with zinc-rich paint or bitumen Replace wall ties with stainless steel
Wrought iron structural ties	Radiating cracks indicate movement is still occurring	Indication of past trouble	Assess loading of walls
Arches and lintels	Distorted arch Cracking	Lack of properly formed abutments Excessive deflection and lintel over opening	Reconstruct arch and abutment Replace lintel and brickwork
Bonding and tying-in failures	Local bulging in exterior face of wall adjacent to window reveals Lack of junction between structural walls (common in terrace houses)	Inner skin not bonded to outside skin Inner structural walls not tied into external structural walls	Cut out cracks by stitching across with new brickwork: block bonding, if bonding at every course not possible Rebuild inner skin with wall ties
Sulphate attack on cement based mortars	Progressive expansion causing horizontal cracking Mortar joints assume whitish appearance with narrow cracks Spalling of surface, mortar becomes friable and weak	Presence of water	Remove sources of water If to be rebuilt, use sulphate resisting cement
Reinforcement corrosion in mortar joints	Corrosion of ($\frac{1}{8}$in $\times$ 1in) wrought iron strips laid in bed of brickwork		Cut out corroded iron, replace by galvanised steel and make good mortar joints

2.3 Stone

Element	Defects	Reasons	Comment and remedial treatment
External walls, natural stone	Weathering: face or edge of stone worn or eroded, loss of detail on moulded and sculptured stone Surface deterioration: split faces of individual stones Accumulation of dirt unevenly distributed (not washed by rain)	Principally atmosphere pollution, frost action, crystallisation of soluble salts Pollution results in deposition of sulphur dioxide and other chemicals which dissolve in rain: mechanism of attack depends on the stone	Decayed surfaces restored by specialist firms (crushed stone cement and resin binders buried in) Decay in depth, cutting out and replacing
		Frost failure is not common, but results in pieces breaking off If large part of exposed face flakes off the stone has not been laid on its quarry bed	Applying a colourless water proofing treatment needs careful consideration Protect back faces of stone with bitumen

Table III   Guide to building defects and treatments—*continued*

3 Floors and ceilings

3.1 Floors: timber

Element	Defects	Reasons	Comment and remedial treatment
Boarding	Stained and/or damp	Leak in sanitary fitting Rot in floor to be suspected (see below)	In all cases; remove cause Allow to dry out
Suspended timber	Collapse, sponging, sagging, uneven	Fungal attack, wet or dry rot Insect attack Exceeded floor loading (also substandard timber or inadequate sections) Notching of service pipes in joists Sleeper walls dropped due to ground movement (ground floor only)	Use preservative particularly on built in joist end If insect attack, check remaining timber elsewhere in building Dry rot needs special treatment (see section 5) Replace or add strutting
Boarded floor	Gaps between boards	Shrinkage and warping of boards, affects finish	Refix, plane and sand or take up and recramp Adequately nail

3.2 Staircases: timber

Element	Defects	Reasons	Comment and remedial treatment
Treads	Squeaking underfoot	Could be nailed not screwed Blocking pieces and wedges defective	Attention to timber work and carpentry, soffit (if any) NB check for insect attack and remove cause
	Bottom riser split string	Check rot over solid under floor or outside wall	

3.3 Floors: concrete

Element	Defects	Reasons	Comment and remedial treatment
Concrete floors	Excessive deflection and side effects Failure to provide continuous partition support Horizontal crack at base of partition	Poor design and workmanship Overloading Excessive shrinkage of concrete	Each case to be dealt in accordance with situation (structural engineer required)
	Lifting and cracking Movement of perimeter walls at or near dpc level	Settlement or ground movement Sulphate attack from hardcore (shale), chemical wastes, bricks and gypsum plaster) transferred to concrete by ground moisture attacking Portland cement	Removal of concrete floor and screed Polythene dpc on ground and up sides Slight lifting, possible to cut through and fill gap with compressible material Cut out damaged area and select resistant floor finish
	Disintegration of concrete finishings and slabs particularly industrial floors caused by liquid spillage	Portland cement attacked by acids and food products	

3.4 Floor screeds

Element	Defects	Reasons	Comment and remedial treatment
Screeds	Hollowness, lifting, curling	Poor preparation, cleaning of base, unsuitable mix Poor workmanship, too rapid drying	If not excessive, cut out and replace worst areas
	Cracking, breaking up, unevenness	Incorrect mix poor quality aggregate incorrect curing	Remove and relay and/or cut out and patch

3.5 Clay floor tiles

Element	Defects	Reasons	Comment and remedial treatment
Clay floor tiles	Lifting or arching	Irreversible expansion of tiles due to absorption of moisture from air or water Thermal movement if screed is cold and contracts more than tiles Insufficiently dried screed which has shrunk	Take up loose tiles and relay Incorporate movement joint

3.6 Thin tiles and sheeting

Element	Defects	Reasons	Comment and remedial treatment
Thin tiles and sheeting	Lifting and edge deterioration	Water made alkaline which attacks adhesive Excessive water or spillage	

3.7 Plaster ceilings

Element	Defects	Reasons	Comment and remedial treatment
Plaster ceilings on lathing	Cracks around perimeter of wall and ceiling junction	Differential shrinkage between materials	Unsoundness located by tapping (hollow sound) Fill before redecorating If loose, remove and replace
	Long straight cracks across from wall to wall Ceiling bellying below general level	Deflection of supporting structure due to loads above Timber laths off key with supporting structure	

Table III Guide to building defects and treatments—*continued*

4 Drainage

Element	Defects	Reasons	Comment and remedial treatment
Drainage	Blockage Leaking of liquid out of inspection pit Appliances do not empty Staining	Cracks in pipes cause ingress of silt below and above ground; may be caused by tree roots	Use specialist help Rodding etc Replace broken pipes by those more capable of withstanding load Prune tree roots
Ground	Subsidence or marshy area	Check for leaks; if without symptoms listed above and does not satisfy test, look for cracks in damaged pipes or via joints	Repair pipes and possibly introduce new manholes for access

5 General defects

5.1 Timber decay

Element	Defects	Reasons	Comment and remedial treatment
All timber	Dry rot (*Merulius lacrymans*) Early – musty mouldy smell Later – presence of red brown dust and flat mushroom growths Finally – timber bulges and becomes light in weight, loses strength and crumbles readily into cubical pieces	Timber remaining moist over long periods (eg from brickwork) Lack of adequate ventilation	Use specialist help; at a particular temperature ascertain cause and eliminate Burn all timber showing signs of decay (thoroughly and systematically) Treatment to include areas of plaster work and brickwork Clean before applying fungal poison Repair remaining timber and treat with preservative
	Insect attack (woodworms) disfiguring of timber surface by small circular/oval shaped holes, gradual reduction of strength	Untreated timber	Remove affected wood and if extensive add strengthening pieces; treat by insecticide (usually liquid)
All timber but usually ends of joists and rafters and in window frames	Wet rot; timber becomes dark (most common) in colour, cracking less deep than dry rot	Timber is exposed to rain or in contact with wet material (walls)	Use specialist help; ascertain cause and eliminate Cut out decayed timber and burn Replace with preserved timber particularly where damp/wet conditions cannot be totally eliminated

5.2 Dampness

Element	Defects	Reasons	Comment and remedial treatment
Basements	Dampness observed, water seen leaking through	Depends on construction; causes may include: Ground water pressure if excavation for basement was in impermeable subsoil which acts as a sump, trapping surface water Natural path of water interrupted by excavation Natural high water table Damp penetration from subsoil through cracks Condensation – humid air precipitating moisture on cold walls	Depends on inconvenience and new conditions required Sump in floor, pumped out as necessary Water path can be diverted by additional drainage Cracks and faulty joints plugged and sealed by pressure grouting or internal rendering work carried out by specialist Normal damp penetration may also require pressure grouting and internal waterproof rendering Condensation cured by raising surface temperature of walls and floor by additional insulation and better ventilation
Walls	Dampness showing on internal wall up to 750mm, or higher if outside covered by protective finish If dry, film of salts seen as fluffy crystalline growth	Check presence of dpc and condition If dpc present check whether it is bridged by earth outside or mortar dropping in cavity wall Failure of dpc, eg blue bricks vertical joints are open	Incorporate cpc – wall injection, electro-osmosis (special treatment) If bypassed, remove cause Repair or replace dpc; alternatively use lining out of contact with wall
Associated with rainfall; solid walls	Damp patches appear on inner face of walls exposed to driving rain	Wall not resistant to rain deterioration of mortar pointing Render may have perished Leaks from down pipes (large amounts of water)	Choice of rendering or claddings to outside Repair all cracks Put in inner lining on treated battens

3.02 Guide to defects in structural materials

Before the Industrial Revolution made iron cheap and readily available, the commonest building materials were stone, brick and timber. The choice would depend on the social standing and wealth of those who were to occupy the building.

These materials have, of course, continued in use up to the present day, with the gradual tendency for elements to become thinner and more highly-stressed as structural understanding and manufacturing quality control have improved. But they have been supplemented by others such as cast iron, wrought iron, steel, concrete (plain, reinforced or prestressed) and the designer should be aware of the possible element types and forms of construction that he may encounter in a particular building.

Table IV identifies particular problems that may need to be studied in assessing the structure for reuse. The advice of a structural engineer may be necessary, particularly when dealing with metal or concrete-framed buildings or with the many types of timber and composite trussing forms that have been built in the past. Figure 1 illustrates some typical traditional structural elements and weaknesses.

Table IV Guide to defects in structural materials and remedies

1 Timber

Form of construction	Defects	Reasons	Comments and remedial treatment
All timber (including timber piles)	Rot, insect attack		Total replacement Selective replacement Proofing treatment
	Splitting		Total replacement Strapping
Roof trusses	Defective joints		Total replacement Strapping/tying
Attic trusses and partition trusses (see 1.1 table III)	Failure and collapse	Diagonal bracing cut by later openings	Total replacement Strapping/tying

2 Brick and stone

Form of construction	Defects	Reasons	Comments and remedial treatment
All (including foundations)	Decay of masonry and/or mortar		Total replacement Grouting Vacuum impregnation
Walls, piers, etc and foundations	Cracking	It is essential to establish the cause(s) of cracking whether 'live' or dormant, before considering solutions. The causes must be dealt with if 'live': they could include Settlement Overloading Moisture/thermal effects	Total replacement if very severe Cutting out and refilling Grouting Pointing with soft mortar or mastic No action (if structurally and visually acceptable)
	Bulging or leaning	As above, but additional causes include: Soil creep Inadequate lateral loading Spreading of rubble in filled walls Unbalanced thrusts from arched floors or roofs Incipient overall instability	Total replacement Fixing tie-rods and wall-plates to arrest movement Tying rubble-filled walls across and grouting Adding lateral restraint (buttresses to floor and roof bracing etc) No action if structurally and visually acceptable
Brick arches, particularly jack arches (see table III)	Spreading	As above but can be caused by removal of jack-arch tie-rods: this should never be done without engineering advice	As for cracking and bulging
Brick vaults under pavement	To be abandoned	Local authority require voids to be accessible (risk of gas build-up, vermin, etc)	Clear out all organic matter Fix with weak concrete or compacted gravel to local authority approval
Stone flagstone and steps	Failure	Deterioration of strength	Calculation, load testing

3 Cast iron

Form of construction	Defects	Reasons	Comments and remedial treatment
All cast iron	Cracking or splitting	Overloading Lack of maintenance and rust Faulty casting	Presence established visually or by ultrasonics Total replacement (especially if in tension zone of beam) Welding (needs care) Strapping
Circular columns	Cracking or splitting	Non-concentric casting (determined by ultrasonics or careful drilling of small holes)	Some irregularity usually acceptable In extreme cases total replacement or strengthening, eg by rc casing
	Vertical splitting	Vertical splitting between two halves of casting on joint line	Welding (needs care) Strapping As for cracking or splitting, see above
	Cracking	Caused by freezing of water in column used as down-pipe (common)	

Table IV   Guide to defects in structural materials and remedies—*continued*

4 Wrought iron

Form of construction	Defects	Reasons	Comments and remedial treatment
All wrought iron	Corrosion	Especially where watertraps in riveted girders	Total replacement Extra plating bolted to wrought iron, casing in rc The corroded section may still be structurally adequate after cleaning and protection against further corrosion

5 Steel

Form of construction	Defects	Reasons	Comments and remedial treatment
All steel	Corrosion	As above	As above

6 Concrete

Form of construction	Defects	Reasons	Comments and remedial treatment
All types of concrete	Surface damage (leaching out of cement, staining, spalling, crazing, etc)	The cause of damage must be ascertained; could include Overloading Over or under-rich mix Acid attack Reinforcement corrosion, etc	Appropriate surface treatment (renders, epoxy mortars, sealants etc) Removal of cause of damage The cause must be dealt with if 'live'
	Cracking	See above; causes could be Settlement Dynamic loading Design/construction defects	Total replacement in extreme cases Local cutting out and either grouting or pointing with mortar or mastic No action if risk of reinforcement corrosion slight and appearance acceptable
High alumina	Failure and cracking	Deterioration of concrete strength and condition	Cutting of core from lightly-stressed areas for testing (and chemical analysis if high alumina or calcium chloride suspected) Visual inspection Non-destructive testing (rebound hammer, upv etc – need skilled operators and interpretation)
Reinforced and prestressed concrete (table III)	Failure and cracking	Determination of reinforcement present and its condition	Covermeter survey to locate position and spacing of bars and tendons Careful chasing at selected points to establish size and condition Sampling of lightly-stressed samples for testing
Reinforced and prestressed, including 'breeze' and 'clinker' concretes and filler joint construction	Corrosion of reinforcement	The cause must be established and, if practical, arrested. It could be: Insufficient cover in aggressive environment, Under-rich mix; Harmful chemicals in aggregate; Excessive cracking (see above) etc	Total replacement or strengthening if corrosion severe and continuing Surface treatments (renders gunite, epoxy mortars, etc) to enhance cover to steel
	Reinforcement failure	'Odd' bar shapes (star-shaped, strip, figure-of-eight, etc) common in early patented rc systems	Investigation as above not totally avoidable, but search for documentation (patent specs, brochures, articles) may be fruitful and simplify assessment
Prestressed	Failure and collapse	Any alterations to prestressed members risks 'explosive' collapse	Seek expert engineering advice
Composite construction (two or more structural materials used in combination)	Examples: trussed beam, (see 4) table III roof trusses, (see 5) table III flitched beams, (see 6) table IV steel beams and concrete slab	Problems associated with particular materials used: see above as appropriate. Calculation of strength	See above as appropriate Structural engineering advice desirable

4.00   Assessment of structure as it stands

4.01   Establishing a sound structure

The structural survey represents the information on which decision and structural costs for a new use will depend. Having this information, the designer is in a position to assess the existing structure. In this task he may well seek the advice of a structural engineer. In practice, the designer will often be aware of a new use already proposed for the building and the requirements that this will generate are probably known, at least in broad outline. While these should be borne in mind in assessing the structure (eg to avoid devoting unproductive time to considering elements which are to be removed anyway), it is equally important to be dispassionate in appraising the existing fabric. A fundamentally unsound structure will require expensive repairs irrespective of whatever alterations are to be made.

Many possible defects will have become self-evident in the course of the survey – rotting timber, leaning walls, structural failures or excessive deflection. Measures to deal with

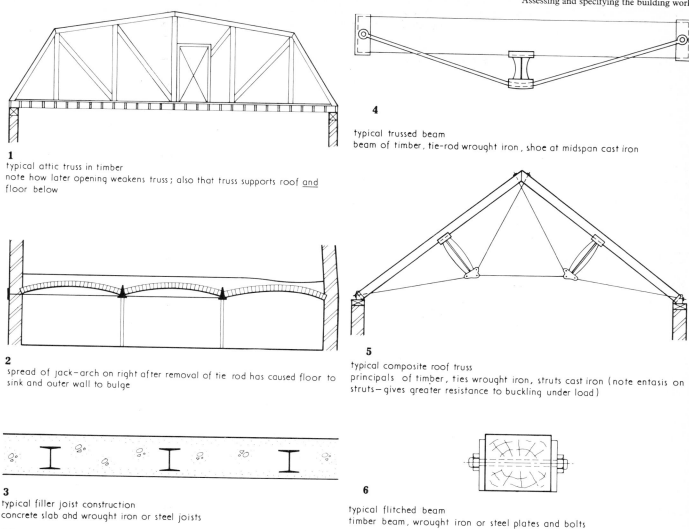

1
typical attic truss in timber
note how later opening weakens truss; also that truss supports roof *and* floor below

2
spread of jack-arch on right after removal of tie rod has caused floor to sink and outer wall to bulge

3
typical filler joist construction
concrete slab and wrought iron or steel joists

4
typical trussed beam
beam of timber, tie-rod wrought iron, shoe at midspan cast iron

5
typical composite roof truss
principals of timber, ties wrought iron, struts cast iron (note entasis on struts – gives greater resistance to buckling under load)

6
typical flitched beam
timber beam, wrought iron or steel plates and bolts

Figure 1   *Typical traditional elements and weaknesses referred to in the checklist*

these will often be equally self-evident, generally involving replacement of affected elements and, if appropriate, remedial work to prevent spread of recurrence of the problem.

In general, the structural assessment should supply answers to the following questions, in order of importance.

1 Is the structure generally sound and stable? If not, reuse for any purpose is unlikely to be feasible.

2 Are there any signs of continuing distress? If so, these must be diagnosed to establish the cause, and remedial measures considered.

3 Are there signs of past distress? Their treatment must be considered.

5.00   Assessment of structure for new use

5.01   Implication of conversion

Structural adequacy broadly consists in the structure possessing sufficient stability, strength and stiffness for its intended purpose. Having established the state of the existing structure, it is now necessary to consider the implications of the new use it is to serve.

5.02   Ensuring stability

The major removal of existing walls or frames may jeopardise the ability of the structure to withstand wind and other lateral loads. Removal of floors and/or roof, even temporarily, could produce instability of walls and columns which they restrain. Removal of individual elements may take away support, either vertical or lateral, from the elements. Each of these possibilities must be considered, and if necessary, measures to cope with the problem – either temporary or permanent – must be devised and incorporated in the scheme.

5.03   Meeting new load requirements

Change of use calls frequently for an increased loading capacity and the existing structure must be assessed for its ability to support this. If found to be inadequate, then it will be necessary either to strengthen what is there or to replace it. Particular attention should be given to the effect of openings, both existing or proposed.

An alternative to strengthening or replacing is to restrict the loading to be applied, but this may not be possible for the intended use. It should be remembered that future occupiers may not be aware of this restriction unless the intending owner is informed of it.

5.04   Stiffness

The structure must have adequate stiffness to function satisfactorily under service conditions. The prime consideration is that floors and roofs should not deflect under load to the point at which this movement generates problems. These could include malfunctioning of machines sensitive to movement, ponding of water on roofs, possible collapse of high-stacked goods and damage to finishes. Dynamic effects should not be ignored. Out-of-balance machinery, fork-lift trucks etc can increase deflections substantially above those due to a static loading.

In the low-rise buildings that are the commonest subjects of reuse, lateral stiffness under wind is not likely to be a problem if stability and strength have been shown to be adequate.

5.5   Other considerations

The above considerations relate exclusively to the satisfactory performance of a structure in terms of its capacity to support normal loading. It should not be forgotten that other requirements may be generated by the new use. Among these may be the need for increased fire resistance, acoustic insulation, thermal insulation etc. In general, these can be met by applied finishes or treatment if the existing structure cannot achieve them, although it must be remembered that these measures in turn will increase the loading and must therefore be taken into account when assessing the structure.

6.00   Work required on the fabric

6.01   Categories

Work on the fabric breaks down into the following categories, which are interconnected, but for convenience are considered separately.

Repair Repair or renewal that is required because of the poor condition of the building due to lack of maintenance, or a particular element having come to the end of its life.

Upgrading Work on upgrading finishes or structure that is required to satisfy the regulations, eg means of escape, or fire protection that may be required because of change of use.

Improving the space efficiency Work related to replanning the interior spaces and improving the spatial efficiency by additional subdivision, linking buildings or strengthening upper floors.

6.02   Strategies

If there are limited funds, or the length of the building life or the lease is short, the building work should be evaluated against a strategy of doing nothing in each category unless it is really necessary. Working out the minimum specification with options for better standards is a useful check. This will have the following advantages:

Money is not wasted if the building has a limited life or short lease
Upgrading to a better standard can take place later
Work can progress in step with available finance.

The standard of repair work will range from complete preservation and restoration, to rectifying defects and replacing sufficient elements to allow the building to continue functioning.

Urgent elementary work to keep out the weather and improve the stability of the structure may well be necessary. It is unlikely that economic considerations will allow such scope for a conservation approach. Emphasis will be placed on designing around defective elements of the fabric, often providing an alternative structure rather than an expensive repair. For example, it may be better to box around openings rather than rebuild arches, unless the budget allows.

There is less latitude in varying the standard of upgrading, because the requirements of the building regulations and other legislation must be met. Upgrading finishes which are not demanded by statutory considerations will be decided by cost and desirability.

Work on buildings, which are subject to patching and short-life strategies, demand methods different from those for traditional design. This could cause difficulties for the conventional designer who is used to thinking sequentially and envisiging a well-defined end product.

7.00   Specifications

7.01   General

Generally the initial project feasibility examination will be biased in favour of buildings with more facilities and working services, as less conversion work should be required and costs should therefore be lower. The amount of building work and, ultimately, costs will depend on:

Original use and configuration of the building
Client's and users' financial policies
Existing condition of the building, its resilience, and how long since it has been maintained
Length of life and durability of the building
Proposed new uses and their implications for fire and health regulations
Phasing and construction programme
Degree of finishes required, ranging from an empty shell to fully equipped units
Level of specification required (see below for categories).

7.02   Background knowledge

In addition to carrying out a formal investigation of the building fabric, the designer will need to draw on a wide knowledge of traditional building construction techniques and materials as an aid to interpret the survey findings and write future required specifications to include:

Historic development of building techniques
Wide knowledge of traditional building materials
Historic development of building types
Modern conservation techniques
Archive material, such as measured drawings which may not only provide plans and elevations but also give an insight into methods of construction.

Traditional aspects of building materials
For the type of building considered in this book, the designer and builder should be well acquainted with the following aspects of materials listed below. More detailed references on specifications and materials are regularly listed in the technical press; some are covered in existing British

Standards, Codes of Practice. The better trade literature, specialist directories, and product data are increasingly devoting their attention to the growth of refurbishment.

Timber
Traditional construction
Traditional and present-day timber types
Methods of felling, conversion, seasoning
Traditional carpentry and joinery
Weathering
Timber pests and fungi
Methods of repair and strengthening timber
Window construction.

Roofing
Tiling and slating
Repair and renewal.

Metalwork
Metallurgy and development in buildings
Structural cast iron
Wrought iron, steel
Modern repair techniques.

Plasterwork
Development of lime and gypsum plastering
Repair techniques.

Paints/decoration
Internal and external decoration, preservation paints
Protection and decoration finishes.

Stonework
Geology of building stones
Quarrying and masonry techniques
Walling techniques
Static and dynamic construction
Weathering and decay
Renewal
Dentistry repair
Chemical treatment
Availability of replacement building stone.

Brickwork/masonry
Clay building materials
Bricks, tiles and terra cotta, traditional craftsmanship
Bonding, mortars
Weathering and decay
Repair and renewal.

7.03 Measuring extent of building work
There are five categories of work (previously outlined in chapter 8. A being the most expensive and E the cheapest.

A: major structural alterations, additions and new services
B: general repairs to fabric, fire proofing and services
C: no structural partitions, upgrading finishes, overhauling services
D: upgrading finishes only
E: no work at all.

Typical example
The premises now occupied by working communities mentioned in chapter 17 para 3.02) required work in categories B and C. A typical list of required work in each case included:

Minor repairs to the building, where maintenance had lapsed
Some major repairs to the roof and a lift (in one case)
Complete refitting of the electrical system, power and lighting
Provision of mains services, some new lavatories
Fire proofing of structure between compartments, an additional fire escape
Subdivision: provision of partitions and basic finishes.

7.04 Preparing detailed specifications
Detailed specifications for the work can be grouped under the categories in paragraph 6.01: repair, upgrading: improving space efficiency. These categories will be useful in assessing the priorities of the work, especially when budgets are low. Repair and upgrading work will need to be done first, while improving spatial efficiency can sometimes follow later. In practice a decision on change related to space efficiency should be made, if it means disturbing earlier work of repair and upgrading.

Table V shows typical building adaptations which fall into the specification level of categories A and B, listed above. They can also be used as a check-list to test the effectiveness of the planned solution. Old buildings possess existing facilities and arrangements of spaces which can be a rich resource when upgrading is being considered. The building's particular arrangement can often allow for an increase in (figure 2) capacity, or suggest ingenious and unexpected solutions for reuse.

8.00 Specification of structural work

8.01 Consultation with the local authority
Before a binding specification of structural work is prepared, it is highly desirable that the building control officer (district surveyor, building inspector etc) be approached with the results from the survey and assessment. The interpretation of the condition of existing structures frequently entails some subjective judgements and it is important that the designer and the building control officer see eye-to-eye on what is considered to be necessary. Particular areas in which agreement is essential are permissible bearing pressures on foundations and permissible stresses in old masonry, and in iron, steel, and reinforced concrete construction. Once these have been agreed, it is possible to define the extent of work to be carried out.

8.02 Scope of works
The structural work necessary for buildings covered in this book is unlikely to be greatly different from that applicable to other rehabilitation work, although the scale of operations may well vary.
For work on structures of masonry or timber construction, reference should be made to the *Housing Rehabilitation Handbook*. (Architectural Press 1980).

For work on structures of iron, steel and reinforced concrete the advice of a structural engineer will probably have been sought at the outset and he will therefore be available to prepare the structural specification.

8.03 Establish realistic solutions

It is not intended to review here the many techniques that may be applied for the strengthening and consolidation of existing structures. But it is emphasised that the designer should satisfy himself that the end product required can be achieved by the methods proposed, taking account of matters such as stability of the structure while the work is taking place and feasibility of operations (phasing, adequate working space, accessibility etc.)

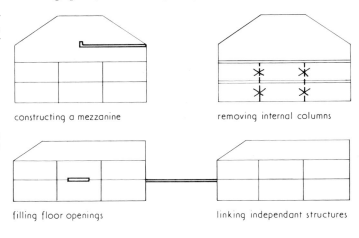

constructing a mezzanine   removing internal columns

filling floor openings   linking independant structures

Table V Typical building adaptations and specifications

1 Providing access

● Closing road, replanning yards, demolition of outbuildings	These strategies are covered in more detail under Chapter 13. 'Planning the space', where extra space can be gained by extending the sphere of operations beyond the building being considered.
Fitting new lifts internally and externally ● Use of hoists; use of vertical shaft of a mill building for gravity feed of goods	Provision of a new lift in a strategic place can usually allow the existing space to be more efficiently used. Sometimes an existing shaft can be utilised to allow better transport of goods within the building. Additional builders' work will be required to protect the lift shaft. Useful hoists/gantries often exist on industrial buildings.

2 Improving means of escape

● Demolish internal partitions, replan interior layout, create new internal corridors, staircase, separate basement stairs, external fire escapes, links to adjacent buildings by balconies.	Chapter 10 Statutory requirements' describes the requirements for which these changes may provide solutions. Tortuous circulation may have grown up when the building was in industrial use, alternatively an existing building can have existing facilities which are at present under-utilised.

3 Increasing capacity (see fig 2)

● Linking structures, horizontal extension of building, adding on the roof, building in an enclosed space, constructing a mezzannine or an intermediate floor, removing internal columns	These strategies are particularly appropriate in buildings where there is excess structural strength in the existing materials (walls and beams).

4 Altering volumes

● Altering the top floor, altering floor levels, altering floor openings, internal subdivision	There is a possibility of increasing the spatial efficiency within the existing outline of the building. An earlier industrial process may have caused an irregular alignment of floors or required deep space which can now be better utilised. Brick walls and timber floors can allow these changes to be simply effected; unskilled labour could be used.

5 Increasing strength

● Strengthening foundations on an upper floor, rebuilding upper floors	These measures are covered in detail in 'Assessing the structure' which follows. Technical advice form a structural engineer will be needed.

6 Sound insulation and security

● Relying on fixtures and fittings, using solid partitions, special doors and locks, building a screen wall	Each building will be considered on its merits; it may possess a useful set of elements which can be reused or relocated.

7 Fire protection

● Removing dangerous materials, relying on excess structural strength or existing sprinklers, lining the walls, cladding structural elements, painting or spraying structure	Chapter X Statutory requirements' provides requirements. Table shows typical forms of construction which are deemed to satisfy the regulations. Making a case for continuing to use large sectioned timber beams uprotected, by relying on their excess structural strength, provides a simple and cheap solution which involves no building work. Calculations from an engineer will be needed.

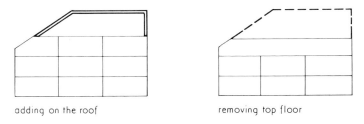

adding on the roof   removing top floor

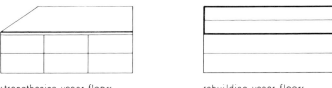

strengthening upper floors   rebuilding upper floors

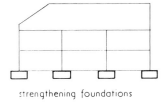

strengthening foundations

Figure 2 *Some options for increasing capacity and altering volumes.*

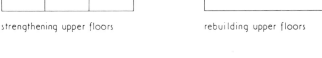

8.04 Specialists

Many specialist firms are now capable of undertaking work of this nature but again their experience and suitability for the particular task should be assessed. Where a guarantee is offered by such a firm, the designer should be clearly aware of the terms under which it is available, to ensure that these do not conflict with the client's other rights under a contract.

8.05 Contingencies

In specifying the extent of work required, it must be recognised that – however thorough the survey – some contingency should be allowed for work for which the need becomes apparently only after the contract has started. Nevertheless, it should be possible to define with reasonable accuracy many items such as underpinning, replacing areas of floors and strengthening of members. Less precisely quantifiable activities, such as making good cracked masonry, should be treated as provisional items.

8.06 Temporary and sequential works

Particular attention must be given to specifying temporary works necessary to maintain stability of the structure during building operations and where the work has, of necessity, to be performed in a certain sequence then this too must be clearly pointed out in the specification to avoid later contention.

9.00 Conclusions

The need for an individual approach

Each building will require special treatment, and generalisations about upgrading and improvement measures are difficult to make. Precedents from case studies can be very useful, as they will act as a framework. Architects and designers can help by giving general guidance on techniques which will establish the level of work expected.

Work on the fabric will be dictated by the nature of the building, assessment of the building's opportunities and problems and the client's short and long-term needs. A realistic approach will be through careful phasing. Essential works such as providing basic services and making the building watertight can take place in the first phase. Bringing tenants into the building early will produce income to pay for the building work. This could have the double advantage of allowing the upgrading and servicing to be tailored to users' needs, with the users themselves contributing by helping to manage the project.

13 Planning the Space

1.00 The planning process

The process of planning the space for a project can be divided into three levels of investigation (table I):

Planning the site
Planning the building
Planning individual tenancies.

1.01 Planning the site
An evaluation of the site will establish the optimum set of buildings to be retained and will consider any advantages to be gained from selective demolition or rebuilding to plan for efficient access for goods and people.

1.02 Planning the building
The building must be planned to meet the changing requirements of an organisation over a period of time. For an individual organisation this entails making strategic decisions about the location of circulation, service points and common facilities which will allow for activities to be relocated and the new activities to be accommodated. For buildings being developed to provide units for rent the space should be planned to allow for different tenancies, varying in size between 20 sq m and 100 sq m.

1.03 Planning individual tenancies
Within a building or unit, individual firms may wish to adapt the space to meet their particular requirements.

Site
Step 1 — Establish access for deliveries and the amount of car parking to be provided

1.1 — Decide on number and type of deliveries and amount of car parking generated (table III)

1.2 — Establish strategy for providing access and parking space (table II)

Building
Step 2 — Zone uses to the buildings available

2.1 — Decide on the types of use to be accommodated in each building (table II)

2.2 — Decide on strategy for organising tenancies (table IV)
2.3 — Test the subdivision capacity of the building (use the building plans)

Step 3 — Establish the adaption required to meet statutory requirements (chapter X)

Step 4 — Decide on the allocation of common facilities

4.1 — Sanitary requirements (table VI)

4.2 — Tenant/staff amenities (para 3.04)

4.3 — Service standards for the building (table VII)

Step 5 — Tenancies

5.1 — Test the rental units proposed against different user types (chapter 14 table I)

Step 6 — Plan individual tenancies

6.1 — Decide on the type of function and layout required (fig 4)

6.2 — Decide on future requirements (by interview and consultation)

6.3 — Develop space requirements (chapter 14 tables II & III)

6.4 — Draw up floor plans

Table I *Checklist of the steps to be taken in planning the site, buildings and tenancies.*

Table II A critical constraint on the re-use of older industrial stock will often be the difficulty of providing adequate access for vehicles. Ways to avoid this are given below

	Planning	Traffic control	Clearance	Layout	New construction
1 Terraced workshop L loading 40 per cent site coverage	Combine pairs of streets	Eliminate on street parking.	Create way through to rear.	Locate storage on ground floor.	
2 Mill L loading ■ lifts 40 per cent coverage		Allow space for vehicles to turn.	Clear out buildings and gate-houses.		Install new lift on yard site and create loading bays.
3 Factory L loading ■ lifts 60 per cent site coverage.		One way circulation system.	Clear outbuildings and enlarge entrance and exit points.	Locate storage functions away from road.	
4 Warehouse complex L loading ■ lifts 60 per cent site coverage.	Block by block planning essential.	Eliminate on-street parking and allow space for vehicles to turn.	Open up rear loading bays to the yard at ground level.		Install hoists on yard side.
5 Inner city block L loading ■ lifts 100 per cent site coverage.	Close off cross streets for parking and delivery.	Signage system.		Relate service roads to existing delivery points.	Define parking and delivery areas with change of road surface.

2.00 Planning the site

2.01 General
The site may consist of one or more buildings and vary in its intensity of site coverage. Sites which consist of a number of buildings normally have a mix of building types, eg factory, boiler house, gatehouse etc, which provide the possibility of a mix of uses. The strategic decisions in planning the utilisation of a site cover access for delivery vehicles, car parking provision, the degree of clearance or rebuilding required and provision for future expansion.

2.02 Accessibility for delivery vehicles
Table II describes some possible strategies for dealing with access and delivery on differnt types of site. Sites may be zoned according to the size of delivery vehicles allowed, eg for articulated lorries there may be direct access to 20 per cent of the units, with access for small vans to all the site (figure 1). The critical dimensions for turning and parking of a range of delivery vehicles are shown in figure 2.

2.03 Provision of car parking
Each planning authority has its own standards for car parking provision. In some authorities the amount of car parking required reduces the larger the floor area of the unit. A scheme wishing to provide for very small units (50 sq m to 150 sq m) may face a more stringent requirement for parking provision than schemes providing for large units (500 sq m to 1,000 sq m). Table III presents the parking standards for offices and industry for a county council and a central city planning authority.

2.04 Degree of demolition or new building
This will depend upon:

• How far the demolition of outbuildings will improve the circulation, parking and yard space on site. In the disused mill example (table II type 2) the demolition of single-storey sheds could lead to more vehicle space for upper floor tenants in the remaining structure, which could command more rent overall despite the loss of floor area.

• The utility of each building, given the expected range of user types, the rental levels anticipated and the costs of rehabilitation; keeping a building empty costs money.

• Whether the construction of new buildings would improve the stock of available space. A row of new 'nursery' units could bring in a different type of tenant whose rents would contribute to the financial viability of the total project.

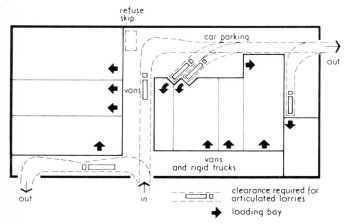

Figure 1 *Site planning where vehicle access is restricted.*

2.05 Providing for future expansion
Providing speculative accommodation for small firms invariably entails a risk factor, and the developing agency will wish to minimise its commitment at the early stages while it is testing the demand. Site development should allow for the work to be completed in stages, without compromising the functioning of the scheme at each phase.

Table III Parking standards

Spaces per floor area	Inner city	Suburbs and rural
Distribution		
Heavy goods vehicles	1 per 1000m²	1 per 500m²
Light commercial vehicles	1 per 1000m²	1 per 500m²
Cars	1 per 400m²	1 per 1000m²
Light industry		
Heavy goods vehicles	1 per 4000m²	1 per 2000m²
Light commercial vehicles	1 per 1000m²	1 per 500m²
Cars	1 per 200m²	1 per 50m²
Office space		
Light commercial vehicles	1 per 1000m²	1 per 500m²
Cars	1 per 150m²	1 per 30m²

These standards are typical for the uses and types of location specified and apply to developments where the needs of a group of tenants are pooled in communal parking areas. They do not apply to special or unusual uses, nor do they necessarily apply for individual units taken on their own, nor do all planning authorities necessarily operate the same standards in development control.

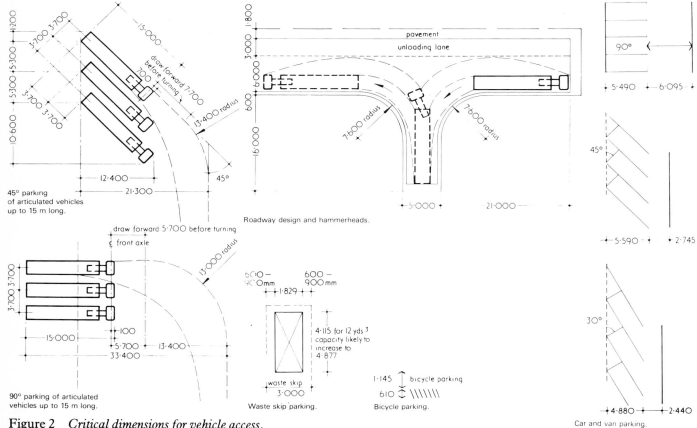

Figure 2 *Critical dimensions for vehicle access.*

3.00 Planning the building

The ways in which the planning of the building should respond to the type of user and the type and size of tenancy have been discussed in chapter 4.

3.01 Subdivision strategies

Table IV presents alternative approaches to subdividing different types of building into multiple tenancies. The size of the tenancies to be provided will be affected by:

● The location of fire escapes.

● The depth of the building – for effective interior planning very small individual tenancies should have a proportion of frontage to depth of not more than 1:2.

● Sufficient frontage being available to provide for perimeter cellular offices.

3.02 Allocating uses to upper floors

A major article of faith with factory estate developers is that manufacturing and warehousing space should be in single-storeyed buildings, which allow for flexibility of layout, modern materials handling techniques, and ease of servicing. However, there are many processes that are labour intensive, high value added, and create small end products which are very suitable for location on upper floors (figure 3). When converting multi-storey structures it is important to plan the use of the building in three dimensions, allocating uses to the upper floors according to their needs for access, the size of items produced and the density of employment.

3.03 Meeting statutory requirements

These are covered in detail in chapter 10.

Special efforts should be made by the architect/developer/building owner to negotiate specific relaxations which suit the particular contingencies of:

A building's special historic value
The needs of trades most likely to use the building
A phased programme of financial investment
A short term occupation.

Local branches of relevant employees' federations/trades councils may be able to assist in this if they have intimate knowledge of existing local examples of trade traditions.

3.04 Common facilities

Common access arrangements

In multiple user buildings other than the direct access type, entrances, stairs, lifts, loading bays and corridors will be shared, and various management problems can arise if the design is not adequately considered.

● Entrance areas. These are to be used by visiting vehicles, should allow space for an inquiry desk/porter's cabin readily visible to traffic from the road or parking area.

● Stairs. In most cases the arrangements made for fire escape will be adequate for other purposes.

● Lifts. Various types are available (table V) each with their

Table IV Subdivision strategies for providing self-contained tenancies

advantages and disadvantages. The choice of lift system is one of the most important decisions to be made in developing a redundant building, as it affects both initial cost and cost-in-use. If there is inadequate capacity, some tenants may attempt to appropriate the facility for their own use to the exclusion of others. In extreme cases it may be necessary for the building owner to employ a lift operator or set up an internal service company to act as collector and distributor of goods.

• Loading bays. The same considerations apply as for lifts. In a large development it may be wise to allocate groups of users to particular bays as a means of rationing their use of a valuable amenity.

• Delivery parking. When lorries and vans have unloaded and are waiting their next consignment, they can be moved to a nearby parking area.

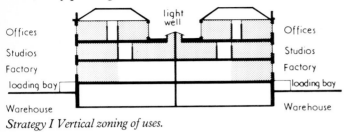

Strategy I Vertical zoning of uses.

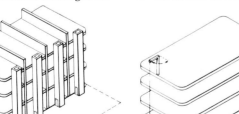

Strategy II Horizontal zoning of space types.

☐ zone of natural light and ventilation

Figure 3 *Strategies of zoning for mixed use.*

Table V   Approaches to lift installation

a *Single loading area*

c *Restricted access (type 1).*

Goods lifts serving a large group of tenancies: central management may be needed to maintain free use of lifts at peak times.

Passenger lift may be used by small firms manufacturing light goods (eg theatrical costumes).

b *Alternative loading areas*

d *Restricted access (type 2).*

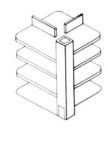

A number of goods lifts, each serving a small group of tenancies, who must co-operate on its use.

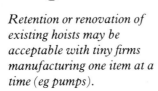

Retention or renovation of existing hoists may be acceptable with tiny firms manufacturing one item at a time (eg pumps).

• Corridors. These must be wide enough to accommodate hand operated pallet trucks etc. (up to 2.00m wide).

Common user facilities

The following common spaces have to be provided for the building as a whole or, in the case of a major tenant, for the unit itself:

• Washing facilities. These must be provided. A special guide *Cloakroom accommodation and washing facilities in factories* is issued by HMSO. Recommended standards are shown in table VI.

• First aid rooms. Should be provided and in some cases are required (together with ambulance rooms).

• Eating areas. These are normally optional but if a process is carried on which gives rise to dangerous fumes, there must be a separate space outside the work area where people can eat.

• Creches and nurseries. These are desirable where local industry employs a high proportion of female labour.

In addition, common facilities may be provided for meetings, reception, display and for office support services such as printing, reprographics and telex.

Common building services

Typical levels of specification are given in table VII. In most situations main supplies will be provided at or near a stairwell, or in main corridors, or with a branch taken into one corner of each tenancy. The tenant himself will then be responsible for the expense of fitting and running his own services, which will be metered at his particular tap-off point. The exceptions to this rule are:

• Open-plan layout. Where lighting and heating have to be shared to a common standard.

• Some working communities. Where facilities such as sinks, kilns and dark rooms are installed by the community as a common resource.

The design provision of services is discussed in more detail in chapter 14.

Table VI   Sanitary requirements for industrial units

Persons of either sex	Wcs (no urinals)	Washbasins	Males (where urinals are provided)	Wcs with urinals	Urinals
1 to 15	1	1	1 to 15	1	0
16 to 30	2	2	16 to 30	1	1
31 to 50	3	3	31 to 45	2	1
51 to 75	4	4	46 to 60	2	2
76 to 100	5	5	61 to 75	3	2
Over 100	5 of each plus one per 25 or part		76 to 90	4	3
			90 to 100	4	4
			over 100	4 of each plus 1 per 25 of part with at least ¾ of the additional appliances to be wcs	

The Factories Act standards are not generally considered adequate by many authorities and the slightly higher office standards are usually required.
The table above shows three standards. Where occupancy is not known, one person per 25m² for factories and one person per 12.5m² for offices may be assumed based on gross area. Calculations should be based on a range of occupancies from a predominance of men to a predominance of women.

Table VII   Service standards for the building

Service	Details
Electricity	Each unit to be provided with separate 415 V three-phase supply including provision of a main distribution board sited normally within the production area. The distribution board shall be of adequate capacity for the normally anticapted unit need of about 70kva* and shall be fitted with a fused switchboard. Lighting circuits to be provided within offices and wcs in appropriate locations. Power socket outlets to be provided in offices. Fused switch socket outlets to be provided in wcs where electric hot water storage heaters are used. In offices, lighting wiring should follow likely office subdivision and should finish with fluorescent fitting, but in wcs and cloaks should have a batten ceiling type fitting. External flood lighting should be provided to the rear of the building over the service door wired to each individual unit to illuminate the rear service area, and this may be supplemented by street lighting where layout permits. Note. No provision to be made in standard specification for lighting trunking 13 amp ring main in production areas.
Telephone	Underground service duct to be provided into ground floor to allow ease of cable connection.
Gas/gas central heating	Service to be carried into the building and sealed off in production area. Supply capacity to be designed to permit provision of central heating to production and office areas to normal working standards. Central heating to be provided only when required at Corporation's cost which may be in office areas for larger units using conventional hot water radiator system incorporating provision for hot water for domestic purposes. Boiler to be sited in production area.
Water supply/plumbing	Cold water supply to be carried into building to serve domestic needs only. Tenants' process or sprinkler requirement is not allowed for and supplementary service will have to be laid if excessive need is indicated. Cold and hot water supplies to be connected to all wash basins etc with hot water supplied from either wall mounted electric 3kw storage heater (54 litre capacity) or from a central hot water cylinder (if more economic) having a capacity of approximately 35 litres per basin or sink. All storage tanks to be adequately insulated.
Drainage	Surface water drainage down pipes should have access traps accessible from ground floor level and should be located in positions to avoid accidental damage. Ample external surface water gullies should be provided in the service yard to avoid water standing and grid channels and should be provided across service door entrance where levels of the yard could permit surface water to run off into the building. Foul drainage should allow for domestic demand and a sealed gully in the production area for process effluent. It is recognised that a trade effluent certificate will be required for individual tenant trade needs.
Ventilation	Mechanical ventilation to be provided to wcs only where layout is impractical to allow natural ventilation. All offices should be naturally ventilated and production areas need only have separate provision for manually controlled roof mounted extractors where heating provision is not intended in a form which will achieve this result. Any extraction fans to be completely weather proofed and capable of being serviced at roof level.
Fire alarm	An alarm system to be installed throughout office/production areas to each unit. The system to be electrically operated with manual initiation. Commerce supplementary brief to advise if provision is to be made for sprinklers, smoke detectors or emergency lighting. Hosereel points only to be provided where required by Building Regulations or other statutory provision.

*70kVA units in the range of 1000m² and upwards require separate load calculations.

a *Straight line.*

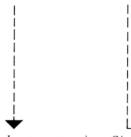

Goods in and out on opposite sides of plant.
Common in medium-sized firms.
Requires building with good access on both sides.

b *Overlapping.*

*Similar to type **a** but with a much larger type of firm.*

c *U-shape.*

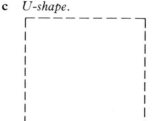

Goods in and out on the same side of plant.
Common with very small firms.
Possible in building with only limited access.

d *Convoluted.*

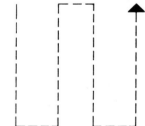

Goods in and out on the same side of plant.
Sometimes necessary for large firms when accommodated in building with restricted access.

Figure 4   *Production line patterns.*

4.00   Planning individual tenancies

4.01   Deciding on the type of layout
The machinery in a small manufacturing firm may be organised into separate zones for each process (process type layout) or to allow for a production line (product line layout). Where the maximum flexibility is required a mixed layout may be used.

Process type layout
Most suitable to unit or batch type production because of its extreme flexibility in producing a wide variety of products with the same equipment. The greatest advantage of the process type of layout is its flexibility, a number of different products being manufactured at the same time with the same machine. New products can be introduced and unprofitable products can be discontinued without replanning the layout. The disadvantage is that additional space is required for storage of materials in process, and it is difficult to obtain a full utilisation of machinery.

Product line layout
Most suitable for a firm where a limited line of items is produced (figure 4). This form of layout may result in lower handling costs between operations, lower inventory of materials-in-process, steady flow of materials and a high utilisation of machinery. The disadvantages are the lack of flexibility in being able to adapt to new products, and the higher initial investment in plant.

131

4.02 Planning for growth and change

When deciding on the internal planning of an individual tenancy, an assessment should be made of the degree of expansion or change that may be expected within the firm over, say, a five year period. The evolutionary stages in a firm's development are discussed in chapter 2. Firms may be typecast into three groups.

1 Satellites. These are dependent on larger companies for trade. Their equipment and productive capacity will change with the fortunes of the companies they serve, eg component suppliers in the automobile industry.

2 Specialists. These have the most precise and fixed plant, and survive on selling a particular skill to a well-established market. These firms will tend to be well established and static.

3 Marketeers. Marketeers compete openly with the larger firms by being innovative and being able to react promptly, eg small electronics firms. They need to be able to grow or contract, and to alter their product or change the process completely at short notice. They are most suited to the process type layout.

Given that the amount of growth can be estimated, it is helpful to predict a time factor. Firms can be considered as fast-growers or slow-growers.

Fast growing firms will need to increase their space-use but will have less cash to do it. They are unable to predict far into the future. They adapt as required by making capital investment only when necessary and provide additional space by moving or leap-frogging into additional space close by.

Slow growing firms tend to be well established and can plan ahead. A high proportion of their money will already be in fixed assets, so any expenditure will need to be justified by prospects of business improvements. Their adaptation strategy is to provide for expansion by sub-leasing space additional to immediate requirements and to reorganise space, production processes so as to use less space more efficiently. When considering a policy for growth and change, firms should consider the following options:

Subletting space they use inefficiently
Sharing facilities they use only some of the time
Using their existing space more efficiently by reappraising the production layout
Expanding into adjacent premises
Adding space by new building
Moving.

Chapter 4 table V sets out a 'premises ladder' showing accommodation likely to be required by firms at different stages in their growth.
Every company and their professional advisers should ask the question: what will requirements be in five years' time? The answer to this question should be reviewed annually. Although the volume of production and staff numbers may increase gradually, the increase in equipment and space requirements will happen in jumps.

Expansion strategies such as subleasing and allowing for additions should be related to the steps encountered when new equipment is required.
To help future planning an ideal layout should be agreed to which all moves conform. This layout may be reviewed and revised as conditions and objectives change.

4.03 Allocating space requirements

An accurange knowledge of space requirements is dependent on an understanding of the production process.

Preparing a lists of operations
The following steps will provide the basic information needed to allocate space for each section of the factory and developing demands:

List of products or components manufactured
List operations required to complete each item
For each operation for each machine, output per hour and special equipment required (dimensions etc)
Decide on type of production (process or product line).

Computing production area requirements
The following steps are used in the calculation:

● The daily production desired divided by the production per hour per machine gives the net machine hours required.

● The net machine hours per operation plus total of estimated down time and allowance for delays equals the total machine hours required per day.

● Total machine hours required per day divided by the number of net working hours per day equals the number of machines or workplaces required.

● A number of workplaces required times area of each workplace plus total of aisle space equals production area required.

Providing support areas
An additional area will be required for non-productive space

● Office space: reception, sales office, managers' offices, accounting and order processing area.

● Plant maintenance: the area where equipment can be serviced.

● Testing and inspection area: set aside for checking production before preparation for shipment.

● Receiving storage and shipping: receiving and shipping may be at opposite ends of the process, or at the same end of the building (figure 4).

● Employee facilities: in addition to the normal sanitary facilities, other facilities may be provided within the building to attract personnel, such as cafeteria, recreational facilities, and a creche or a shop for those with domestic responsibilities.

14 Equipping and Servicing the Unit

1.00 Introduction

Having dealt with the broad strategies of planning the space for a unit or individual tenancy, this chapter discusses the particular spatial requirements of equipment and servicing for common types of small firms. The information will be useful for the building owner and architect and will guide the prospective tenant in making the most suitable and effective use of the space available.

1.01 Layout of the workplace

In planning a workplace, allocate space for:

The machine or workbench

The servicing of the machine

The working space; sufficient space being allowed for the worker to perform the tasks and handle large and unwieldy parts (eg timber for joinery)

Tools

Raw materials, parts and assemblies

Space for the finished product

Special requirements, such as fume extractors or noise absorbers may need to be taken into account

Dangerous operations may require additional space for safety fences.

Dimensions for commonly found equipment are provided in table IV.

2.00 Planning guide

2.01 Purpose

The following tables provide a checklist to enable the designer to inter-relate the particular requirements of each work activity to be accommodated in the building. It is impossible to suggest 'best' layout examples as each firm is an individual operation and the spatial variations in different buildings are enormous. The information which follows is intended as a net, enabling the problem of planning the space to be solved in a number of interlinked ways. Our research has shown a great variation in the efficiency of the use of space in small workshops. Checks on the space standards provided should help the tenant avoid serious errors.

2.02 Contents

The information consists of five tables and a series of exam-

ples. Tables I–V set out the general characteristics of seven types of space: craft rooms; workshops; factories; repair shops; store rooms; cellular offices and open plan offices. The examples (figures 1–10) show a craft room, three types of workshop, a factory and a repair shop. It should be noted that the nomenclature between space types such as craft-rooms and workshops is blurred. Table I space budgets analyses the percentage of floor area devoted to the activities, giving an overall check on space available in unit.

3.00 Servicing

3.01 Services brief and criteria

There are two interlinked stages for which information must be collected.

1 Survey the existing services (para 3.02)

2 User needs and specialist requirements (para 3.03).

It will be necessary to prepare information for each main service – electricity, water and gas – which may already exist in the building or have to be renewed or replaced. The information must be assessed with conclusions drawn for each item, so that a services brief can be established. These should be considered with specialist help, taking account of all factors before a final assessment is made.

The preliminary appraisal of building services should yield sufficient information to enable the architect to enter into preliminary discussions with statutory undertakings. The guide given below (para 4.00) will give an early indication of the size of the necessary services equipment.

The system for each main service must fulfil the following criteria to satisfy the client/building owner:

Start cheaply, with allowance for upgrading later, as funds permit and space expands

Allow for specialist requirements

Satisfy the minimum level of specifications for safety, convenience and workability

Allow for monitoring (metering and controlling) individually, without great cost. Alternatively, consider what disadvantages and lack of flexibility would be incurred if it is controlled communally. (*Text continues on page 138*)

Table I Space budgets

Space type and typical small firms	Per cent floor area	Display	Desk space	Bench space	Machine space	Assembly area	Delivery and storage	Amenities	Circulation
1 Craft room	30								
Pottery	25								
Glass blowing	20								
Timber furniture	15								
Film production	10								
Studios	5								
2a Workshop – **bench orientated**	30								
	25								
Furs, skins	20								
Film processing	15								
Electronic recording	10								
Engraving	5								
2b Workshop – **bench and machine** **orientated**									
Toys, musical	30								
instruments	25								
Metalwork, plating,	20								
casting	15								
Clothing	10								
Shoes	5								
2c Workshop – **machine orientated**	30								
	25								
Light engineering	20								
Valves, tools	15								
Desk accessories	10								
Plastics	5								
3 Factory	30								
Printing	25								
Manufacturing	20								
stationery	15								
Brewing	10								
Spinning	5								
4 Repair shop	30								
Repair of	25								
electronic and	20								
electrical	15								
equipment	10								
Theatrical props	5								
5 Store room	30						60%		
	25								
Audio-visual	20								
distributors	15								
Fashion packaging	10								
and dispatch	5								
6 Cellular office	30		70%						
	25								
Scientific	20								
research	15								
Professional	10								
consultancy	5								
7 Open plan offices	30		75%						
	25								
	20								
Insurance broking	15								
Business services	10								
Design	5								

Table II Space types

Type	a Diagrammatic layout	b Plan proportions width : depth	c Maximum unit size	d Module for lettable units	e Minimum column spacing	f Floor-to-ceiling heights	g Area covered by typical services outlet	h Relationships with exterior
			m²	m²	m	m	m²	
1 Craft room		1:1 to 1:2	80	20	5.00	2.700 min 3.300 max	9	Telephone system View to exterior or rooflighting Corridors 2 m Small goods/passenger lift Car parking Van parking
2 Workshop		1:2 to 1:3	360	40	5.00	3.300 min 3.600 max	18	Telephone system View to exterior Corridors 2.5 m Goods/passenger lift Car parking Rigid truck access to loading bay
3 Factory		1:1 to 1:5	560	80	10.00	4.200 min 5.400 average 6.600 max	18	Telephone system Corridors 3 m Large goods/passenger lift, or separate goods and passenger lift Car parking Articulated truck access to loading bay
4 Repair shop		1:1 to 1:2	160	40	10.00	2.700 min 3.600 max	9	Telephone system Corridors 2.50 m Goods/passenger lift Car parking Rigid truck access to loading bay
5 Store room		1:2 to 1:10	560	40	4.60	3.600 min (2 pallets) 7.800 with hi-lift trucks 9.300 max	30	Corridors 3 m Ground level recommended Articulated truck access to loading bay
6 Cellular office		1:1 to 1:2	40	10	2.50	2.700 min 3.300 max	3	Telephone system View from work place Corridors 1.50 m Passenger lift Car parking
7 Open plan offices		1:1 to 1:4	560	20	3.75	2.700 min 3.600 max	1.5	Telephone system Passenger lift Car parking Van parking

floating benches
▨ storage   × equipment   --- circulation

Table III   Environmental requirements for typical small firms

Column key (a–n):

- **a** — Access for visitors: important / Access for vehicles: daily / weekly
- **b** — Goods need wide corridors for horizontal movement / Goods need hoist for vertical movement
- **c** — Process produces noise (or vibration) / Process affected by noise from others
- **d** — Normal security / High security
- **e** — Preferred lighting: north light / natural / artificial
- **f** — Preferred heating level: 16 C to 19 C / 19 C to 22 C / 22 C to 25 C
- **g** — Water services needed: cold / hot / Sink cannot be shared
- **h** — Waste disposal: domestic drain / industrial drain / solid material / paper and packaging
- **j** — Electricity: three phase needed / Gas normally used
- **k** — Telephone: own line needed / could share
- **l** — Preferred plan: self-contained / open plan / partly enclosed
- **m** — Required room sizes in range (m²): 5·00 × 3·75 to 5·00 × 7·50 / 10·00 × 3·75 to 10·00 × 12·50 / 15·00 × 7·5 to 10·00 × 12·50
- **n** — Floor loading: up to and including 3 kN/m² / up to and including 5 kN/m² / over 5 kN/m²

Type and common uses:

1 Craft rooms
- Pottery
- Glass blowing
- Timber furniture
- Film production

2a Workshops — bench orientated
- Furs, skins
- Film processing
- Electronic recording
- Engraving

2b Workshops — bench and machine orientated
- Toys, musical instruments
- Metalwork, plating, casting
- Clothing
- Shoes

2c Workshops — machine orientated
- Light engineering
- Valves, tools
- Desk accessories, plastics
- Food processing

3 Factories
- Printing
- Manufacturing stationery
- Brewing
- Spinning

4 Repair shops
- Electronic repairs
- Motor car repairs
- Bicycle repairs
- Theatrical props

5 Storage
- Audio-visual distributors
- Fashion packing and dispatch
- Art gallery storage

6 Cellular offices
- Scientific research
- Professional consultancy
- Solicitors

7 Open plan offices
- Insurance broking
- Business services
- Designers
- Photographic studio

Examples of unit workshop internal layouts
To be read with tables I and III

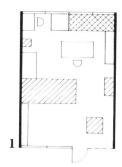

1

Type 1. Craftroom: timber furniture (two workers)

This firm uses a 'nursery unit' run by a local authority. Of the two partners, one makes pine kitchen furniture in the workshop, the other drives the van, collects materials and orders and delivers the finished goods. The corporation have arranged for one typist/telephonist/secretary to a group of ten firms like this (figs 1, 2).

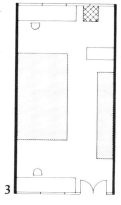

3

Type 2a Workshop: fur skins (two workers)

Two brothers do identical work cleaning and cutting small skins. Each has a bench against a window but on opposite sides of the space. Storage is mostly on the floor with little use made of the volume available. (figs 3, 4)

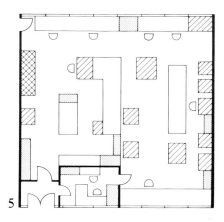

2

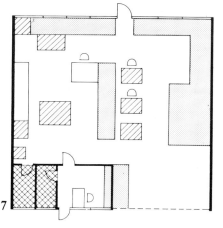

4

Type 2b Workshops: die sinker, engraver (nine workers)

A manager works mostly in the office, six skilled workers operate various tools and two sort and pack. A noisy, dirty environment with something always on the move. A simplified flow line is in operation and this gives a functional organisation to the visually chaotic space. (figs 5, 6)

Type 2c Workshops: printer (four workers)

Occupying a ground level factory unit, this printer employs three youths working small lithographic presses. Plates can be made; folding and simple bindings are also undertaken. The space is not intensively used and the owner is actively seeking smaller, cheaper premises. (figs 7, 8)

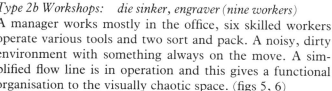

5

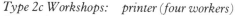

7

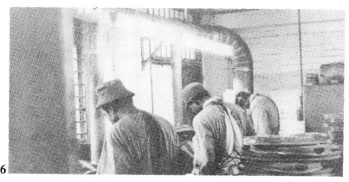

6

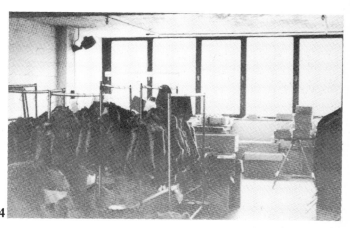

8

Type 3 Factory: trouser manufacturer (64 workers)
This manufacturer of ladies' slacks has expanded over about six years from a simple workshop to what is in effect a small factory. At second floor level, the space has been carefully organised and is intensively occupied. (fig 9)

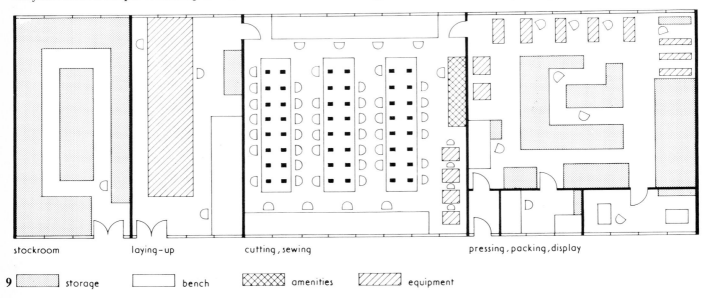

stockroom   laying-up   cutting, sewing   pressing, packing, display

9 ▨ storage   ▭ bench   ▨ amenities   ▨ equipment

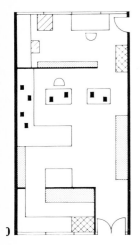

Type 4 Repair shop: electrical instrument repairs (two workers)
Two partners operate a rudimentary division of labour; one undertakes most of the detailed wiring and electrical work; the other takes on associated metalwork, packaging etc. They have partitioned off some space for an office but spend little time in it. (fig 10)

3.02 Survey of existing services
If the building and its services have been in operation for 10 years or more, the services can be said to have reached two-thirds of their useful life. The service system would need to be reviewed on its merits. There is a balance to be drawn between replacement and renewal. It is possible to spend half the cost or more, on replacement, to bring services up to a good standard.
The client must be convinced that his limited capital is put to the best use and therefore running and maintenance costs must be considered in conjunction with replacement cost to reach a 'cost effective' conclusion.
Factors to consider are:

Life expectancy and existing condition
Access and size
Maintenance records (eg for boiler, mechanical equipment)
Possibilities for extension (service capacity and space available)
General requirements of local statutory authorities
Standards applicable under the Health and Safety at Work Act:

1 Safety margins for maintenance (working platform, properly protected permanent access)
2 Height of light fittings above working level
3 Length of leads from socket outlets limited to 2m.

3.03 User needs and special requirements

Evaluation and assessment
Plans should have been made concerning the management of the building, which will include the responsibility for metering electrical and gas services. The statutory authorities may insist on one person or occupier being responsible for payment. A discussion will be required on whether to select subcircuit metering, which could involve additional management and installation costs, or whether each tenant should pay a pro rata contribution based on the space occupied. A large space user, taking 30 per cent to 40 per cent of the total space, would require subcircuit metering. This decision should be made when the scale of the operation is more fully established and individual requirements are known. Table VI shows an example of the main requirements for typical users.

Factors to consider
These fall into three categories:
Existing services

Will the existing services suffice?
Does the system comply with the relevant standards? (Offices, Shops and Railway Premises Act 1963)
Can subcircuit metering be accommodated?
Can service layouts accommodate replanning studies?
Will any increase in capacity of plant require new incoming supplies and structure?

Specialist requirements
Lighting
Small power and three-phase power

Table IV   Equipment requirements for principal inner city industries

Activity type	Equipment in common use	Working space per item (m)★	Special needs
Metal work	Machining centre	6.0 × 4.0	
	Jig boring and milling machine	3.0 × 3.0	
	Turret drill	2.6 × 3.2	
	Surface grinding machine	2.6 × 2.2	Dust extract or collector
	Capstan lathe	3.0 × 4.0	Dust extract or collector
	Bar and billet shears	2.5 × 3.0	
	Press brake	3.0 × 6.0	Anti-vibration mounting or solid floor
	Engraver	2.2 × 3.0	Natural light
	Die sinker	1.8 × 2.2	Anti-vibration mounting or solid floor
	Welding plant	1.5 × 3.0	Gas cylinder storage
Plastics	Extruder	2.0 × 7.0	Water chiller
	Vacuum-former	2.8 × 2.8	Water chiller
	Blow-moulder	3.0 × 4.5	Water chiller
	Acrylic saw	3.0 × 5.0	Dust extract or collector
Woodwork	Band saw	3.0 × 5.0	Dust extract or collector
	Circular saw	3.6 × 5.2	Dust extract or collector
	Surface planer	2.6 × 5.0	
	Knot hole drill	2.2 × 4.2	
	Milling machine	4.0 × 5.0	
	Slot boring machine	2.2 × 5.0	
	Dove-tailer	2.2 × 4.3	
	Belt sander	4.4 × 4.8	Dust extract or collector
	Veneer press	5.0 × 4.2	
	Lathe	2.0 × 3.0	Dust extract or collector
	Polisher	2.2 × 2.6	
	Carpenter's bench	3.0 × 4.5	
Printing	Lithographic press	2.5 × 5.0	Anti-vibration mounting
	Plate maker	1.5 × 1.8	Industrial drainage
	Folder	1.2 × 1.5	
	Drill	1.2 × 1.5	
	Guillotine	1.5 × 3.0	
	Glueing belt	2.0 × 4.2	Fume extract
Photographic	Developing tank	2.4 × max length print	Black-out, industrial drainage
	Enlarger	1.5 × max length print/2	Black-out
Clothing	Laying up machine	7.0 × 14.0	
	Sewing machine	1.2 × 2.2	Overhead power supply
	Steam press	2.0 × 2.0	
	Ironing bar	2.0 × 2.0	
	Steam boiler	1.2 × 1.2	Water supply, three-phase power
Footwear	Nailer	1.5 × 2.2	
	Sole press	1.5 × 2.2	
	Heel press	1.5 × 2.2	
	Shaping machine	2.0 × 2.5	
	Leather cutter	3.0 × 3.5	
	Pattern stamper	1.5 × 1.7	Anti-vibration mounting or solid floor
Electronics	Instrument bench	1.5 × 4.5	
General	Compressor	0.75 × 1.2	Anti-vibration mounting or solid floor
	Dust collector	1.5 × 2.0	Ducting to machinery concerned
	Furnace	1.5 × 3.0	Three-phase power
	Hot dip tank	1.7 × 2.2	Water services, drainage
	Drying cabinet	2.0 × 7.0	Three-phase power
	Upholstery press	2.5 × 3.5	

★These dimensions should allow preliminary workshop-floor layouts to be prepared for typical users. It defines the area required for operating an average-sized machine of each type, allowing a minimum of on-the-spot storage and room for the operative to move about. It would not permit general circulation on any scale nor for maintenance to sides of the machinery which are normally placed against a wall.

It is essential to obtain a schedule of equipment
Local authority approvals are required for:

1 Exhaust dust and fumes (Public Health)
2 Emergency lighting (Fire Officer)
3 Safety at Work Act (Factories Inspectorate)
4 Statutory undertaking requirements, ie Gas Board (1972 Gas Act), Electricity (IEE regs), Water (storage etc)
5 Drainage (Public Health)
6 Means of escape (Fire Officer and Local Authority)
7 Telephone requirements (special requirement for PABX room)
8 Petroleum licence of flammable liquids stores, toxic waste (Petroleum Officer)
9 Noise (Public Health).

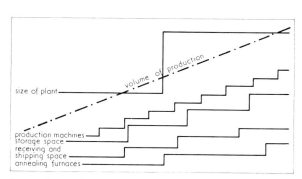

Space demands of various types of equipment vary considerably. These demands are not met gradually as production increases but periodically as it becomes necessary to add another production unit.

Table V Design considerations for the movement of people and goods

Type	Suitability			Requirements			
	Passengers	Heavy goods	Light goods	Machine room	Pit	External fittings	Access
Electric elevators	yes	yes	yes	yes	yes	yes	3 sides
Hydraulic lift	yes	yes	yes	no	yes	yes	3 sides
Manually operated lift	yes	no	yes	no	yes	yes	3 sides
Platform hoist	no	yes	yes	no	no	yes	2 sides
Electric service lift	no	no	yes	no	no	yes	3 sides
Scissors lift	no	yes	yes	no	yes	no	4 sides
Dock leveller	no	yes	yes	no	no	yes	2 sides
Electric belt conveyor	no	yes	yes	no	yes	no	2 sides
Gravity conveyors	no	yes	yes	no	no	yes	2 sides
Electric winch	no	yes	yes	no	no	yes	4 sides
Manual winch	no	no	yes	no	no	yes	4 sides
Manual floor crane	no	no	yes	no	no	Mobile	Mobile

Legislative requirements covered by Factories Act 1971, sections 22 to 27; hoists, lifts, chairs, lifting tackle, cranes.

plan dimension (mm)	underside of deck from ground (mm)
800 x 1000	130 – 150
800 x 1200	
1000 x 1000	
1000 x 1100	
1000 x 1200	

Standard pallet sizes-plain

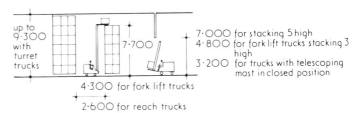

up to 9·300 with turret trucks

7·700

7·000 for stacking 5 high
4·800 for fork lift trucks stacking 3 high
3·200 for trucks with telescoping mast in closed position

4·300 for fork lift trucks

2·600 for reach trucks

Storage of goods. Use of fork lift trucks.

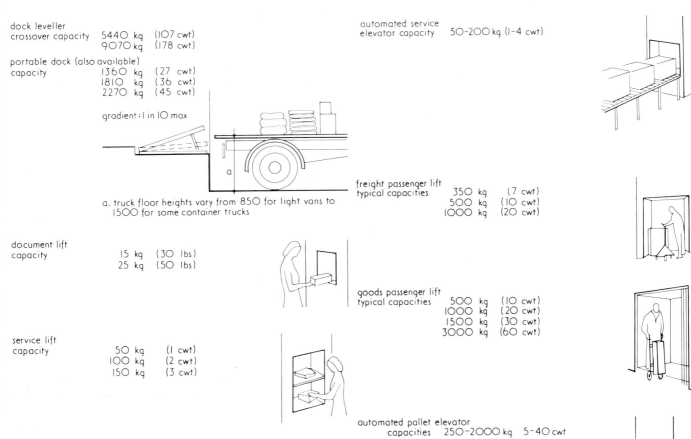

dock leveller
crossover capacity   5440 kg   (107 cwt)
    9070 kg   (178 cwt)

portable dock (also available)
capacity   1360 kg   (27 cwt)
    1810 kg   (36 cwt)
    2270 kg   (45 cwt)

gradient : 1 in 10 max

a. truck floor heights vary from 850 for light vans to 1500 for some container trucks

document lift
capacity   15 kg   (30 lbs)
    25 kg   (50 lbs)

service lift
capacity   50 kg   (1 cwt)
    100 kg   (2 cwt)
    150 kg   (3 cwt)

trollivator
capacity   150 kg   (3 cwt)
    250 kg   (5 cwt)
    350 kg   (7·5 cwt)
    500 kg   (10 cwt)

automated service
elevator capacity   50-200 kg (1-4 cwt)

freight passenger lift
typical capacities   350 kg   (7 cwt)
    500 kg   (10 cwt)
    1000 kg   (20 cwt)

goods passenger lift
typical capacities   500 kg   (10 cwt)
    1000 kg   (20 cwt)
    1500 kg   (30 cwt)
    3000 kg   (60 cwt)

automated pallet elevator
capacities   250-2000 kg   5-40 cwt

Methods of changing level.

Table VI   Service requirements for typical users

	General requirements	Local power	Lighting	Hand tools	Air extract	Air supply	Heating	Gas	Notes
Jewellery	Small single phase	Yes	General and task	Small electrical	None	None	Radiators	Yes	Possible furnace requirements
Woodworking	Three phase	Yes	General	Electrical	Yes dust a problem	None	Unit heaters	Yes	May need to comply with Public Health Regs
Light engineering	Three phase	Yes	General	Electrical	None	None	Unit heaters	Yes	Safety at Work Act needs panic buttons
Car workshops	Single and three phase	Yes	General and task	Compressed air	Yes car exhaust	Yes	Unit heaters	No	May need petrol interceptor and local authority licence for oils, etc
Pottery	Three phase	None	General	Yes	Yes	None	Different options	Yes	Possibility for kilns
Clothing	Single phase	Yes	General and task	Electrical	None	None	Radiators		Occupier comfort and lighting important

Client information
He must be made aware of limits of systems
He must be aware of management costs (maintenance etc)
Running costs must not make the building uneconomic
Diversity of users (scale of operation and working hours).

3.04   Implementation
The methods of organising the installation of services are related to those generally adopted for building work, chapter 15.

Contractor – design and construct package
This type of contract may be competitive or negotiated. The main disadvantage is the absence of close design supervision which may lead to higher costs. The cost of design is not usually itemised in the contract sum.

Consultant design
This involves obtaining competitive quotations where close design supervision is available, with careful cost checking and site control.

Client organises a series of individual subcontracts
The service engineer will advise. The main disadvantage is the lack of control and the risk of prolonging the contract time, but the cost to the client could be less where he is putting in his own management time.

4.00   Servicing guides

4.01   Purpose
The following guides are intended to give the designers an early indication of the size of equipment which may be needed. The data does not take into account the variations one may expect with different types of system (ie steam, electrode boilers for convectors and does not consider the age and condition of the systems. There is obviously no hard and fast condition of the system analysis in any build-

ing, and designers should always seek expert advice once they have made the initial appraisal.
The following subjects are covered:

● Energy management.

● Heating services.
Analysis of building types and sizing data
Hours of operation and annual rent required
Factors leading to choice of fuel and hence annual costs
Running costs
Plant room sizes.

● Lighting services.
Lighting levels.

● Ventilation services.
Ventilation routes in buildings.

● Electrical services.
Factors leading to the establishment of electrical load
Size of substation switch room.

● Telephone services.
Plant rooms sizes.

● Generators.
Plant rooms.

4.02   Energy management
Without accurate survey information, it is not possible to define where money is best spent in reducing energy and running costs. Generally the following summary can be used as indicative of the rate of energy usage for most types of building.

Heat loss, percentages:
1 Roof   20
2 Windows   15
3 Floor   15
4 Walls   15
5 Infiltration 45

Table VII Hours of operation and annual heat required

Building fabric	8 hour day/5 day week equivalent hours per year
large glazing curtain walling solid partitions and multi-storey	1,200
large glazing no partitions	1,750
normal glazing none or light partitions	1,950

Therefore net annual heat required $= \dfrac{\text{equivalent hours} \times \text{heat loss kW} \times \text{sec/hr}}{10^6}$

This figure used in conjuction with fuel tariffs will give the annual running costs for a particular type of system.

The greatest area where control can be made is in effective control of infiltration. These infiltration percentages are:

Table VIII Factors leading to choice of fuel and hence annual costs

Calorific values		Efficiency	
Fuels	Calorific values	Fuels	Seasonal efficiency
natural gas	41.37MJ/m^3	gas	65%
electricity	——	electricity	95%
class D oil	45 MJ/kg ($\times$ 0.835)	oil	65%

The efficiencies give are for typical installations and are for average types of installation complexity.

Therefore annual fuel required $= \dfrac{\text{net annual heat required}}{\text{calorific value} \times \text{seasons efficiency}}$

therefore annual costs = annual fuel required $\times$ tariff.
The table gives the last output for a given quantity of fuel together with anticipated losses due to the method of burning heat.

1 Window seals	30	3 Controlled ventilation	15
2 Door seals	35	4 Other	20

Table IX Properties of the simpler low-cost heating systems available

Type	Description	Advantages	Disadvantages	Emission range
Radiant radiant panel	Consists of steel tube or cast-iron water ways attached to a radiating surface. Back may be insulated to reduce rear emission or may be left open to give added convective emission. Particularly useful for spot heating and for areas having high ventilation rates (eg loading bays), the radiant component giving a degree of comfort in relatively low ambient air temperatures.	No moving parts, hence little maintenance required; may be mounted at considerable height or, in low temperature applications, set flush into building structure.	Slow response to control; must be mounted high enough to avoid local high intensities of radiation, eg on to head.	350 W/m^2 to 15 kW/m^2 of which up to 60% may be radiant.
Radiant strip	Consists of one or more pipes attached to an emissive radiant surface. Is normally assembled in long runs to maintain high water flow rates. The back may be insulated to reduce rear emission. When using steam, adequate trapping is essential together with good grading to ensure that tubes are not flooded. Multiple tube types should be fed in parallel to avoid problems due to differential expansion. Hanger lengths should be sufficient to allow for expansion without lifting the ends of the strip. Heating media may be steam, hot water or hot oil.	No moving parts, hence little maintenance is required; may be mounted at considerable height or, in low temperature applications, set flush into building structure.	Slow response to control; must be mounted high enough to avoid local high intensities of radiation, eg on to head.	150 W/m to 5 kW/m of which radiant emission may be up to 65% of total.
Natural Convective Radiators	Despite their name, 70% of the emission from these devices is convective. Two basic types are available, column and panel. The column type give a higher emission per unit length but project from the wall more than the panel type. Column radiators, mostly being cast iron, are heavier than the pressed steel panel type. In application they should be set below windows to offset the maximum heat loss and prevent cold downdraughts.	Cheap to install; little maintenance required.	Fairly slow response to control. With steel panel radiators there is a risk of corrosive attack in areas having aggressive water, often accentuated by copper swarfe left in the radiator. This leads to rapid failure unless a suitable inhibitor is used. Not suitable for high temperature water or steam.	450 to 750 W/m^2
Natural Convectors	These give high emissions from fairly small units. Often fitted with damper to reduce output when full emission not required; usually to about 30% of full output. Heat exchangers normally finned tube. United may be built into wall of building.	May be used on high temperature hot water or low pressure steam without casing temperature becoming dangerously high; fairly rapid response to control.	Take up more floor space than radiators. Likelihood of fairly high temperature gradients when using high temperature heating media.	200 W to 20 kW
Continuous convectors	These have a shallow depth with a fairly high emission. Give a smooth continuous run and are able to telescope to fit wall to wall. Can be fitted with a damper or local output control, which reduces the emission to approximately 30% of the full output. They should be placed at the point of maximum heat loss, usually under windows. The wall behind the unit should be well insulated to avoid wasting heat. As elements are long finned tubes they can be used as builders' work casing if required.	Take up relatively little space; give even distribution of heat in room. May be used with medium temperature hot water or low pressure steam without casing temperatures becoming dangerously high. Return pipework may be concealed within casing.	May produce large temperature gradients on high temperature heating media if poorly sited.	500 W/m to 4 kW/m

On assessing the economic level of insulation, the following priority should be given to upgrading insulation levels:

1 Roof
2 Walls
3 Glazing
4 Floor.

4.03 Heating services

Analysis of building types and sizing data
There are five basic types of building likely to be encountered:

1 Single storey with 50 per cent glazing 50m × 50m plan
2 Multi storey 10m × 10m plan
3 Multi storey 50m × 50m plan
4 Multi storey 100m × 100m plan
5 Internal zones 7.5m from perimeter.

It should be remembered that perimeter zones vary in heat gain level whereas internal zones are constantly in heat gain. It is not possible to determine exactly the equivalent full load operation of any building. Table VII is intended as a guide for equivalent hours of operation which, when used in conjunction with calorific values and plant efficiency, will give a guide to annual running costs.

Heating equipment
A detailed analysis of the different types of heating equipment available is outside the scope of this brief guide. Advice should be sought from a specialist service engineer.

Running costs
It is not possible to give an accurate indication of running costs due to likely increases in prime fuel costs. Table X is produced as a guide to prime fuel costs. The figures take into account working efficiencies of the systems and are not direct prime fuel cost comparisons (current 1980).

Table IX Properties of the simpler low-cost heating systems available—*continued*

Type	Description	Advantages	Disadvantages	Emission range
Skirting heating	There are three types of skirting heating; convective, radiant/convective and radiant. The convective type is a finned tube heat exchanger in a sheet metal casing, usually with provision for a return pipe within the casing. The other two types are of cast iron, the radiant/convective having a convective air passage within the casting. The sections clip together with inserted bushes to make a continuous length. Water flow rates must be kept fairly high to avoid reduction in emission.	May be used on water or low pressure steam. Give low temperature gradients in the room. All pipework concealed.	Relatively low output per metre of wall. More work involved when installing in existing building as existing skirting has to be removed.	Convective: 300 W/m to 1.3 kW/m Radiant/convective: 280 to 800 W/m Radiant: 130 to 500 W/m
Forced Convective				
Fan convectors	These units give a high heat output her volume of space occupied by the unit, together with the ability to distribute the heat over a considerable area using directional grilles. Air can also be supplied through stub ducts to heat several rooms. May be used to bring in heated fresh air for room ventilation. Leaving air temperatures should be above 35°C to avoid cold draughts, hence low entering water temperatures (below approximately 50°C) should be avoided. Where mixed systems of radiators and fan convectors are installed it is advisable to supply fan assisted units on a separate circuit to avoid control problems. To minimize stratification, leaving air temperatures above 50°C should be avoided. Must not be used on single pipe systems. Care must be taken at design stage to avoid unacceptable noise levels.	Rapid response to control, by individual thermostat. By use of multispeed motors rapid warm up available on intermittent systems; filtered fresh air inlet facility.	Electrical supply required to each individual unit.	1.5 to 25 kW
Warm air units	These are a variant of the above with a more powerful fan to enable them to supply a whole or part dwelling through ductwork. They are generally of square shape to be built into cupboards. Suitable for industrialised building techniques. May be fitted with charge metering based on hours run by fan. Must not be used on single pipe systems; care must be taken at design stage to avoid unacceptable noise levels.	Rapid response to control, by individual thermostat; by use of multispeed motors rapid warm up available on intermittent systems; filtered fresh air inlet facility.	Electrical supply required for each individual unit.	2 to 25 kW
Unit heaters	A unit fitted with a large propellor or centrifugal fan to give high air volumes and wide throws. Louvres direct the air flow in the direction required. May be ceiling mounted, discharging vertically or horizontally or floor mounted. Can be used with fresh air supply to ventilate buildings. Large units may be mounted at a considerable height above the floor to clear travelling cranes etc. May be used with steam or hot water but care should be taken to restrict leaving air temperatures, usually 40 to 55°C to avoid reduction of downward throw and large temperature gradients in the building. The air flow from the units should be directed towards the points of maximum heat loss.	Rapid response to control, by individual thermostat; by use of multispeed motors rapid warm up available on intermittent systems; filtered fresh air inlet facility.	Electrical supply required for each individual unit.	3 to 300 kW

Source: Extracts from IHVE *Guide Book 8* 1970.)

Table X Comparative prime fuel costs

Gas	Oil	LPG (Liquid petroleum gas)	Electricity
100	100 + 75	100 + 50	100 + 100

Therefore for comparison

1 unit cost gas	1.75 unit costs oil	1.5 unit costs LPG	2 units costs electricity

Table XI Floor space requirements for plant rooms of various capacities

Heating	Cooling
50 kW = 7m^2	100 kW = 7.5m^2
100 kW = 13m^2	200 kW = 9m^2
200 kW = 22m^2	300 kW = 18m^2
300 kW = 28m^2	400 kW = 21m^2
400 kW = 33m^2	500 kW = 24m^2
500 kW = 37m^2	

Table XI is intended as a guide to designers to allow floor spaces for plant and equipment for various building sites. The areas indicated assume an average height of 3 metres.

4.04 Lighting services

Lighting levels
Table XII is intended as a general guide to aid designers in assessing lighting levels for various categories of buildings.

Table XII Lighting levels for various activities

Industrial buildings	Illumination lux	Glare index
Assembly	400	25
Printing	400	25
Jewellery workshops	900	16
Leather working	600	22
Paint and spray	900	22
Potteries	600	19
Offices and shops		
General offices	400	19
Drawing office	600	—
Shops	400–600	—
Showroom	600	—
Computer unit	600	19

Definitions:
Lux Unit of illuminance, equal to one lumen per square metre.
Glare The discomfort or impairment of vision experienced when parts of the visual field are excessively bright in relationship to the surroundings.
It is not possible within the context of this summary to give a complete analysis of light fittings. Reference may be made to the Interior Lighting Design Handbook (Lighting Industry Federation Limited).

4.05 Ventilation services

Building Regulations require, where a space has no openable windows, mechanical ventilation to provide a minimum of 8 litres per second per person.

These minimum ventilation rates may on occasions need to be supplemented particularly when large extract volumes are needed for process equipment or the internal heat gains to the space are such that the temperature may increase to unacceptable levels.

4.06 Electrical services
Factors leading to establishment of electrical load:

Lighting   40 watts/metre^2
Small power   10 watts/metre^2
water heating if not central boiler = 10 watts/metre^2

To the above load should be added:
External lighting
Cooking
Fans, pumps etc
Computer.

Size of sub-station/switchboard
Main switchgear: if the load is more than 100 kW there is a possibility that the Electricity Board will request substation facilities. This is more likely if the site is remote or the local network is already heavily loaded. It is unlikely to receive such a request for loads smaller than 250 kW.
The substation obviously needs access from outside 24 hours a day and, although this is not always possible, should be at street level.
The size will be approximately:

up to 500 kW 20m^2
500–1200 kW 35m^2
1200–2000 kW 45m^2

4.07 Telephone services
Modern PABX equipment is microprocessor based and hence a smaller room is required than for the old cross-bar machines. Plant room sizes are as follows:

200 extensions 15m^2 (5)
300 extensions 20m^2 (7)
400 extensions 25m^2 (9)
The figures in brackets are for a separate externally ventilated battery room which will be required.
Much larger rooms are required for computer-based equipment, (eg IBM), together with false floor, air conditioning and statutory diesel generator. Ventilation will be required, usually provided by louvres, of 0.1m^2 per 100 kW.
The main switchroom should be beside the substation and obviously requires separate access. The size is determined by the type of switchgear to be provided (the cheapest not being the smallest). Obtain advice on new equipment (p. 156). The following will give a rough idea:

up to 250 kW 15m^2
250–500 kW 20m^2
500–1200 kW 30m^2
1200–2000 kW 40m^2

4.08 Generators

Plant rooms
Diesel generators are not usually considered necessary for office buildings unless the computer facility is large or the client indicates otherwise.
Care should be taken to house the plant room as close to the switchroom as possible, bearing in mind the problems of the exhaust, room ventilation, noise and fuel storage.
The approximate size of the plant area required is as follows:

up to 50 kW   9m^2
up to 100 kW 12m^2
up to 250 kW 15m^2

15 Managing the Conversion Project

1.00 Introduction

1.01 Each project is unique
There is a bewildering array of ways of setting up and managing projects for reusing redundant buildings, each demands a different development response. Many did not have a conventional start; but grew out of the determination of some group not to allow a building or group of buildings to be destroyed.

Clearly, professionals, architects, engineers, surveyors and cost consultants have an important role to play in the rehabilitation of old building stock, but how best can they help? Particularly when clients are small enterprises, often without capital, and the building problems are little more than repair and maintenance. By looking at a range of projects, it is possible to see a pattern of use of professional services in converting redundant buildings.

2.00 The variables

2.01 Pattern of variables
Each project can vary according to a number of factors.

Size of the project
Largeness does not necessarily mean complexity. Usually, the need for different professional skills, structural, engineering, design, quantity surveyor etc is a function of size.

Condition of the fabric
Elderly structures often have inherent problems caused by building elements and materials reaching the end of their useful life. These problems are often compounded by the fabric not being properly maintained.

Quality of the end result
Some new uses for old buildings demand a higher specification than others either because of statutory demands or because of the users' needs. Activities needing a dust-free environment, or extensive structural fire protection, will be more expensive to accommodate than, say, light engineering workshops.

Type of tenure
Single, mixed or multiple use as well as the length of tenure can each throw up unique problems.

Amount of end user involvement in the decision-making process
A high degree of user involvement can take place, owing to either demanding requirements or the participative character of the enterprise or because of the need for common areas.

Amount of work being left to the end user
Often an enterprise will provide only the more basic facilities leaving the end user to complete his space to meet his own needs. This has obvious attractions from the point of view of project management.

Methods of funding
There are various sources of funding open to enterprises. Some of these may demand the use of qualified professionals as a condition of commitment and, later in the project, certification, as a condition of release of the money.

Successful project management depends on balancing the competing demands of each of these factors. Does, for example, the release of money depend on the certified completion of stages of the work? Or, in a mixed or multiple use project, are the end users making a capital contribution or paying enhanced rentals, and if so, how do they have a stake in the decision-making to safeguard their interests?

3.00 Methods of approach

3.01 Professional services
The type of project management to be adopted can be described in terms of the extent of involvement of the traditional professions: architects, engineers, surveyors and cost consultants. Basically, there are four different approaches which an enterprise can adopt. These are as follows:

Full professional service
Professional consultants
Main contractor
RIBA plan of work and stages.

Table I   Selection of appropriate services for project variables (see 2.01)

Project variables	Full professional service	Partial service	Client building team	Do-it-yourself
Size and complexity	Big or complex. Full service probably advisable	Even on a complex project this could be the best way of working if control of building work within house team	Not advisable as sole means of management for complex building projects	Only for relatively simple projects
Condition of the fabric	Very bad condition will probably result in full range of different professions being needed	Very bad condition will probably result in full range of professional inputs being required	Good for keeping on top of the minutiae of small building work items	Only for relatively simple projects
Quality of the end result	Quality of work depends as much on good specification as good supervision. Use full service if high quality result is needed	Strategic input may preclude detailed specification and supervision	Not critical	High quality difficult to achieve
Type of tenure	Not critical	Not critical	Helps establish sense of user control	On small projects could help
Amount of end user involvement in decision-making process	Full service will ensure project has a momentum of its own which may make client input difficult	High degree of end user involvement will probably make partial service attractive	Gives end users good access to project team	On small jobs high degree of involvement. Work together
Amount of work being left to end user	Not critical	Could be attractive	Could be attractive	Probably the best way on small project
Methods of funding	Funding from outside bodies may be dependent upon independent certification	May be in conflict with funding methods	Could be attractive if work funded out of revenue	Could be attractive if work funded out of revenue

Table II   Services according to specification categories

Category of specification	Full professional service	Partial service	Client building team	Do-it-yourself
A Involving major structural alterations, additions, new services etc	Use full service if these alterations are extensive and if affect most of other building elements	Could be a disadvantage if work is complex	Not advisable as sole means of expertise	Not advisable
B General repairs to fabric, additional fireproofing and services	Full service could be an unnecessary financial burden	Probably the best approach	Could be a good approach if used with partial service of technical suppliers and subcontractors	Depends on client skill level
C Non structural partitions, upgrading finishes, overhauling services	Should not be required	Could be required for services	Probably best approach	Depends on client skill level best approach for small and simple projects
D Upgrading finishes only	Should not be required	Should not be required	Depends on how much resources are required	Probably the best approach

Partial service
Professional consultants providing strategic inputs
Several possible contractual arrangements.

Client/building team
Project management provided by client
Mainly direct subcontracts, sometimes labour-only contracts
On small-scale, low-complexity projects client may have traditional professional skills on call
Exploiting the technical expertise of suppliers is a feature of this approach. Often this arrangement goes hand in hand with a partial service.

Do-it-yourself
End user(s) completely involved at all stages, with random profession input.

Table I compares the types of service available with the

possible variations, noting which type of service may be best.
Table II compares the types of service with the different levels of specification which could be adopted (see chapter 8). Four categories have been used as a convenient way of showing that the quality of the initial building fabric and the quality of the end result can have a bearing on the most suitable professional service. The fifth category, no work at all, has not been included.

4.00   Organising the building work

4.01   The traditional way
Normally, when an architect is involved there will be a contract between the client (employer) and the contractor which is administered by the architect. The contract will normally be the Joint Contracts Tribunal (JCT) Standard form of building contract or the agreement for minor build-

ing works. There are several references books explaining how to run building contracts under these forms of contract. Some of the key points to watch are listed below.

Experience
Make sure that the proposed contractor has had experience of similar work by going to see examples.

Resources
Try to establish that the proposed contractor has sufficient financial and manpower resources to tackle and complete the job. In particular, consider major problems that could be met. For example, could the proposed contractor cope with reproofing or shoring up collapsing structures, should it be required in an emergency, without having to call in specialists.

Rates
Particularly if preliminaries are not priced in the tender, it is important to establish rates so there is a basis for negotiation if there is an overrun or extensive charges to the scope of the works.

Balance
Ensure that the contractor's price is not front-loaded so that an incentive remains to complete the work.

Dayworks
Most conversion works, particularly to redundant buildings will involve a daywork element. Establish what these rates are. On small contracts, particularly those with a Clerk of Works, it will demand extra vigilance in keeping and scrutinising records of times expended.

4.02 Other ways
Frequently, enterprises seeking to convert redundant buildings have aims of a social or community nature. They are often commited to finding alternative ways of achieving the end result. For example, they may wish to use voluntary or unskilled labour or gifts of materials. Listed below are some of the issues which can arise and can cause problems. The list is not exhaustive but it is typical of projects which employ partial professional services or none at all.

Dealing with statutory authorities
Sometimes it is as simple as discussing problems with the building inspector or, in London, the district surveyor. But much more frequently applications supported by drawings and calculations will be required for the planning, building control, environmental health and fire authorities.

Insurance
There are three types of insurance to consider in a typical building contract.

● Liability to third parties. Under both the minor and standard forms the contractor must carry third party liability as a condition of the Employer's Liability (Compulsory Insurance) Act 1969. Cover is normally up to £250,000.

● Liability to neighbouring property. Under both forms of contract this is the responsibility of the main contractor. Cover is normally up to £500,000 on any one claim.

● Insuring the works and materials. This applies to materials on or near the works against fire and Acts of God, but not theft.

Under the minor works form responsibility rests solely with the employer to ensure whether the works are new or existing. Under the standard form new works may be insured by either the contractor or the employer whereas existing structures must always be insured by the employer. In a small DIY project, insurance may be difficult to effect.

Project manager
In the client/building team approach, a project manager is often appointed to be responsible for the day-to-day running of the site. It is vital to ensure that the limits of his delegated authority are described, particularly in relation to:

Appointment of supplier and subcontractors
Hiring of labour
Signing cheques
Site security
Continuous cost control
Access to the client for decisions
Payment of wages
Dealing with statutory authorities.

Administrative overheads
The client/building team is in effect a contracting organisation and has to provide all the normal administrative support provided by a contractor. Setting up and equipping for this job can be expensive and should not be underestimated. If the building task is complex, or the timetable extended, administration costs will rise.

Building costs
There are many reasons which can make building costs rise above original estimates. Some are more forgivable than others. There is some evidence to show that labour costs are more volatile than material costs and contingency means to cope with this will be required. Typical problems are:

● Increased specification to meet requirements of statutory authorities, planning, fire etc, and also of incoming tenants which is not properly monitored.

● Unforeseen contingencies such as the difficulties of drain connections in areas where there are existing but unknown services.

● Use of unskilled labour leading to the need to redo work.

Site supervision
Supervising the quality of work on a site where many of the detailed design decisions have been left to be resolved on the job causes many problems, even with the use of skilled labour. These problems are compounded when unskilled or voluntary labour is employed or where gifts of materials or second-hand materials are to be used.

On the following pages are two case studies, one at Rotherhithe, London, the other at Hull, where different management methods were employed.

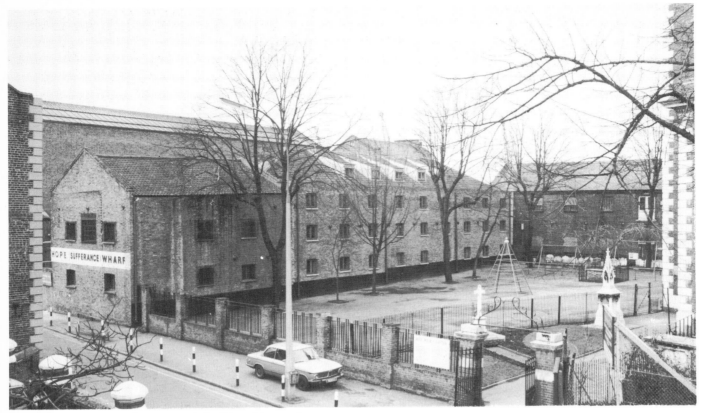

From left no. 61a, the Granary and the Riverside warehouses.

5 Case studies

5.01 Hope (Sufferance) Wharf, Rotherhithe, London
The project at Hope (Sufferance) Wharf was to convert several warehouses to workshop use. The large warehouses date from the eighteenth century. The whole site is in an outstanding conservation area. The developer was the Industrial Building Preservation Trust in association with the London Borough of Southwark. The trust had a management council which consisted of various professionals and craftsmen who were to be eventual tenants.
Originally, the project intended to raise most of the finance required from long-term commercial loans at favourable rates. In practice, grants from charitable foundations were the main source of capital income owing to:

Delay in securing a long lease or the freehold
Reluctance of financial institutions to invest in conversion of older buildings to multiple uses
Cutbacks in local government expenditure, which forced the local authority to reduce its financial support.

The management council opted for a partial professional service backed up by an on-site team with a project manager which, acting on professional advice, administered a series of separate contracts for the work which, for all but the last phase, exceeded £100,000.
The project ran into debt because capital grants and loans did not keep pace with expenditure. Eventually the project was handed entirely over to the London Borough of Southwark. Although the initial aims of the project have been successfully achieved, the way of achieving them changed. There is now a thriving community of craftsmen at Hope (Sufferance) Wharf.

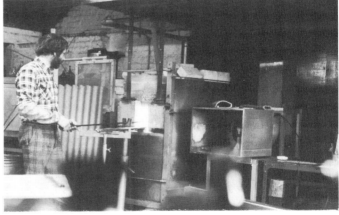

The glass blowing workshop.

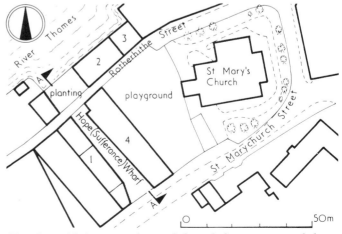

Site plan with 1 community workshop, 2 three-storey workshop, 3 single-storey glass blower, 4 three-storey Granary converted to provide craft workshops.

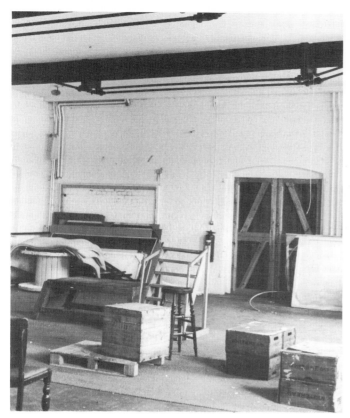

Theatre workshop.

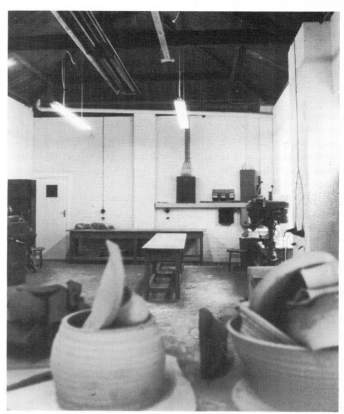

Workshop for use of local community.

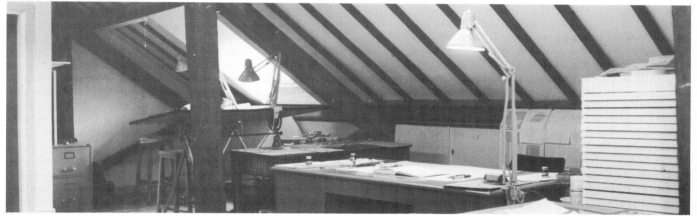

Silk screen design studio.

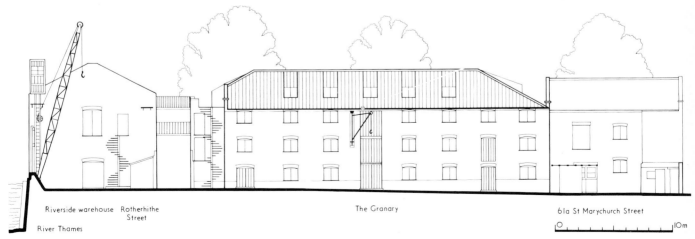

Riverside warehouse   Rotherhithe
                       Street

River Thames

The Granary

6Ia St Marychurch Street

River Warehouse housing the theatre workshop, glass blower and other workshops, and the Granary, converted to craft workshops, silk screen studio and exhibition gallery.

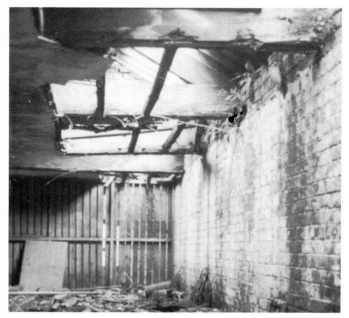

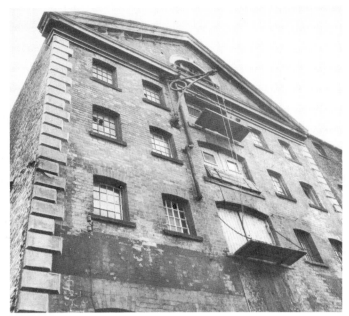

Inside the Hull project before work began: this highlights the neglect these buildings have suffered.

Posterngate frontage.

5.02 The waterfront development, Kingston-upon-Hull
The waterfront development is essentially a 'do-it-yourself' operation with very minor professional input. It is a good example of what can be achieved by an energetic entrepreneur. The warehouses are situated in an outstanding conservation in the old town of Hull. No 22 Princess Dock Street was built in 1831 and is a class II listed building. The adjoining warehouses were built later. All had been empty for at least 12 years. The previous use appeared to have been for fruit and nut warehousing.

The buildings were acquired on a 99 year lease from Hull City Council, who gave planning permission for conversion to a nightclub and restaurant, arts and crafts workshop and 12 residential units with associated car parking. Phase 1, the nightclub and restaurant is complete and trading successfully.

Funding in the main was provided privately, only about 10 per cent of the value of the work to the building being provided in grants. Hull City Council provided a small 'start up' grant and the Historic Buildings Committee gave a grant on completion of the work to phase 1, which took about one year from gaining planning permission to completion.

The owner hired direct labour: bricklayers, joiners, roofers etc, as these skills were required. He started with one person and, when a licence was granted, built up to a labour force of seven.

On phase 2, the hotel, income from phase 1 is being ploughed back into the project. From his experience of the first phase, the owner draws certain conclusions.

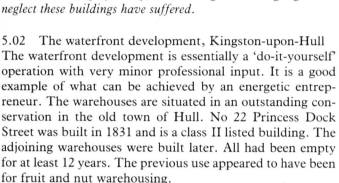

• He did it the best way, starting cheaply and slowly building up momentum.

• Generally, labour costs exceeded estimates, whereas material costs were less than predicted. This is mainly attributed to the use of second-hand and recycled materials.

• Even for simple building operations with skilled labour, extensive supervision and trouble-shooting is required.

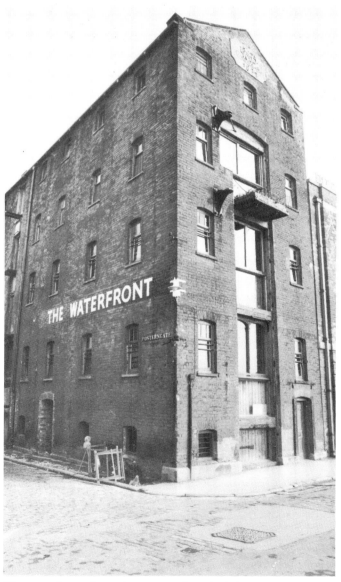

The quay front, the main entrance is to the left.

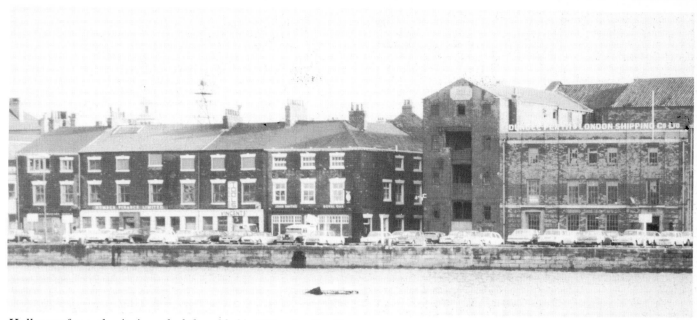

Hull waterfront, the site is on the left and behind 'Dundee Perth'.

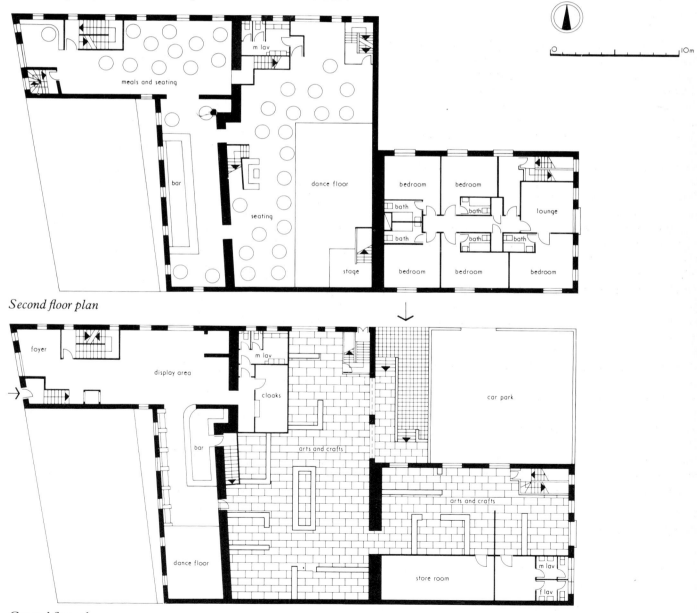

Second floor plan

Ground floor plan

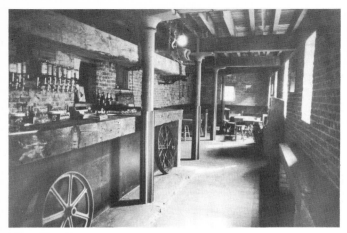

Chandlers Bar.

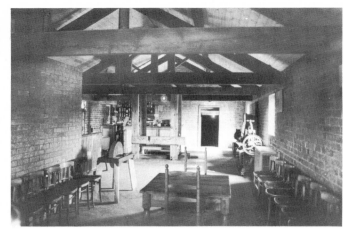

Winch Bar.

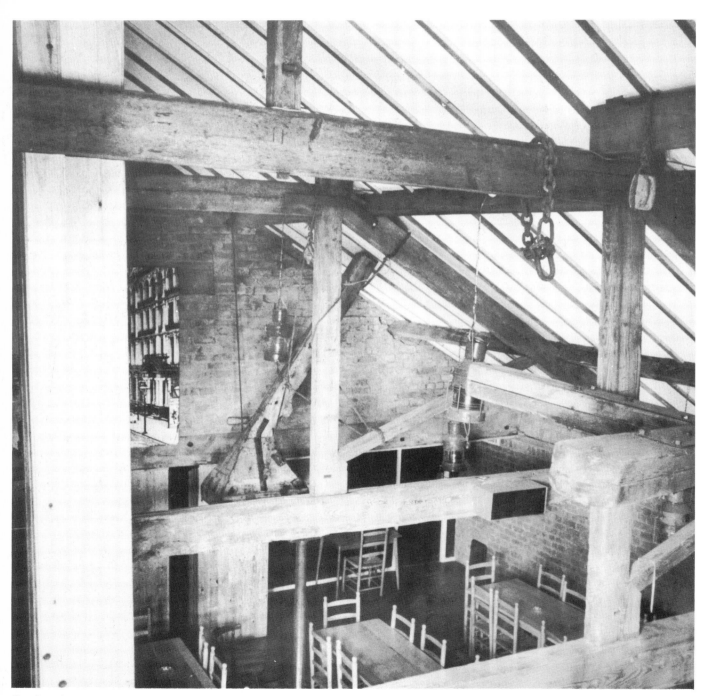

Roof garden restaurant.

16 Managing the Building

1.00 Introduction

Careful management of a complex of activities within a single building can never be underestimated. In a building project designed to function as a whole unit with a number of component parts, the building manager is the essential member of any client group. In chapter 1 working communities were seen as a fresh concept of building management and services. This new initiative has been brought about by the on-site manager who provides active administration support for the tenants. Together, they can influence the quality and type of services offered, the mix of tenants and the running of the building. The working community operates under a particular form of legal and organisational structure and depends greatly on the extent of the occupants' involvement and the drive and personal charisma of the organisers. Building management approaches to multiple-use buildings can embrace both orthodox multi-occupation and that of the working community. Tables I and II summarise the main features of working communities and compares the facilities provided in a building for the latter and orthodox multi-occupation. Each project and development will tend to evolve a different form of management and support structure with appropriate services and facilities.

2.00 Legal structures

The options for legal structures covering the management of the buildings are:
Private limited company
Public limited company
Company limited by guarantee
Common ownership
Charity
Building preservation trust
Association of occupants.
It will be seen from the following paragraphs that one project could embrace a number of these options simultaneously. The prime object in selecting an appropriate legal structure is to eliminate or reduce the personal liability of the principles of participants for any losses in the event of the enterprise winding up.

A building run as a non-profit enterprises for the benefit of the participants will, in addition, require a legal entity that allows voting powers for each of its members. On the other hand, a building run as a profit-making enterprise will frequently be part of the operation of an existing company, although in certain circumstances it may be advantageous for tax purposes that each enterprise be run by a separate subsidiary company.

A useful by-product of deciding the nature of the legal structure and formulating a memorandum of association for a project is that the objectives of the enterprise are clarified ensuring a consensus view of the aims of the enterprise and the way it will function.

Table I Summary of the features of working communities

Advantages	Commitment only to required size of space but with potential for expansion.
	Economies of scale resulting in real savings.
	More facilities than if in isolation.
	Less capital outlay on premises, releasing money for other uses.
	Saving principal's time in dealing with building and services.
	Reduction in staff required.
	Payment of more items in lump sum resulting in less purchasing and accountancy.
	Premises and services budgeted in advance.
	Possibly better environment in building terms.
	Improved morale in being with other small firms.
	Business generated by forming work links with other firms.
	No capital outlay for conversion, nor dilapidations on removal.
	Can move without needing to find new occupant.
Disadvantages	Individual firms suffer some loss of identity.
	Having to compromise in taking into account other firms' needs.
	Contributing to some services which may not be used.
	Building and joint services not under principal's sole control.
	Being 'featherbedded', when moving additional resources will have to be acquired.
	Difficult to retreat into one's own 'empire' – have to be good neighbours.
	Possibly noise problem if space not compartmentalised.
	Apprehension about security.
	Will not be able to sublet or assign at a profit or use premises as collateral.

Table II   Comparison of facilities provided by multi-occupation and working communities

Type of organisation	Classification	Examples of facilities
Orthodox multi-occupied building	Basic	Lighting, heating, power. Water, telephone (direct line). Lavatories, goods lift, refuse collection. Fire alarms.
	Initial phase (based on real or anticipated needs of participants)	Building maintenance and management, cleaning. Telephonist/receptionist; telex; security guards. Secretarial service; reprographics; bookkeeping. Display area; conference rooms. Materials storage and handling; goods delivery and messenger service. Social activities; canteen.
Working communities	Development phase (capitalising on full potential of co-operation when confidence is established)	Joint marketing and public relations. Information sources and library. Production planning; quality control; prototyping and workshop. Computer terminal and computer access; accountancy system. Microfilm equipment for records; audio visual presentation; word processing. Export packaging. Sharing production machinery; bulk buying. Staff to cope with overload or holidays. Photography and dark room; interpreters; insurance; leasing.

2.01   Private limited company

The individual members of a limited company set up for a project, do not have personal liability for the debts of the company. Because of this building landlords often require personal guarantees, unless the limited company to which the lease is being granted is well established and of 'good covenant'. In turn, working communities may well require personal guarantees from individuals taking space in the name of a limited company.

A private limited company provides a method of raising money from participants for conversion and working capital to operate the building, by the sale of shares. They are restricted to a maximum of 50 members, and are appropriate where the property is:

● Owned by the leaseholder or freeholder who is letting space to several tenants for profit.

● To be jointly owned by less than 51 members sharing space and services on a non-profit basis who need to raise share capital.

A limited company is not difficult to form; specialists exist who set up 'off the peg' companies with stereotyped aims, objects and articles of association at economic cost. Alternatively, most solicitors will assist in these routine procedures. It is possible to take over a defunct company that has ceased trading, providing the existing memorandum of association allows the new owners to carry out their intended function. Sometimes an advantage can be derived by inheriting a tax loss which can be set against future profits:

In the event of liquidation those involved do not have liability for the company's debts and therefore the personal assets of the individuals involved in the company are preserved.

It enables control of the company to be in the hands of the shareholders by giving them voting rights at annual and special general meetings (in working communities shares can be issued on the basis either of one share to each member firm, or pro rata to space occupied). If certain members have agreed to act as guarantors to the lease then an additional block of shares can be allocated to them in order to give them a controlling interest in the company and thus protect the risk situation they have assumed.

2.02   Public limited company

Basically, public limited companies are those that offer shares for sale on the open market. It is still possible to restrict the sale of shared to the occupants but this would require a 'statement in lieu of prospectus'. These are appropriate where the property is:

● Owned by the leaseholders or by freeholders who are letting space for profit and who wish to raise capital by issuing shares on the Stock Exchange.

● To be jointly owned by 51 or more member firms sharing space and services on a non-profit basis, to whom shares are issued to give voting rights and raise capital.

This is probably unsuitable for a new venture which has yet to prove itself.

The latest Companies Act (1981) seeks only to distinguish between a private and public company, in that the company declares that it is either one or the other and all reference to the number of members is dropped.

2.03   Company limited by guarantee

This is appropriate where the company is to be jointly owned by member firms sharing space and services on a non-profit basis.

These firms require voting rights, but do not need to issue shares to raise capital (although their nature does not preclude the possibility of issuing shares if this is considered desirable).

In the event of the company winding up, the members may each be called upon to contribute an amount up to a predetermined maximum. There can be various categories of membership which could allow any members guaranteeing the lease to protect the risk they are assuming. There are restrictions on the number of members. The members have the same voting rights as in a limited company.

2.04   Common ownership

In common ownership all the occupants regardless of their formal status as employer or employee have an equal interest in the firm and share in the profits (or losses!). They all have equal voting rights at special or annual general meetings. The company can be any of the legal entities previously described except those that issue unequal allocation of shares or shares on the open market; however, a company limited by guarantee is the best choice.

Common ownership is appropriate to buildings:

• Where the occupants have decided to totally merge their separate businesses.

• Where firms interested in changing to or forming a common ownership company have got together to both trade and share premises and facilities on this basis.

It is unlikely that a common ownership project will cover both the service company operating the building and extend to cover the activities within the building. One of the strong points of a working community is that participants, while enjoying the benefits of collaboration, do not surrender any of their precious independence. One can, however, also consider a building occupied in the main by single artist craftsmen already (or planning to become) integrated to the extent of sharing common marketing and publicity, who decide to merge their separate businesses. In this situation common ownership would be the obvious type of legal structure. They can also be registered under the Industrial and Provident Societies Act.

2.05 Charity

Where the objectives of the enterprise can be very clearly seen to be of benefit to the community at large, there is a possibility of registration as a charity. A service company running a building exclusively occupied by charities has a possibility of qualifying, but not if the occupants are commercial. A recent court case decided that an association of craft firms was a charity only if it maintained a library and a collection of tools, which were also open to the public. The fact that the Charity Commissioners approve registration as a charity does not necessarily mean that the Inland Revenue will be of the same mind. Negotiations with the Charity Commissioners will take some time.

2.06 Building preservation trust

If the building being rehabilitated is a listed one and the object of the company is to conserve it, then a Building Preservation Trust can be formed. As such it can be registered as a charity. This scheme is administered by the Civic Trust at 17 Carlton House Terrace, London SW1 (01 930 0914)

2.07 Association of occupants

This is not an entity in the legal sense, no more so than a residential tenants' association, but nevertheless it will require a formal structure and terms of reference in order to operate.

The building in which the occupants have a formal landlord and tenant relationship will find it useful for both parties to set up an association for occupants. This is beneficial to the landlord in that it provides a corporate body with which he can negotiate, and reduces the matters in which he has to deal with each tenant separately, saving management time. It is useful to the tenants in that they have more muscle in dealing with the landlord, and a method by which they can decide on the scale of services they need.

A working community which has formed a company to run

the building will already have a ready-made structure, so the individual members' views can be represented via the management board. Directors will be elected by general vote and there is an annual general meeting to which the board are answerable, at which members can raise any pertinent matters.

The landlord may find it advantageous to turn his building into a working community, offering small serviced spaces with a wide range of available facilities decided on by an association of occupants. This is a marketing feature which can keep his building fully occupied when the property market is in decline.

The tenants in a building where none of the services (listed later) are provided could well get together and form themselves into an association of occupants, purely to organise these services themselves and enjoy the advantages of them.

3.00 Occupants

An essential element in any community who share a building is that the activities of the participants should be generally compatible in order to offer work links between members and maximise the potential of shared facilities. Therefore the general composition of the occupants should be planned in relation to the following:

• In addition to the compatibility of occupants there needs to be a mix of firms of various sizes for the planning, design and economic reasons outlined in earlier chapters and in the 'nursery' function below.

• In order to cover the risk it is necessary to have a base of well-established firms in addition to new firms.

• Applicants need to provide bank and trade references to establish their credit-worthiness – in the absence of a track record guarantors may be required.

• The temptation to accept all comers to fill vacant space should be avoided. Information on finding and selecting tenants is contained in paragraph 10.05 following, on letting.

3.01 The working community

While the sharing of services is a readily appreciated advantage, the invisible assets of being part of a group of like-minded people are difficult to quantify. Members of a working community will admit that while the original attraction was primarily economic, in time the 'friendly atmosphere' was the most appreciated feature. There is an informal relationship between all the members, which at one level is good neighbourliness, and at the other the exchange of information and co-operation on joint projects. The result is a better morale among people with a common bond who formerly had an isolated existence working from home, small offices or workshops.

3.02 The nursery function

There is a proven market for small units of space both for self-starters and for established small firms in a growth position. As the working community idea spreads, more people will consider this a valid use for a building. Either 'consumers' will get together to fill their own needs or the 'supplier', in the shape of a landlord or developer will seek to meet the demand. In meeting the needs of the small firms, the nursery function of the working community must be accepted. In order to provide a variety of different sized units, so a firm can expand within the building there will be a turnover of occupants. Some new firms may not make the grade and others will outstrip the size of accommodation that the building can provide.

4.00 Management staff

The following skills will be required to form the basic management team. If the building is very small it could be possible to run it with only two people, but, if larger, greater support will be required. Initially it is important to have a full-time executive, with part-time help.

Chief executive-Initiator manager

He (or she) should have had some experience at running a small business himself, for not only is the operation of the building services company a small business in its own right, but also the past experience will have given him valuable insight and understandings of the small firm. The manager's most important role, regardless of whether he is employed by the occupants or by the landlord, is his ability to develop relationships with the people in the building. He will be heavily engaged at first, but will progressively make the work routine and hand it over to be managed by the administrative secretary, leaving him free to expand the operation and initiate new projects.

Administrative secretary/workshop manager

The administrative secretary should be chosen, not so much for special secretarial skills but as a potential workshop manager with the ability to handle tenant negotiations face-to-face and to undertake simple book-keeping. He or she should be fully involved in this work from the outset to ensure continuity.

Maintenance foreman

The maintenance foreman should be chosen for his willingness and ability to turn his own hand to any building maintenance problems and to oversee minor works undertaken by local tradesmen. It would be of great advantage to choose a person who is already familiar with a multi-storied building and to engage him at an early stage so that he can assist the project team and be familiar with the modifications made as work progresses. He could also be a tenant.

Security man

The security man should be chosen for his friendly and willing disposition and preferably should be able to live very near the site, to provide an informal security presence.

Cleaner

It is preferable to employ a specific person for this job, possibly the wife of the caretaker, rather than contracting it to a specialist firm. In smaller developments one person may cover all these functions as manager.

5.00 Finance

The financial outgoings will be:

Rent
Rates
Maintenance
Running costs of services
Adaptations
Administration of shared services.

5.01 Financial control

Firm control and monitoring of the finances is vital and must be entrusted to someone with at least a basic knowledge of accountancy.

Future expenditure should be forecast and budgets prepared; when approved these can form the basis of a system of budgeting control. Each category of expenditure should have an annual budget figure which cannot be exceeded by a large margin. The control can be exercised by either a method of analysis built into the accountancy system which can be regularly reviewed, or approval of priced purchase orders against a periodic financial allocation. Should the building and its facilities be the sole concern of a single company, then the same person may be responsible for the financial control.

5.02 Meeting commitments

Obviously a friendly relationship should exist between administrators and the occupants. In the interests of the occupants as a whole, a hard line must be taken in ensuring that members meet their financial commitments. Members should be discouraged from using delayed payment as a means of financing their business rather than paying interest charges on an overdraft. To this end the company should consider writing a clause into any lease or agreement to apply a punitive surcharge on any outstanding payments.

6.00 Shared services

The advantages to the participants of shared services lies in enjoying the benefits of facilities which would be either more expensive or prohibitive for them to provide on their own. This can be achieved by the provision of those services imperative to the functioning of the business and those non-essential services that enable the business to perform more efficiently and competitively.

A small building will only support basic services. On the other hand, one of the large industrial buildings that abound in the decaying inner city areas of our cities that could house, say, 100 small firms, could for an extra £10 per week provide some quite sophisticated facilities with the £52,000 pa raised.

6.01 Examples

Prices given on the next page are correct for new November 1983 rates, but relate to one piece of equipment, in one area only. The structure of telephone charging has become more varied, and for a larger, collaborative system the cost per extension might well be lower: but it is no longer easy to discover how much lower. Equipment is available on lease, or by outright sale. Costing has become complex and is now governed by several factors which include locality and a wider range of equipment, so that although some packages are available, representatives of the Telephone Manager will have to be contacted for individual quotations.

In isolation	£00.00
2+4 Ambassador switching system (connection charge £90) annual rental	15.60
2 lines @ £88 (connection charge each £85)	176.00
4 telephones (connection charge each £33) @ £16.40	65.60
Nominal broken time answering telephone at £5.00 per hour (ie 1 week pa)	200.00
	£457.20

Note: answering machine costs additional: charges quoted above are quarterly rates

NB More firms involved means more constant use of lines available and therefore less lines are required pro rata to the extensions provided.

The three examples following, illustrate the scope and extent of collaboration in shared services which could be applied in a variety of circumstances. The first is applicable to any building and the remaining two are examples of areas of collaboration by specific activities.

1 A building shared by several firms
Management; building maintenance; heating, lighting; interior cleaning; window cleaning; refuse collection; fire and security alarms; fire equipment; building and individual insurance; private branch telephone exchange and switchboard; internal communication telephones; telex; message taking; ceefax; secretarial service; bookkeeping service; press relations; canteen; games room; rest room; medical facilities; safety at work.

2 A building shared by service industries (office function)
Conference rooms; library information service; photocopying; offset litho printing; advertising and public relations; computer terminal on shared time; word processing; hire of furniture and office equipment.

3 A building shared by light engineering industries (manufacturing function)
Van contract hire; drivers; despatch and delivery scheduling; warehousing; centralised goods reception; stock control; material handling; packing/export packing; specialist production equipment not fully employed by any one firm; security; quality control and testing; prototyping and tool making; marketing/export marketing; sales promotion; exhibitions; public relations and advertising; safety at work.

6.02 Service charge
The service charge, as distinct from rent/licence fee and rates, covers the cost of the basic services detailed above. Like the sharing of rent it can be based on a square footage or per head basis. It should be paid weekly, monthly, quarterly or annually in advance. The cost of all the services to be provided should be estimated and then a proportion added to allow for inflation and unforeseen contingencies. It should also include any interest charges on loans to purchase equipment.

Any surplus at the year end can be returned to members or, conversely, if there is a loss then members may be called upon to pay their share. Without making the service charge too much of a burden, it is obviously better to perform below budget and make a refund to members.

It is good practice to embody a clause in the lease/licence outlining the services to be provided and the member firms' responsibility for their share of the total cost, or this can be the subject of a separate agreement.

6.03 Shared benefits and costs
There must be common consent that these services benefit the users of the building as a whole, and that member firms are happy to support them, realising that they may use some services more heavily than others while those services they seldom use may be important to other firms. A service that a firm rarely uses could still be valuable, merely because of its availability eg no clients using the telex, but the presence of a telex number on their letter leading may be a contributing factor in gaining orders from a potential client who does use telex.

The cost of those services that only benefit a few members can be split among those using them and be separately charged. Viability will need to be tested.

7.00 Building handbook
It may be useful to draw up a checklist relating to the management of the building which can be expanded as information is gained from the briefing stage to the time when the building is let. Table 3 draws on the experience of the management of industrial estates and working communities. A separate promotional leaflet could also be prepared based on the section headings.

8.00 Caring for the building

8.01 Cleaning
To ensure the maintenance of standards, window and space cleaning require constant vigilance, either by the supervisor if a contract cleaner is appointed or by the responsible person if cleaners are employed directly. Even in the best regulated circles things slacken off. To avoid any misunderstanding a schedule and the scope of daily, weekly and periodic cleaning should be drawn up and agreed, which can provide a reference. The 'periodic' cleaning is important and is often overlooked. Items such as light fittings can either form part of the routine cleaning, or a periodic 'spring clean', can be undertaken as a one-off job.

8.02 Maintenance
An observant person in charge, who becomes aware of faults when moving about the building, is the key to successful day-to-day maintenance. It also depends on a good relationship between this person and the occupants, who can feel free to mention any matters needing attention. Periodic

Table III   Required contents of building handbook

Headings	Items to be covered
1 Introduction and objectives	• Principal motivations of why the project was started and how it has reached this stage (history, founders, particular advantages and benefits of this organisation, etc) • Policy of the company and structure • Method of application for units • Public relations/promotions/marketing for the benefit of tenants/licensees
2 Building manager	• Named individuals, including directors, managers and those responsible for maintenance (services), cleaning, caretaking close-down and night/weekend security • Form of organisation (eg service company) • Communication methods with the management, maintenance requests, complaints, notice boards, etc • Exhortations on 'communal good', 'management can't know everything'
3 Agreement	• Licence, membership, fixed fee, lease
4 Finance	• Fees and charges (including rates and services) to be paid with arrangements for payment, date due, action on arrears • Distinguish between communal (essential) and individual service charges • Deposit, conditions or return • Method of reviewing fees and charges

NOTE Policy on fees could vary if unit is already connected to services or subdivided. Rate of charges for providing new services.

Headings	Items to be covered
5 Building complex description	• Total and type of accommodation provided, number of floors, yard space. General arrangements on zoning spaces and circulation, means of escape, range and number of units (date) • Form of subdivision, type of tenancy, direct or indirect, equipment provided • Policy for allowing change within the building shell
6 Services available	• Heating, lighting, water and waste. Power, gas, telephone (public and private) • Special facilities (piped gases, gantries, fume cupboards, special floor loadings) • Methods of metering • Restrictions on use • Control of thermostats and switches etc
7 Opening hours	• Weekdays, weekends • Special arrangements for access to building or site • Security alarm policy, bells etc
8 Entrance areas, security arrangements and key policy	• Reception, arrangements for visitors, messengers, mail (pigeon holes), collection and delivery of production materials. Domestic deliveries (post, milk). Staffing of porter's cabin/reception • Responsibility for licensees'/tenants' locks (spare key left with management) • Master key to front door and policy when lost, deposits etc. Entryphone • Fire escape keys, yard/loading bay access key, lift/hoist key • Security is joint responsibility of management and keyholders • Licensees' procedures for visitors • Possible use of security pass and its presentation. Policy towards strangers in building or site
9 Facilities	• Location and provision of communal facilities: meeting rooms, display, Information area (booking arrangements), canteen or refreshments, first aid and medical rooms or facilities, crèches or nurseries, welfare or learning facilities • Location of toilets (male and female) • Special services, printing, telex, reprographic, secretarial and book-keeping • Communal furniture and scenery, company consultation on standards and change
10 Communications within building	• Policy on reception facilities • Signposting of units and their locations (unit door, entrance area, externally) • Notice boards, location and type

Table III   Required contents of building handbook

Headings	Items to be covered
11 Parking	• General situation locally • Relation to yard or access space • Policy towards motor and pedal cycles
12 Insurance	• Overall insurance cover of the building fabric by the management or service company (included in fees) • Licensees/members/tenants to make own arrangements for their individual firm space, internal improvements, special equipment and contents relating to fire, theft, public and employees liability, loss of income, bad debts.
13 Cleaning, refuse etc	• Responsibility for common areas, extent of brief • Location of rubbish disposal, special arrangements for bulky refuse (additional charges) • Disposal of liquid wastes
14 Fire precautions	• Alarm system and fire drill • Location and managements of fire fighting equipment (types etc) • Individual extinguishers for each unit's activities (bought or hired) • Location of fire escapes and staircases leading to exits (list required) • Avoid location of rubbish and stored goods in public circulation routes • Workshop waste containers to be metal and lidded
15 Transfers and moving out procedures	• First refusal on vacant units for existing users of building • Length of notice when moving out • Financial arrangements, deposit, charges • Procedures and responsibilities with unwanted equipment, partitions etc • Keys
16 Useful general information	• List nearest letterbox, post offices, banks, libraries, shops, public transport stops – bus, rail, leisure facilities, police station, DHSS, hospital/clinic • Useful organisations related to interests of licensees/tenants: small firms, information, transport hire etc • Area map • Predominant activities in the area

routine maintenance inspections by the person responsible for the building, possibly accompanied by the architect or surveyor, are essential. This should be done with a critical eye, as familiarity with a building can often make one unaware of the slow deterioration which takes place, particularly with decorative finishes.

8.03   Improvements
Capital available for the initial installation is often limited. It is in any case an established fiscal policy to achieve a low capital expenditure even when funds may be available, but in either circumstances accountants recognise the necessity of having an adequate budget to cover maintenance and improvements. For the aim should be not only to keep pace with deterioration but to progressively improve the building, undertaking those works which were not covered in the beginning. This should be funded out of income. An amount should be reserved annually for improvements in order to build up an improvement reserve and avoid the total cost falling on those in occupation during the year the improvements are undertaken. Short-life buildings are a problem and the extent of improvements has to be related to the potential period of occupation or the possibility of the lease being renewed.

9.00 Assessing the needs of potential occupiers

The checklist in table IV is intended for the use of the management team needing to assess potential users. It will be prepared at the stage when the site and location of the units within the building are known but before the planning of individual tenancies has been considered in detail.

Table IV   Assessing potential occupiers

1 The firm
Name of particular organisation

Which of the following is the firm/organisation?
Partnership
Limited company
Subsidiary of a large group
Sole ownership
Job creation or charitably based

Number of years firm has been in operation

Date of arrival in present location

Brief description of function of the firm
Type of goods handled
Activities undertaken

2 People (including respondent)
Total number of employees

Breakdown by male/female, full time/part time

Employees in each category
Professional
Managerial
Skilled
Semi-skilled/apprentices
Unskilled

3 Present accommodation
On which floor level(s) are you accommodated now?
Is this important?

Approximate size of unit occupied (sq ft/m²)

Into how many main spaces is your unit subdivided?

What types of workspace are they?
Shop (display area) (approx size sq ft/m²)
Office (cellular or open plan)
Studio/craft room
Light industrial workshop/repair shop
Warehouse/storage area
(bracket together uses occupying a single space)

Has your floor area expanded recently?
If so, please specify when and by how much (approx)

How much additional space would you need?

4 Planning
What kind of tenancy type required?
Direct access
Indirect access
Open plan (shared space)

What kind of design of separation?
Self-contained unit
Shared space
Partly enclosed

Access for people and vehicles (cars, vans, trucks)
Importance of visitors generally
Deliveries; daily/weekly, of goods/services
Parking and loading bays
Special requirements (outside working hours etc)

Goods movement
Can goods be manhandled?
Special equipment required
Corridors for horizontal movement
Hoists/lift for vertical movement (if upper floor)

Noise
Process produces noise or vibration
Process affected by noise from others/needs to be vibration-free

Table IV   Assessing potential occupiers

Planning continued

Degree of security
For whole workspace
For tools and equipment
Bulk material storage away from workspace
Items relating to special insurances

Demands on fabric
Particular nature of operation sequence
Floor loading required (special equipment) KN/m²
Use of trolleys
Spillage (oil, liquids)
Particular floor finish required

Safety and hazard
Nearness to escapes important
Are processes dangerous?
Are materials toxic, explosive?
Any waste inflammable, toxic, explosive?
Do you use a naked flame?

Communal facilities desired
Personnel (cafeteria, recreational, creche, shop etc)
Business services (secretarial, reprographic, book-keeping)

Linkages
Trades, and works of other firms existing/future preferred
Trades on which there is dependence for servicing or support

5 Services

Visual conditions
Natural and artificial light, essential/desirable
Do you use task lighting?

Environmental conditions
Is temperature critical? preferred range 13–16°C, 16–18°C, 18–21°C
Is humidity critical?
Is mechanical extraction required?

Requirements for
Water supply, hot, cold, both
Wastes, drainage (plumbing, sinks, etc)
Electrical supply, single or three phase, number of points required
Gas
Telephone, own line needed/could share
Fire alarm/security
Any special requirements (ducting etc)

10.00   Particular management requirements for a working community

10.01   Amateur management
Where the users are highly involved, the building may not only be occupied but also run on a joint basis. A management committee from the most interested and motivated users can share the various tasks between its members. In some situations this can involve everyone in the building and then the job would be a voluntary contribution. In buildings where these tasks are only undertaken by a proportion of the members, they should be adequately compensated for their loss of 'production' time.

As an alternative, one member might take over the management role on a part-time basis, adequately compensated for his time, with or without assistance from other members, providing his business can continue to function efficiently under his part-time control.

10.02   Professional management
Where the occupants' work in terms of manhours which give a high return, it is obvious that their time will be more productive in pursuing their main job and they should employ someone else to take the running of the building off their hands. The occupants are probably specialists skilled

in their particular activity and should appreciate that the running of the building also demands a certain type of experience and personality.

10.03   The manager as catalyst

It is clear that, as with residential flat dwellers, a certain amount of superficial contact between users will take place spontaneously but it does not follow that the interaction will evolve automatically without some social engineering. The manager's role is crucial. He cannot make the members mix but he or she must endeavour to create an environment in which informal interaction can take place, acting as a catalyst by having some knowledge of the members' work and sensing the possibilities of mutual interest and co-operation, as well as by organising activities in which members can participate.

10.04   Need for on-site personnel

It may be that the manager will have responsibility for several buildings, be they working communities run for the members or properties as part of a profit-making enterprise. There is, however, no real substitute for a presence permanently based in the building to attend immediately to the problems of the building or the occupants when they arise. A comparison with another building type – residential – is pertinent: the experience gained from the shortsighted policy of having high-rise flats without caretakers, resulting in rapid deterioration and a breakdown in the relationship with tenants. The role could be carried out by a high calibre of cleaner/caretaker, security man or handyman, willing to become involved, using his initiative, and getting on well with people.

10.05   Letting

Using estate agents

If estate agents are employed, they should be fully briefed so that they appreciate how a working community differs from the conventional building with several occupants, ie in the former criteria for selection is crucial and potential members may have to be vetted. They also need to be fully aware of the 'sales appeal' of the total package offered making the most of marketing possibilities. Letting is not a one-off but a continuous operation, because of the nursery function of working communities, with embryo firms outgrowing the building. Generally, estate agents will not be accustomed to dealing with this unorthodox situation and, due to extra work involved in the continuing commitment, most working communities have dealt with the letting themselves.

Promotion of the project

Working communities have found that even though there is a great shortage of small spaces, they still have to 'sell' the community idea. The most effective way of doing this is through a sustained public relations exercise; since it is newsworthy and topical there should be no difficulty in getting local coverage. This not only brings the idea to the notice of potential members but has long-term benefits in building up the image of the working community.

If the operation of the working community is spelt out in advance, potential members are quite clear on what basis it is intended to operate so a 'self screening' process will occur. Applicants without the goodwill to co-operate will not be attracted by the concept and not pursue their enquiries.

Care in selection

The problem of a really unsociable occupant causing problems to all the other members is difficult, and some form of majority vote to evict the member could be the answer, but if he has a legal entitlement to occupy, this is impossible. It might be avoided if a representative committee of the members can 'vet' the potential member and form their own conclusions on how he will fit in.

10.06   Security

Security is a particular problem for firms contemplating joing a working community, particularly if planned with mostly office activities, on open plan principles, which allows flexibility in the use and rearrangement of space. There can be a situation where there is no separation of individual spaces. However, when firms are in occupation this fear is quickly dispelled, as a mutual trust generally develops from a vested interest in preserving the security of their own and others spaces.

A working community is in effect a large/medium sized company and in matters of security individual member firms should consider themselves as departments in a large company. Such companies seldom require security between each department, but are concerned with external and internal security.

External security

Access from outside should be channelled through one entrance, visitors always encouraged to report to the reception. This avoids visitors or messengers arriving in an unattended space unannounced and allows members to screen their visitors.

A security officer for day or night work may be of value to member firms or alternatively a contract with a security firm can be arranged. The police and fire services will need to know who to contact in an emergency.

Internal security

Like any firm with employees a shared building has to guard against pilfering. The modern attitude is that providing it does not assume large proportions a certain loss is acceptable, as the price of totally eliminating is more than the losses. In practice, as the loyalty of employees of small firms is generally greater, this is generally not a problem. Of course, in any situation where there are items of high value there has to be lockable storage or a safe. There are advantages in providing one secure strongroom for all member firms, where all items can be checked in and out by a responsible key holder.

Part III
Learning
from Experience

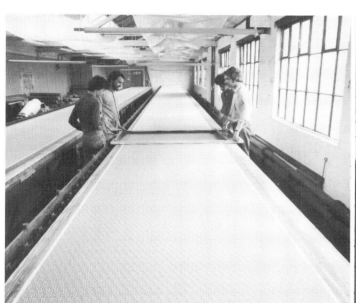

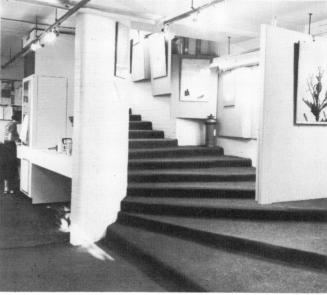

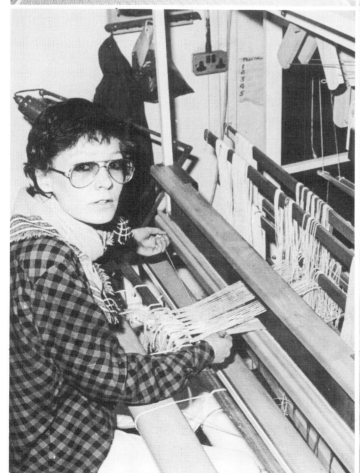

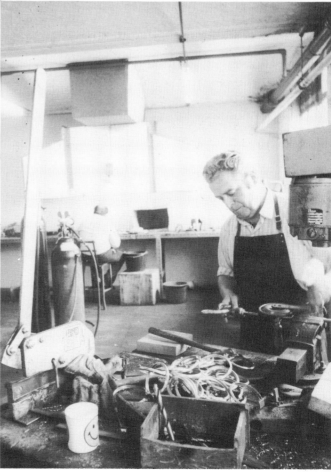

Previous page: industrial rehabilitation as a working reality.
Top left: screen printing at the Atlanta Works.
Top right: stairs to shared area at 5 Dryden Street.
Bottom left: weaving at Barley Mow Workspace.
Bottom right: machining at Meadow Mills.

17 Completed Schemes

1.00 Review of experience so far

1.01 Growth of experience

Until the mid 1970's little thought and meagre resources had been put towards the accommodation requirements of small firms. The majority of building effort was directed at new factories on green field sites often for specialised manufacturing processes. Some notable exceptions existed however, such as the GLC's flatted factories in Hackney, developed to provide premises for small firms displaced through comprehensive redevelopment schemes.

The publication of the Bolton report on the small firm sector in 1971 stimulated a concern to support and nurture small firms. This was followed in turn by a number of surveys by local authorities of the general condition of inner city industrial premises which revealed that the problems most consistently reflected about premises were lack of room for expansion, access for delivery vehicles, the constraint of multi-storied buildings, and shortage of storage space.

Successive political parties have realised small firms to be an important factor in any plans for the regeneration of an ailing economy. The national papers recognise them as newsworthy and *The Guardian* provides an excellent forum within its small business page published weekly. Since 1975 through the pioneering work of organisations such as URBED and ARC (Action Resource Centre) grass roots developments to convert old buildings for workshop space and set up community enterprises have steadily increased. Recent years have seen a shift of informed opinion towards the problems of inner city industry. The pioneering approaches of Rochdale's industrial improvement areas with its special powers have been followed up and adopted by other authorities, with support from the Inner Urban Areas Act.

SAVE's commendable campaign to preserve our heritage and recognise the industrial mill towns of the north as assets rather than burdens has focussed attention on the potential of our industrial past.

1.02 Experience of historical precedents

The multiple tenancy of large buildings by small firms, working on a co-operative basis is not a new concept. In the 17th and 18th centuries the lace makers of Nottingham shared workspace in large single buildings. In urban centres it was common for individual craftsmen to work in attic workshops above their homes. During the Victorian era a common city centre building type was the commodity exchange where individual traders had their own offices associated with the common trading area. In the 1920s and 1930s an integral part of inner city redevelopment was the construction of small storage and industrial units with staircase and goods lift access.

Projects such as the working communities at 5 Dryden Street and Clerkenwell workshop have a long pedigree. The success of these schemes has stimulated a number of similar developments, both in London (Omnibus Workshops and Wandsworth Workshops) and the regions (King Street, Bristol).

Many of the large mills of the North West have been in multiple use since the early 1960s as the textile industry began to decline. Meadow Mills near Stockport was converted for multiple letting to small units by a developer who had previously undertaken a number of similar developments during the 1960s. The building accommodates over 500 people and has had few vacancies since inception.

1.03 Experience in funding and development

A number of the schemes included in this study could not rely on traditional funding for the development. Their growth has been dependent on the rents from the first tenancies being used to fund the development of the completed project. The conversion of an old London General Omnibus factory in North Road, Islington, begun in 1979 comprises 5,500m^2 of gross floor area and is being developed in stages as rents come in to support the continuing building work.

The Avon Trading Estate in the London Borough of Hammersmith originally built in the late 1880s as a furniture depository and laundries for Whiteleys, was acquired in 1970 by the Greater London Council for a road widening scheme, which was abandoned in 1975. Until 1980 the site, which covers 1.1 ha and has a net total of 35,000m^2 of floor space, was about 60 per cent occupied. The site has recently been sold to a private developer, who in close liaison with the London Borough's of Hammersmith and Fulham is

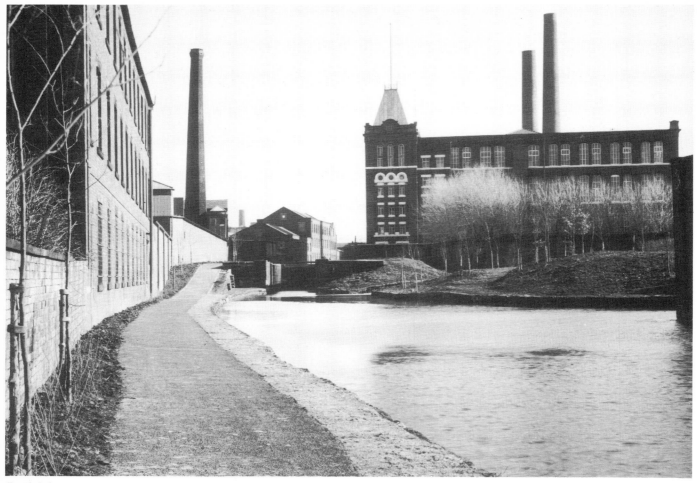

Rochdale industrial improvement area. The importance of industrial relics was recognised by a SAVE report in 1980. Canals are used by many pleasure boats.

developing a mixture of new and converted premises to provide a variety of unit sizes and rental levels. Like North Road, the Avonmore site will be developed over a number of years, gradually building up confidence and improving conditions so that established firms can continue to be accommodated and new firms brought in.

1.04 Experience gained from feasibility data

In parallel with the continuing number of schemes being completed and occupied, a body of data is continuously accruing in the form of feasibility studies. The feasibility study may be scribbled on the back of an envelope, relying on the insights and experience of the developer who will undertake the work, or may consist of a formal feasibility report forming the focus for fund raising and attracting potential tenants. Whichever the case, the early feasibility work is critical to the success of the project. The success of the majority of the schemes described has been dependent on the choice of suitable buildings, an accurate assessment of the potential market, and a precise understanding of the type of building work required related to the funds available.

Funding for these initial studies is difficult to obtain. The work may be undertaken speculatively, which can easily lead to poor decisions; it may be funded by local authorities, charitable trusts, or out of profits from previous schemes. The GLC through the London Industrial Centre, has set up a fund to support development organisations to select potential buildings for subdivision into small units and undertake feasibility studies.

Feasibility studies undertaken by Regeneration Limited with support from this fund have resulted in projects being initiated in Acton, Stratford East, and Wandsworth.

Similar action has been taken by other local authorities. The Merseyside county council has a small unit within its planning department who have undertaken feasibility studies of selected empty buildings or declining areas to suggest alternative uses and provide a spring board for potential developers. In Darlington the amenity society in association with the local society of the RIBA has set up a project to take stock of vacant industrial space in the central area, and undertake feasibility studies of key buildings.

Owners who find themselves with buildings surplus to their needs are beginning, as part of their marketing strategy, to prepare feasibility studies of buildings and sites showing alternative use options, and apply for outline planning permission to enhance the value. The Central Electricity Board has had a marked success with this approach for several of its surplus sites. The Central Lancs Development Corporation have taken a similar approach in their attempt to find new uses and funds for Preston Docks.

Feasibility studies are clearly a valuable source of comparative data on the economic viability of different building types and development approaches. The flow of funds to seed such studies is essential, in conjunction with a 'clearing house' where feasibility reports could be collected and analysed. In many boroughs this work could be co-ordinated by the industrial development officer. The DOE through their Re-use of Industrial Buildings Service may be able to make a grant available for feasibility studies.

2.00 Variety of approaches

2.01 A national survey

The case studies which form the core of this chapter have been chosen to exemplify the variety of approaches that exist. Where successful schemes have been carried through the results have revitalised blighted areas and provided space for small firms to flourish. There are now sufficient completed initiatives available for the opportunities to be assessed, confidence engendered and positive plans formulated on how to reuse vacant buildings and revitalise decaying industrial areas.

The survey which follows is based on information collected by the authors from local planning authorities, statutory undertakers and nationalised industry on over 130 projects for the conversion of buildings for use by small firms. The case studies present a cross-section of the kinds of conversion work taking place throughout the country. The main criteria for including schemes were that they involved the reuse of an existing building, were occupied by at least three firms each using less than 500m^2 and were used for general or light industrial activities. Arts centres receiving substantial grants from the Arts Council or other sponsors were excluded but job creation projects were included.

2.02 Types of development

The types of premises provided for small firms have been broadly divided into four categories:

Community workshops
Working communities
Start-up spaces
Flatted factories.

Community workshops

Community workshops are aimed at encouraging embryo enterprises by developing skills and providing equipment and support. They are normally located within or on the edge of low income residential areas, easily accessible by female labour, young people and the disadvantaged. Community workshops normally have been set up with one or all of the following objectives:

Introducing the unemployed to skills and work through adult education or community activities
Providing the opportunity for a hobby to become a means of livelihood
Providing starter space for community inspired enterprise.

There are a variety of versions of the community workshop concept. Some workshops such as Kingsgate, West Hampstead, have been initiated by voluntary organisations. In other cases local authorities have directly developed space to foster embryo enterprises such as the new enterprise workshops in Birmingham, and the enterprise workshops at Paisley and Hamilton. With support from Manpower Services

Commission grants several community enterprises have been formed with their own converted premises, such as Telegraph Textiles in Lewisham. Others such as 50 Limited in Vauxhall have been set up purely as training centres under the Youth Opportunities Programme (YOP).

Community workshops offer a practical answer to some of the problems of regenerating run-down areas. They can help to mobilise local resources and stimulate self-help. But they need to be properly staffed and funded. This is especially difficult where a wide range of programmes and hence beneficiaries are involved. It would be tragic if cut-backs in public spending make it even more difficult to get projects of this kind going, or keep them running.

Working communities

Working communities are groups of independent small firms co-operating in sharing a building and joint services. The idea is to enjoy a scale of premises and facilities normally only available to larger companies by the use of joint purchasing power, while retaining the intimate relationship and job satisfaction which comes from working in small firms.

Working communities will normally have a full time building manager, and policy of selecting compatible firms where individual tenants can sell or share their services and resources with other firms in the building.

Although working communities can make a contribution towards the current problems of small businesses, inner city decline and unemployment, the long-term influence lies in the social interaction of the people working in the building. The initiators of some of these communities have set out to select members who have something in common, both in the principle that they will get better if there is some link between them and because of the possibility of using each others' skills to mutual advantage. Even if this informal interaction between members is not planned and encouraged it will take place spontaneously and relationships will develop.

The Federation of Working Communities was started by those involved in working communites to share their experience, to assist others in starting similar projects and to promote the concept. 5 Dryden Street, the starting point, has already been an inspiration in the formation of similar ventures at King Street Bristol and Bridlesmith Gate Nottingham.

Start-up units

Start-up units are small, cheap, easily accessible units with the minimum of communal support. Units are typically from 25–100sq m and are aimed at attracting newly formed and expanding firms. Units are rented on short leases or licences to allow firms to move on as they grow and become more established. Unlike working communities or community workshops, start-up units are self-contained with their own access.

British Steel Industries, with Regeneration Ltd acting as consultants are creating start-up units in steel closure areas. Regeneration have undertaken feasibility studies at Clyde, Hamilton, Glengarnock, Teeside, Hartlepool, Blaenau, Gwent and Cardiff. Clyde Workshops is already operating and provides 87 units of between 20 and 800m^2 for 50–60 companies, with central management and advisory services, funded by British Steel Corporation Industries. The heart of the project is 200m² of administration offices, showroom and meeting space with an additional 100 m² of canteen area.

Flatted factories

To meet the problems of relocating small firms who were displaced by comprehensive redevelopment during the 1950s and 1960s the larger municipal authorities constructed multi-storied industrial buildings with goods lift access and corridor access to small individual tenancies. This concept was termed flatted factories. Many of the large multi-storied warehouse and mill buildings that have been converted for multiple use, fulfill a similar function. The characteristics of a flatted factory or 'vertical industrial estate' are that the building is multi-storied with several separate tenancies on each floor with direct access to a goods lift. Spaces tend to have a minimum of services and to be rented on leases rather than licences with the tenant adapting the interior to meet his own specific requirements. Common amenities tend to be minimal, and the management support similar to that provided on a typical industrial estate.

The stock of completed case studies has increased, and the following are a good selection of those completed by late 1981.

3.00 Selected schemes

Community workshops
Telegraph Textiles, Lewisham
Hyson Green Workshops, Nottingham
Kingsgate Workshops, West Hampstead
Castlecliff Workshops, Edinburgh
House of Lambeth, London
St. Leonard's House Enterprise, Lancaster
New Enterprise Workshops, Birmingham
New Enterprise Workshops, Strathclyde

Working communities
5 Dryden Street, Covent Garden
Barley Mow Workspace, Chiswick
401½ Workshops, Vauxhall
Clerkenwell Workshops
Waterside Workshops, Southwark
The Barbican, Penzance.

Start-up spaces
Parsonage Farm, Burwell
Blackdown Rural Industries, Haslemere
Fort Fareham, Hampshire
Rockrome Warehouse, Liverpool
Clyde Workshops, Glasgow
Wincomlee Workshops, Newcastle-upon-Tyne.

Flatted factories
Chadkirk Mill, Stockport
Butt End Mills, Mirfield
Meadow Mills, Stockport
Avon Trading Estate, Hammersmith
Menin Works, Mitcham
Atlanta Works, Fulham.

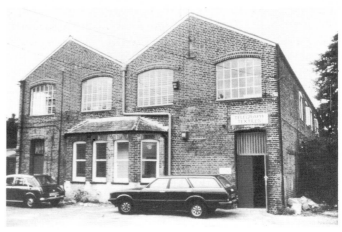

Telegraph Textiles: a conversion but no change of use, as the building previously housed light industry.

3.01 Community workshops

Telegraph Textiles, Lewisham Co-operative Working Community for Women
Age: late 19th century
Location: 8 Hatchem Park Road, Lewisham, London SE14
Date of conversion: 1980
Conversion cost: £94,000
Founder: Telegraph Hill Neighbourhood Council
Gross floor area, number of floors: 1640m² in 3 buildings/1–2 floors
Unit size: 28m²–200m²
No. of units: 7
No. of workers: 20 plus 30 in clothing factory
Rental charge: £2.25/sq ft pa, £0.75/sq ft rates
Service charge: £24.0/m²–£8.0/m²
Features: the project aims to provide employment for local women, especially single parent families, in a clothing factory. A creche is provided and it was hoped to provide machinist training facilities. However, the committee was unable to raise the necessary funds.
History: the buildings were originally used for light industry, therefore major conversion constituted no change of use.
Conversion: Minor structural alterations were made plus repartitioning and upgrading of finishes. New fences and a playground were provided to the creche area.
Funding and tenancy: The Docklands Urban Aid Programme provided capital expenditure and some running costs for the project. A private company holds the lease and sublets to Telegraph Textiles. Part of the premises is then sublet as five workshops which help fund the project.
Management and facilities: the factory is run as a co-operative with its own workers' organisation. The Telegraph Hill Neighbourhood Council acts as a steering committee and currently manages funds for the project. A social worker is employed as building manager and facilities include WCs, canteen and creche.

Hyson Green Workshops, Nottingham
Workshops in new residential garages
Age: 1971
Location: Hyson Green, Nottingham
Date of conversion: 1981

Conversion cost: £300,000 approx.
Founder: Hyson Green Development Tenants' Association
Gross floor area, number of floors: 6,000m², 1 floor workshops, 1 floor plant and exhibition area
Unit size: 20 units 25m², 6 units 50m², 2 units 60m²
Number of units: 28
Number of workers: 70
Rental charge: £30/m² pa let on assignment basis including rates/heating/car parking
Service charge: included in rental charge
Features: the project utilises unwanted newly built garage units in a 700 unit housing complex of 24 five-storey blocks. The garages will provide 28 light industrial units, (six units for training purposes, six larger commercial workshops and fourteen units for new firms).
History: the development association had a long public battle to persuade the council that the 510 garages were underused and satisfy the city and county councils on the ground of noise and traffic generation.
Conversion: only half of the two-storey garage blocks has been converted with workshops on the ground floor, and plant room plus exhibition area on the first floor which also acts as a sound buffer to flats above. There is no natural lighting and the scheme is artificially heated and ventilated.
Funding and tenancy: the inner city budget has paid construction costs. An MSC training workshop for 50 places is proposed using at least six workshops.
Management and facilities: the project is to be run by a limited company with charitable status comprising the city council and tenants. Profits are to be invested in the project. It is hoped to have a team of managers to deal with day-to-day promotions, marketing and the expansion of the co-operative idea. Trent Polytechnic are supporting the project within the small business unit providing advice and help on management of small businesses and on the project itself.
The training services division of the Manpower Service Commission are providing a £14,000 training scheme for 'Start Your Own Business' geared specifically towards tenants in the Hyson Green Area.

Kingsgate Workshop, West Hampstead
Community enterprise craft workshops
Age: late 19th century
Location: Kingsgate Road, West Hampstead, London
Date of conversion: 1977/8
Conversion cost: £35,000
Founder: Camden Industrial Action Group and West Hampstead Community Centre
Gross floor area, number of floors: 140m² 3 floors
Unit size: 15m² upwards
Number of units: 35
Number of workers: 50
Rental charge: £1.80/sq ft pa (1980)
Service charge: 7 per cent rent; electricity and gas metered
Features: the workshops are aimed to assist local craftsmen and artists to establish themselves and hopefully generate employment; also to provide education and training skills through day and evening classes for local residents, especially the young.
History: the project shows how even with a short-life lease and limited finance a community group can bring a derelict factory back into use.

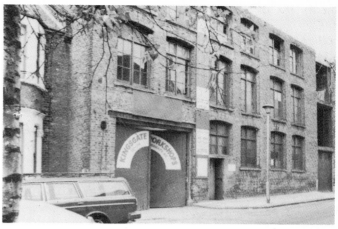

Kingsgate: decline halted, the former depository provides good accommodation on three floors.

Conversion: minimum conversion work was undertaken. It consisted of installing plumbing, electricity and glazing and providing fire protection to the structure and means of escape. The lean of the structure was arrested by employing a honeycomb pattern of partitioning with a central corridor; existing staircases were used. Architects provided considerable advice and technical support.
Funding and tenancy: the secretary of the trustees made available private funds for the conversion which is being reclaimed through rents. Apprentices to craftsmen are paid by the Manpower Services Commission but are treated as normal employees by the firms for whom they work.
Management and facilities: there is one general manager working part-time, a part-time gallery manager and a caretaker. There is a showroom/gallery displaying work of craftsmen and artists in the building which is also available for outside exhibitions.

Castlecliff Workshop, Edinburgh
Youth Craft Training Centre in Edinburgh
Age: 1880
Location: Castlecliff Workshops, 25 Johnston Terrace, Edinburgh
Date of conversion: 1977–8 and 1980 onwards
Conversion cost: Not yet finalised £90–170,000
Founder: Scottish Craftsmanship Association Ltd
Gross floor area, number of floors: 1700m²/3 floors
Unit size: Approx. 20.5m²
Number of units: 54 main units, 24 smaller units
Number of workers: 70
Rental charge: Profits from sale of work ploughed back into project. Building owned by District Council and leased on a repair and maintenance lease to SCA Ltd.
Service charge: Not known
Features: the project houses varied training craft workshops for school leavers under skilled craftsmen and manager. Products include knitwear and articles in wood, including furniture and fitted joinery items.
History: The building was originally built for use as married quarters for troops guarding the castle and its cellular design was adapted for workshop use by trainee labour.
Conversion: Due to the overall design and the stone construction, very little work was required to meet the fire regulations and general requirements of the building

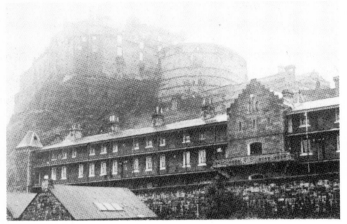

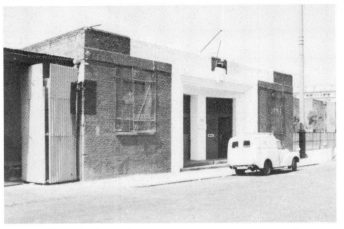

Castlecliff Workshops seen from the Grassmarket. A derelict former barracks until 1977 when it was taken over for unemployed school leavers, it has been transformed into training workshops.

House of Lambeth: behind an unprepossessing frontage 24 formerly unemployed youths find an opportunity to work and develop skills in an area of high unemployment in central London.

regulations, but new plumbing and electrical services have had to be provided throughout. A few openings have been made in walls between 'cells' to architects' layouts. Extensive repair work is, however, still required to secure the roof, galleries, and stonework on a long term basis.

Funding and tenancy: Grants and loans were obtained under the government's former Job Creation Programme, the current Youth Opportunities Programme, from private trusts and companies, and from the Historic Buildings Council.

Management and facilities: A full-time manager was appointed by the Scottish Craftsmanship Association who organised funding. As the project moves into the production phase, additional staff will be brought in to consider marketing and costing the craft work. Facilities include showrooms, exhibition rooms and canteen.

House of Lambeth, London
Woodworking Workshop for the unemployed
Age: 1930s
Location: 220 Farmers Road, London SE5
Date of conversion: 1970s
Conversion cost: £40,000
Founder: Lady Margaret Hall Settlement
Gross floor area, number of floors: 550/m²/2½ floors
Unit size: 550/m²
Number of units: 1
Number of workers: 31
Rental charge: First year rent free, £3.2/m² pa
Service charge: Nil
Features: government grants, local authority co-operation and voluntary effort have combined to provide an employment scheme to produce toys and furniture. People with no previous work record now leave after one year with basic woodworking skills and currently 95 per cent find employment.
History: the GLC purchased the 2½ storey former butter factory for redevelopment but plans were delayed and the building was found lying derelict and vandalised. 2130m² was partitioned off and let to others and the rest converted to a workshop with a three year renewable lease.

Conversion: conversion included very basic cleaning, water proofing, renewal of glass, door locks etc. Some replanning was carried out by removing internal partitions and existing lavatories were replaced in the semi-basement. Recycled materials were used to build extra fire escapes and partitioning, much of which was carried out by the future tenants.
Funding and tenancy: the government granted £70,000 for the inception of the project and private enterprise has donated another £23,000 which financed conversion and the first year salaries. Government grants enabled the Lady Margaret Hall Settlement to bring in a professional manger and send the unemployed people to the London College of Furniture for initial training.
Management and facilities: the first manager was seconded from Rank Xerox for a period of one year and two managers have been recruited subsequently in the normal manner, their salaries being paid by the Manpower Services Commission. At present the factory is able to make enough profit to cover half its costs. It is hoped that in the future the scheme will be converted into a workers' co-operative in which the employees will become sole shareholders. The factory houses workshops, design area, showroom and managers office.

St Leonard's House Enterprise Lancaster
University Laboratories reused as a seed bed for small firms
Age: 19th century
Location: St. Leonard Gate, Lancaster
Date of conversion: 1961 and 1971
Cost of conversion: £200,000 and £9,000
Founder: Lancaster City Council
Gross floor area, number of floors: 2800m²/6 floors
Unit size: approx. 100m² upwards
Number of units: 8 but can be subdivided
Number of workers: 56
Rental charge: £1.82/m² pa + rates and insurance
Service charge: £12.30/m², includes all services with heating, electricity, gas, water, hall porter
Features: benevolent attitude from the city and university has provided start-up units for small scientific, design or technology-based firms.
History: the six storey building was originally a furniture

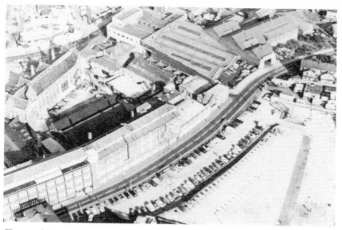

From their origins as a university laboratory the buildings provide an ideal seed-bed for high-technology, science-based enterprises. Lancaster Synthesis Ltd, manufacturing fine chemicals, started in 1972.

workshop. Later bought by the city council, it was used as initial departmental offices and laboratories for the university. Part of it now provides an ideal 'seed bed' for small firms. The rest currently used by the university for storage; a sublet to the adult education department is to be taken over in order to expand the scheme.

Conversion: very little renovation work needed to be done by the present group, except some subdivision and extra fire doors added in 1971. The major conversion and fitting out of benches and services was done by the university in 1961 and was inherited by the present enterprise.

Funding and tenancy: enterprise Lancaster in a joint venture between Lancaster city council and the university to encourage new small firms using the resources of both organisations.

Management and facilities: there is a full manager within the city council and firms who expand beyond one floor (which it is hoped they will) must seek larger premises elsewhere in the city. The management helps new firms with initial office services, business contacts advice and information from university and other sources.

New Enterprise Workshops, Birmingham
Communal facilities to encourage new innovations
Age: 19th century
Location: 99–103 Clifton Road, Balsall Heath, Birmingham
Date of conversion: 1978/9
Cost of conversion: £45,000
Founder: Industrial Development Group of Birmingham City Planning Department
Gross floor area, number of floors: 460m²/1 & 2 floors approx.
Unit size: 25m² plus 80m² workshops
Number of units: 7 workshops, 2 offices
Number of workers: 27
Rental charge: nominal licence fee £5 p.w.
Service charge: nominal licence fee £1 p.w.
Features: in this pilot workshop scheme the emphasis is to encourage innovations in manufacturing new products, modifying old products, providing a service; thus aiming to stimulate local employment. A larger scheme is now under way.

History: the building was formerly two houses with a single storey print shop later built.

Conversion: the main shop was partitioned with breeze walls to a height of 3m (10 ft.) Power, light and heat were provided to each unit. New flooring, air circulation system and power supply were supplied.

Funding and tenancy: financial help was obtained through the probation service and the Manpower Services Commission who initially paid the salaries of the manager, technician and caretaker for six months. Funding has since come from partnership areas scheme. The use of a nursery unit will be available for a period of 3–12 months at a nominal licence fee. Tenants are responsible for puchasing their own materials and special tools.

Management and facilities: help is given in all areas of business from workshop management and professional help from external sources. There are separate nursery units and communal areas for metal machinery, wood machinery, welding and plant spraying. If a business proves viable it moves on to other permanent accommodation. Help is provided from the city offices to find suitable factory units.

New Enterprise Workshops, Strathclyde
Industrial development units
Age: not known
Location: Portland Place, Hamilton, Strathclyde
Date of conversion: 1976
Cost of conversion: not known
Founder: Strathclyde Regional Council
Gross floor area, number of floors: 325/m²/1 floor
Unit size: 8m²–50m²
Number of units: 5
Number of workers: 11
Rental charge: £40 per month rent and rates
Service charge: material and telephone costs
Features: the enterprise workshops facilitate would-be manufacturers to develop new products and allow them to be taken to the point of testing for commercial viability at minimum overheads cost. Facilities are open to employed or unemployed with a good idea which has a possible commercial future in the region.

History: originally a gas works store.

Conversion: the workshop is subdivided into offices and workshops. There is a common area equipped as a small machine shop with work benches for small projects. Additionally there are a number of private workshop units for development of larger items.

Funding and tenancy: the project is organised by Strathclyde regional council's industrial development unit. Users pay a small fee for the use of facilities including the occasional use of machines. Substantial machines are charged on a small hourly rate 10p–15p per hour; materials and telephone calls are also charged.

Management and facilities: applicants are provided with a work bench, vice and possibly hand tools. Experienced advisors are available to give help and guidance where appropriate. In some cases arrangements may be made for part of the work to be undertaken by qualified tradesmen. Facilities are provided for an agreed period of time to develop a prototype. It has been found that the common workshop areas are generally more in demand.

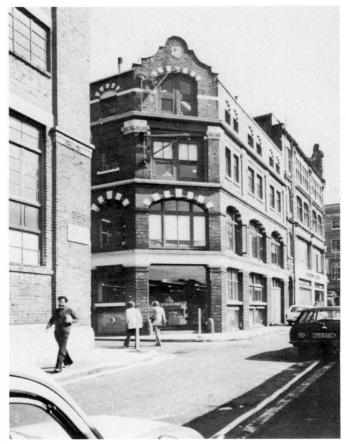

No 5 Dryden Street, Covent Garden: extension of former coach builders' and harness makers' premises.

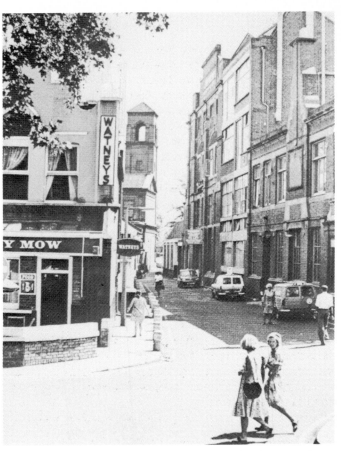

Four-storey building on right is Barley Mow Workspace, housing 100 member firms. Previously a Sanderson wallpaper factory, the building now houses drawing offices and workshops.

3.02   Working Communities

5 Dryden Street, Covent Garden, London
Multidisciplinary design firms housed in warehouse
Age: 1910
Location: 5 Dryden Street, Covent Garden, London WC2
Date of conversion: 1972
Cost of conversion: not known
Founder: architects David Rock and John Townsend
Gross floor area, number of floors: 2000/m^2/4 floors plus basement
Unit size: 5–175m^2
Number of units: up to 70
Number of workers: 180
Rental charge: phase 1 £24.75/m^2 pa, phase II £49.50/^{2} pa
Service charge: workshop average £16.25/m^2 pa
Features: the working space provides office accommodation for designers, engineers, printers and model makers who work in ad hoc co-operation.
History: the building originally housed coach builders, harness makers, then printing works.
Conversion: the building is now sub-divided into open-plan offices, design studios and cellular workshops. The major work was to replace the entrance with a window, install hot water and the French Tekemecanique overhead power and telephone channel system.
Funding and tenancy: funding was through the foundation of a service firm in which members act as shareholders in the building. Amortisation is over the period of lease plus the original rent for the unconverted building.

Phase I   eight year lease,
Phase II   three year lease (since renewed)

Management facilities: All members hold voting shares in the service company that holds the lease and operates the building. There are 3 permanent directors and 3 directors elected annually by an AGM. There is a manager, assistant, reception/telephonist and part-time book-keeper. Games room free tea and coffee, reception, conference rooms, technical library, kitchen and art gallery are provided as communal facilities.

Barley Mow Workspace, Chiswick
Small business communally housed in a former wallpaper factory
Age: 1890
Location: 10 Barley Mow Passage, Chiswick, London W4
Date of conversion: 1976
Cost of conversion: not known
Founders: architects John Morton, David Rock and John Townsend
Gross floor area, number of floors: 3636m^2/4 floors
Unit size: 5/m^2–80m^2
Number of units: 125
Number of workers: 250
Rental charge: £66.6/m^2 pa (studio) £26.9/m^2 pa (workshops)

Service charge: £96.7/m² pa (studio) £81.7/m² pa (workshops)

Features: the aim of Barley Mow Workspace is to provide sympathetic office, design studio and workshop accommodation for small business. Tenants participate in the running of the building through the Workspace Association.

History: Barley Mow Workspace is housed in what was originally Sanderson's wallpaper factory.

Conversion: the building was converted to an open-plan arrangement with space divided by demountable acoustic screens. Services are dropped from a power grid system fixed at ceiling height. Improvements were made to heating and fire escapes.

Funding and tenancy: long term finance was provided by the Cornhill Insurance Company; short term by directors and bank borrowing. There is a landlord – tenant relationship with extensive facilities provided at cost by the landlord as part of the package. These are controlled by the association of users.

Management and facilities: there is a full-time manager, secretary, receptionists, book-keepers, two telephonists and handyman. The use of coffee and restaurant areas, showers etc is included in the service charge. Individual member companies provide printing, computer, restaurant, xeroxing and other services and there is also considerable traffic between member firms.

401½ Workshops, Wandsworth, London
Workshops for artist craftsmen
Age: 19th century
Location: 401½ Wandsworth Road, London SW8
Date of conversion: 1970
Cost of conversion: not known
Founder: Private individual
Gross floor area, number of floors: 1000m²/2 floors
Unit size: 100m²–500m²
Number of units: 23
Number of workers: 50
Rental charge: £8/per week including services
Service charge: not known
Features: open-plan and enclosed workshops are provided for craftsmen designers on a non-profit making basis.
History: the ex-warehouse was converted with minimum alterations.
Conversion: minor repairs, fire-proofing, electrical refitting, servicing and partitioning were carried out and the project was managed on a do-it-yourself basis.
Funding and tenancy: funds for the conversion came from personal capital and membership fees.
Management and facilities: the building is managed through a tenants' co-operative with a membership scheme. A dyeing room, kiln, dark room, printing room and use of light industrial machinery are available as communal facilities.

Clerkenwell Workshops, London
Local industries communally rehoused
Age: turn of the century
Location: 31 Clerkenwell Close, London EC1
Date of conversion: 1976 onwards
Conversion costs: approximately £300,000

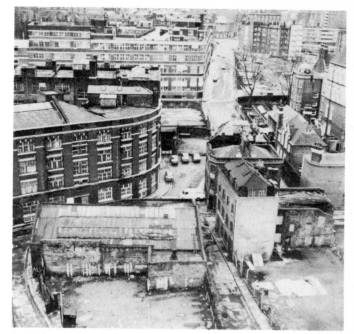
Clerkenwell Workshops.

Founder: four private individuals
Gross floor area, number of floors: 6000m² in 2 linked buildings/5 & 7 floors
Unit size: 15m²–150m²
Number of units: 130
Number of workers: 350
Rental charge: £34.90/m² pa (mid 1980)
Service charge: included in rental charge
Features: accommodation is provided for the rich range of skills from the Clerkenwell area including metal work, printing, instrument making, weaving etc. Firms often utilise each others skills. The buildings which originally provided employment for 40, now houses 350 workers.
History: the building was a mail-order warehouse until it fell redundant. Its reuse was initiated by four individuals anxious to establish an economically viable but socially responsible working community for local firms. The workshops received a 1976 Business and Industry Award.
Funding and tenancy: the four directors formed a limited liability company and funds for the scheme. These were a £5,000 charitable grant; £4,000 charitable loan, £5,000 overdraft; £5,000 personal capital. All remaining funds were taken out of income. The building had an initial 5 year wind and water lease which has now been extended for another 25 years. Letting is on a monthly licence.
Management and facilities: the founder-directors still manage the building through a standard registered company with informal contact with a workshop users' association. A salaried manager and receptionist are planned, although at present only two out of four directors draw a small salary as company employees. Canteen, storage, teaching and 'newstart' workshop facilities are provided with meeting, rehearsal and exhibition spaces for hire. A linked urban renewal trust was formed to take up the charitable aspects of the work and to prepare for the Workshop's role as one of Britain's 50 demonstration projects during the Urban Renaissance Year of 1981.

Waterside Workshops, Southwark, London
DIY Workshops and theatre in conservation area
Age: 1870s
Location: 99 Rotherhithe St, SE16
Date of conversion: 1975 onwards
Conversion cost: £130,000
Founder: two private individuals
Gross floor area, number of floors: 850m²/5 floors
Unit size: 10–50m²
Number of units: 19
Number of workers: 21
Rental charge: monthly membership rate for basic unit
Service charge: included in rental charge
Features: through a blend of public and private funding, plus individual co-operation and endeavour the Waterside Workshops now house a drama studio and a mixture of small workshops.
History: originally a granary, the building is situated in a dockland conservation area. It was bought by the GLC in 1970 on a compulsory purchase order and left to fall derelict until 1974. Renovation was begun by workshop members on a DIY basis and plans are being made to utilise an adjacent building as a fully fledged theatre.
Conversion: major and minor repairs were carried out plus fire-proofing, fire escape, electrical refitting, servicing and partitioning. The low ceiling heights of 2m have caused restrictions on reuse but a mixture of cellular and open plan accommodation has been provided.
Funding and tenancy: money for the project came from personal capital, tenants' rent and grants, although the lease is still under discussion with the landlord, the GLC. Craftsmen are elected as members to the Waterside and pay a basic monthly membership for the basic unit size with a surcharge for extra space.
Management and facilities: there is a full-time manager and the facilities of tools, van, darkroom, exhibition display, cafe and bar are communal.

The Barbican, Penzance
Craft workshop and gallery in tourist area
Age: 18th century
Location: Penzance harbour, Cornwall
Date of conversion: 1972
Conversion cost: £15,000
Founder: Percy Williams Development Ltd
Gross floor area, number of floors: 600m²–100m²
Number of units: 9
Number of workers: 10
Rental charge: £250–£350 pa for workshops, £1,500 pa for coffee shop, £1,250 pa for gallery
Service charge: rates
Features: this is an example of the modest craft centre, increasingly common in tourist areas. Currently it is used for workshops, coffee shop, aquarium, gallery and exhibition space.
History: originally the building was a fish store and later was used as a grain store. The conversion was initiated by the owners, a local firm of surveyors.
Conversion: the building had been in a very poor condition. Renovation included new foundations, damp-proofing, drainage, concrete stair, fire-proofing of ceilings and doors and renewal of windows.

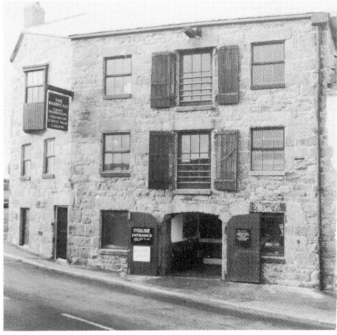

Barbican, Penzance, the main gallery entrance; craft orientated uses for an attractive former storage building on the quayside in a tourist area.

Funding and tenancy: there are four separate tenancies of which the gallery and one workshop form one; the craft workshops another; the coffee shop a third; and aquarium a fourth.
Management and facilities: tenants have their own committee and liaise with the potter who resides next door and acts as building manager.

3.03   Start-up spaces

Parsonage Farm, Burwell, Oxfordshire
Cow shed turned electronics workshop
Age: 17th century
Location: Burwell, Cambridge
Date of conversion: 1977
Cost of conversion: £10,000 approx.
Founder: private individual
Gross floor area, number of floors: 120m²/2 floors
Unit size: 120m²
Number of units: 1
Number of workers: 10
Rental charge: Nil
Service charge: Nil
Features: the electronics factory is housed in an old barn on a commune. The barn is part of a group of listed buildings, and was formerly a cowshed.
History: the commune was originally founded in 1971, and a small business called Delta-T Devices was set up at the same time to manufacture ecologically appropriate scientific instruments. In 1977 the firm needed to expand and chose to renovate and convert the old barn on the site.
Conversion: the design was prepared by a local firm of architects and most of the work was done by members of the commune and the business. The workshop space comprises an electronic assembly room and sound-proofed machine

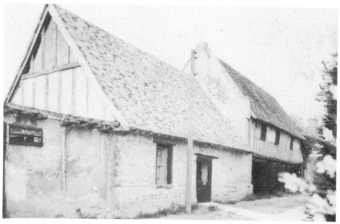

Parsonage Farm, Burwell. A former roofless cowshed (foreground) houses an electronics laboratory with package store over.

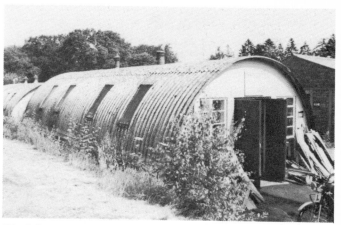

Blackdown Rural Industries; A Nissen encampment nestled in a hollow shaded by trees provides work, but not with the blessing of the local community.

shop on the ground floor, with storage areas above. Adjacent barns on the site are at present used mainly for domestic storage, but there are plans to convert one of them for further expansion on a similar basis.

Funding and tenancy: the capital for the conversion came from the business funds (largely retained profits). The whole site is owned by Parsonage Farm Housing Co-operative Limited. No rent is paid.

Management and facilities: 7 of the 9 commune members work in Delta-T Devices. The business remains financially separate from the commune. Commune and business decisions are made by the members of the respective groups but obviously interests overlap to a considerable extent. Other activities at the commune include a pottery and jewellery-making business. The surrounding garden and grounds are cultivated organically by the commune members to produce food for their own use.

Blackdown Rural Industries, Surrey
Private development of rural site for industrial nursery
Age: 1940
Location: Haste Hill, Haslemere
Date of conversion: 1976
Conversion cost: not known
Founder: private individual
Gross floor area, number of floors: 3200m²/1 floor
Unit size: 40m²–300m²
Number of units: 30
Number of workers: 155
Rental charge: £20.90/m² pa
Service charge: £2.68/m² pa
Features: the site contains 30 Nissen and Quonset huts which have been organised into start-up units for light industry employing many young people.
History: originally a naval research establishment, the land was purchased from the DoE who had intended to create a management training centre. The site was originally bought with a house which, when later sold, covered costs.
Conversion: most tenants could move in straight away although there was some difficulty over fire regulations due to the flame spread hazard of the ceiling tiles. Users installed their own partitioning, some taking two huts and linking

them with a covered way.
Funding and tenancy: this is an example of an opportunistic but benevolent private development. The director acts as informal advisor on business problems and gives support in bank applications for finance.
Management and facilities: the owner aims to have a large complementary mixture of industries on the site and employs a small labour force to help tenants with building conversion and building maintenance. Future plans include an operation to accommodate the post-nursery stages for the firms on a new site.

Fort Fareham Northern Galleries, Hampshire
Disused fortifications as a nucleus for industrial estate
Age: 1860
Location: Fort Fareham Industrial Estate, Newgate Lane, Hampshire
Date of conversion: 1978 to present day
Cost of conversion: not known
Founder: Fareham Borough Council
Gross floor area (including storage), number of floors: 1500m²/single storey
Unit size: 30m²–70m² (not including officers' mess)
Number of units: 25
Number of workers: 100 approx (Northern Galleries)
Rental charge: to be assessed after rent free period
Service charge: infrastructure payment of £750–£1500 depending on size of units (once and for all payment)
Features: the Northern Galleries form part of Fort Fareham, and ancient monument. Part of the fort grounds were leased by local authority for development to house light engineering, car repairs, joinery workshop, builders store, sign maker, electro-plating and the council's architectural salvage store.
History: the fort was constructed circa 1860 as part of a defensive ring around Portsmouth and Gosport. It was finally abandoned by the army in 1960 and suffered at the hands of vandals until 1971.
Conversion: planning permission was obtained by the borough council for light industrial use and the council provided an access road, car parking, street lighting and services to the galley site. Lessees are required to restore the 25

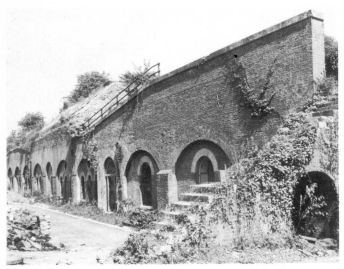

Fort Fareham, Hampshire. The arched bays of the fort's gun emplacement are well suited to the needs of small workshops.

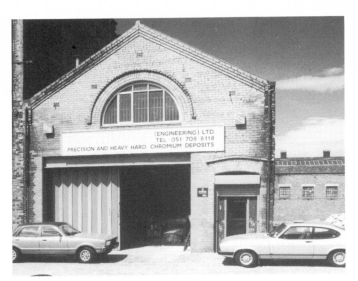

Rockrome, Liverpool. Formerly a transport annexe.

units which make up the galleries in accordance with design prepared by the local authority and DoE ancient monuments division.

Funding and tenancy: the tenants pay a simple payment of £750 to £1,500 for the infrastructure which may be paid over a two year period interest free. Leases are for 25 years with rent free periods ranging from 3 to 5 years depending on works required.

Management: northern Galleries are managed by the borough valuer's section, Fareham borough council.

Rockrome, Liverpool

Single storey warehouse converted by redundant workers
Age: 1880
Location: 11 Cornhill, Wapping, Liverpool
Date of conversion: 1977
Conversion cost: £10,000
Founders: two private individuals
Gross floor area, number of floors: 120m^2/1 floor
Unit size: 120m^2
Number of units: 1
Number of workers: 3–4
Rental charge: £7000 pa
Service charge: not known
Features: Rockrome is a hard chrome plating service located opposite Albert Docks in central Liverpool. If the firm had not started up at least 22 local firms would have had to take their businesses to Newcastle, Glasgow or London.
History: the founders were made redundant in 1976 by the closure of Whitley Ling and Neill, precision tool makers. They had worked all their lives in tool-making and chrome-plating and with their £6000 redundancy pay and the opportunity to buy equipment from the closing firm, decided to set up independently.
Conversion: the partners were offered space in new start-up units in which they would have been unable to dig the two processing pits and which were too flimsy to house the crane necessary. Most of the conversion work was undertaken by the partners themselves.

Funding and tenancy: the partners had difficulties locating a suitable building and were assisted by an interested local business man in negotiations. No money was borrowed for the conversion and the building is now leased from Mersey.
Notes: the original building consisted of little more than a basic shell. Conversion work included installation of basic services (drainage, water, gas, electricity, WCs etc), reception and office.
Management and facilities: the firm aims to take on two or three additional employees and extend at the rear of its property.

Clyde workshops, Glasgow

British Steel Industry instigated workshops for small industries
Age: not known
Location: Tollcross Industrial Village, Fullarton Road, Glasgow
Date of conversion: 1979
Cost of conversion: not known
Founder: British Steel (Industry) Limited
Gross floor area, number of floors: 6500m^2/11 buildings of 1 or 2 floors; site area 8 acres.
Unit size: 20m^2–800m^2
Number of units: 90 units let to 65 companies (including 52 new enterprises).
Number of workers: 580
Rental charge: £13.30/m^2 pa upwards plus rates and electricity
Service charge: included in rental charge
Features: British Steel launched the programme to bring new employment into an area affected by steel closure.
History: originally the site of British Steel iron works, the company instigated start-up spaces for small firms when it closed the site.
Funding and tenancy: the total enterprise is funded by British Steel (Industry) including the lease of the site, consultants' fees, building conversions, site management and management advisory service. There is a monthly licence fee and electricity is metered.

Management and facilities: BSI also help by buying equipment and leasing it to tenants. The project has already proved commercially viable and the initial cost of the project will be in the order of £600 per job created. There are catering, clubs and conference rooms plus on-site free management consultancy and administrative service for tenants. Services include security, waste disposal, street lighting, cleaning and building insurance.

Wincomlee Workshops, Newcastle upon Tyne
Engineers' offices converted to industrial workshops
Age: 1900
Location: White Street, Walker, Tyne & Wear
Date of conversion: 1980
Conversion cost: not known
Founder: City of Newcastle upon Tyne
Gross floor area, number of floors: 2,700m^2/ floors
Unit size: 150m^2–500m^2
Number of units: 10–12
Number of workers: not known
Rental charge: approx £13.00m^2
Service charge: not known
Features: this is one of the few industrial building and refurbishments in the Tyne and Wear district. It is situated one street away from the river in a shabby light industrial area outside the industrial improvement areas.
History: originally constructed as draughting offices for an enginering firm, the building has excellent window lighting. It was subsequently used by Jacksons the tailors before falling redundant. The building is well constructed and has some fine details.
Conversion: the refurbishment to architects' specifications has provided workshops for small light industrial firms such as electricians and clothiers.
Funding and tenancy:
Management and facilities: there is a caretaker and central reception connected to the units by intercom.

Chadkirk Mill, near Stockport
Light industrial workshops in a rural setting
Age: 1870s
Location: Chadkirk Mill, Romilly, Stockport
Date of conversion: 1973–78
Conversion cost: not known
Founder: private individual
Gross floor area, number of floors: 7500m^2/1–2 floors
Unit size: 90m^2–1400m^2; site area 14 acres
Number of units: 24
Number of workers: 150
Rental charge: £6.90/m^2 ground floor pa; £6.45/m^2 top floor pa
Service charge: maximum 10 per cent of rental according to location and services.
Features: this is a set of single and two storey buildings which are located adjacent to a mill pond. They now house light industrial firms of between two and ten people who do work for each other. The popularity of the small, cheap units indicates a real demand in the area.
History: originally a water driven textile mill, the various workshops, laboratories, spinning, weaving and dyeing building were converted to workshops over a five year

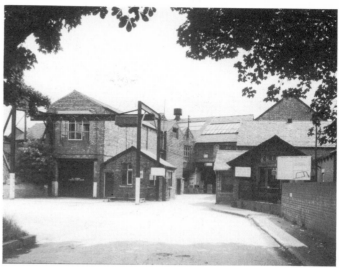

Chadkirk Mill, near Stockport. The main entrance to the former dye works. Signboard demonstrates layout of 24 units.

period. Initial problems with planning authorities concerned the access road, expansion and allowable uses.
Conversion: the ground floor was divided into units of up to 1400m^2 for tenancies such as plastic caravan chassis manufacturers, light wire manufacturers and polythene printing. The upper floors house far smaller tenancies with low fire risks (90m^2–280m^2). A fire corridor had to be built on the top floors and partitioning has been carried out to client requirements by the owner. A temporary access road skirting the mill pond was constructed.
Funding and tenancy: the building was originally bought as an investment, or for possible expansion, by Slimtrue Limited. Two tenants did their own refurbishment for which they were allowed a rent rebate.
Management and facilities: initially a full-time manager on site had responsibility for supervision and conversion work, services and administration and finding compatible tenants. Firms move within the estate as they expand.

Butt End Mills, Mirfield, Yorkshire
Disused textile mills
Age: 1860s
Location: Chadwick Lane, Mirfield, Yorks
Date of conversion: 1977
Conversion cost: indefinable; leases on full repairing and insuring terms, therefore cost partially borne by tenants.
Founder: private individual
Gross floor area, number of floors: 6300m^2/1–4 floors, 22 buildings
Unit size: 100m^2–1600m^2
Number of units: 12
Number of workers: 50+
Rental charge: £4.30/m^2 pa
Service charge: rates, water, gas and electricity are paid independently
Features: the site is adjacent to the river Calder and encloses 22 buildings, mostly single storey. It is divided in two by a railway viaduct, but generous open space allowing easy access was provided by demolishing some of the more obsolete buildings.

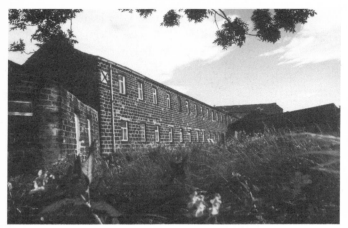

Butt End Mills, Mirfield. In its early stages of development the site was overgrown but there are encouraging signs of revival and enterprise.

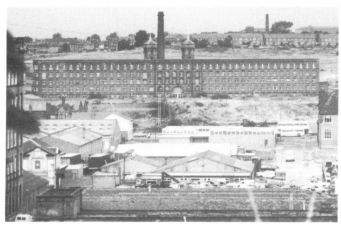

Meadow Mills, Stockport. A former spinning mill over a century old, now over 90 per cent occupied.

History: the whole complex was a former textile mill, parts of which date from the early industrial revolution. The oldest part, the four storey building, is let to a joiner who has done substantial renovation work to the property. The complex is leased in small units and only a single storey building of 1500m² remains unlet due to its large size and bad condition.

Conversion: the amount of work and capital expended on these stone-built, wood floored, slate-roofed buildings depended on their age and character but was usually greater the older the buildings.

Funding and tenancy: the site has been flexibly managed by a firm of chartered surveyors. The 'full repairing and insurance' leases are of three, five or ten years duration. The 200m² units are the most popular size for small firms although a subsidiary workshop of a large car importers uses one unit for body maintenance.

Management and facilities: the only service provided is property insurance by the landlord. Car parking is provided.

Meadow Mills, Stockport
Spinning mill converted into multiple-use units
Age: 1870s
Location: Water Street, Portwood, Stockport
Date of conversion: 1963
Conversion cost: not known
Founder: private
Gross floor area, number of floors: 2200m²/6 floors
Unit size: not known
Number of units: 45
Number of workers: 500
Rental charge: £5.50m² pa ground floor; £2.50m² pa 6th floor
Service charge: £1–£2 per week depending on services used
Features: the mill has the advantage of being close to the centre of Stockport.
History: the mill, originally a spinning mill, is now a listed building. It was bought by a builder for conversion into multiple units in 1963.
Conversion: the building is a long 16m deep block with a central corridor. Conversion consisted of installing large goods lifts, fire escapes and subdividing the space with units accommodating 2–80 people. The surrounding site has been developed for car parking, delivery/access and some new single storey individual units.

Funding and tenancy: the building was converted by a private developer with previous experience in conversion. Units are rented with two year reviews, and are at present fully let.

Management: there is a part-time building manager on site who collects rents and supervises building maintenance

Avon Trading Estate, Hammersmith, London
Furniture despository turned trading estate
Age: 1880s
Location: Avonmore Road, London W14
Date of conversion: 1959, 1981
Conversion cost: not known
Founder: Greater London Council
Gross floor area, number of floors: 30,000m²/floors
Unit size: 280m²
Number of units: 70
Number of workers: 600
Rental charge: negotiable
Service charge: not known
Features: ceiling heights of 12 to 14ft, large windows and medium depth spaces allow for a large range of activities to be housed.
History: the Victorian built depository, laundry and stables have been developed since 1959 to accommodate offices, distribution, display, clothing manufacture and studios.
Conversion: the estate was acquired by the GLC in 1970. The building was divided into 280m² units with four units to each floor around a common lift point. An internal access road with covered delivery points serves the lift shafts and a dead-end allows for three-point turns. There are 600–700 vehicle movements per day and improvements in access are now required.
Funding and tenancy: the GLC is currently offering the estate for sale. Further developments are envisaged to accommodate smaller firms.
Management and facilities: the complex is managed by the GLC surveyor's department and has a full-time caretaker. A common canteen is let as a concession and run as a small commercial venture.

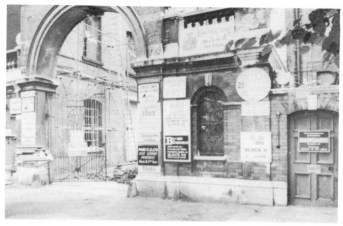

Avon Trading Estate entrance. Note the numerous notice boards.

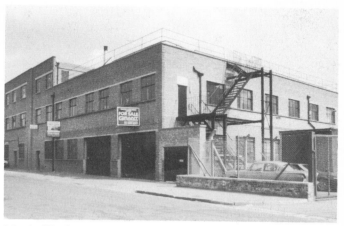

Menin Works.

Menin Works, Mitcham, Surrey
Piecemeal renewal in surplus industrial estate
Age: 1940s
Location: Menin Works, Board Road, Mitcham
Date of conversion: 1966
Conversion cost: not known
Founder: private manufacturer
Gross floor area, number of floors: 7,000m²/2–4 floors
Unit size: 400m²–2500m²
Number of units: not known
Number of workers: 200
Rental charge: £20m² pa
Service charge: 75 per cent of rent
Features: the works is composed of several blocks which have been converted into units for firms in furniture and light industry
History: the site was developed by a manufacturer who having bought out his major competition, found he had surplus factory space on his hands.
Conversion: on each block in turn, new lifts were fitted; stairs and lavatories were upgraded which counted as repair work thus avoiding serious difficulties with local authorities. Outbuildings were demolished to give adequate service access and car parking.
Funding and tenancy: Menin Works is a private company investment run by the managing director. Leases are on a 'full repairing basis' where possible.
Management: there is a full-time caretaker.

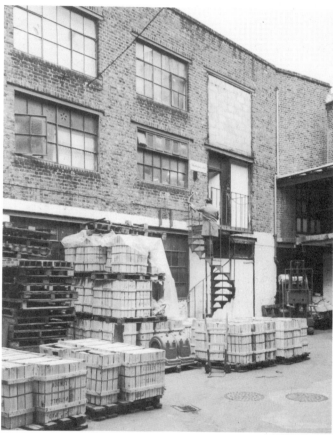

Atlanta Works, London. Light industry having the virtues of shared materials handling and storage.

Atlanta Works, Fulham, London
Paper bag factory converted to workshops
Age: 1902
Location: Atlanta Street, Fulham SW6
Date of conversion: 1974
Conversion cost: £45,000 (1974/5)
Founder: surveyors on behalf of a freeholder
Gross floor area, number of floors: 2400m²/3 floors
Unit size: 90m²–300m²
Number of units: 14
Number of workers: 60
Rental charge: £25–£36.50/m² pa
Service charge: Percentage of expenses of building on a pro rata basis approx £1.50/m²

Features: the building has been converted to house workshops in cellular units.
History: the original use of the building was as a paper bag factory.
Conversion: major repairs were made to the roof and lift; refurbishment, fire-proofing, rewiring and subdivision were carried out. Direct labour was used.
Funding and tenancy: funding was from a private bank loan and letting is by lease with warehouse agreement for ancillay storage.
Management and facilities: there is a building manager assistant who deals with day-to-day administration and warehousing arrangements. The security service, reception and goods handling are communal facilities.

References and Bibliography

Chapter 1. The Challenge Ahead.

1 SAVE *Satanic Mills*. Save, 1979.

2 LANGENBACH, R. *A future from the past: the case for conservation and reuse of old buildings in industrial communities*. Washington: US Department of Housing and Urban Development, 1977.

3 GRIPAIORS, P. 'Industrial decline in London – an examination of its causes.' *In: Urban Studies*, 4. 1977.

4 URBED *Business confidence and the urban environment*: report to the OECD, Urbed, 1980.

5 BOLTON, J. E. *Committee of inquiry on small firms*. CMND 4811. HMSO, 1972.

6 URBED *Space to work*: Report to the Hackney/Islington/DOE Partnership. Urbed, 1980.

7 LONDON BOROUGH OF SOUTHWARK, DEVELOPMENT DEPARTMENT. *Industrial surveys*, 1977.

8 JOINT UNIT FOR RESEARCH ON THE URBAN ENVIRONMENT. *Industrial renewal in the Inner City*. Report to the DOE. JURUE, University of Aston, 1980.

9 DEPARTMENT OF INDUSTRY *Provision of small industrial premises*. A report to the Department of Industry by Coopers Lybrand, 1980. Associates.
See also URBED 'Finding a space for small enterprises in the inner city'. *In: The Inner City*. ed. EVANS AND EVERSLEY. 1980.

10 BOYKIN, JAMES. *Industrial potential of the central city*. Urban Land Institute, 1973.

11 DEGW. *Taking stock* A report for the Department of the Environment/Hackney/Islington Partnership. DEGW, 1980.

12 DEGW/URBED *Accommodating small enterprises in Covent Garden*. DEGW, 1976.

13/14 *Adaptive use: development economics, process and profiles*. Washington: Urban Land Institute, 1978.

15 Working communities. AJ Use of Redundant Buildings' series. No. 15. 6 December 1978.

16 ROCK, DAVID. *The grassroot developers*. RIBA, 1980.

1 Inner city issues (general)

MOBBS, N. *The inner city – a location for industry* Slough Estates. 1977.

McKEAN, C. *Fight blight* Kaye & Ward. 1977.

Inner Area Studies. HMSO. 1977.

JACOBS, J. *Economy of cities* Cape. 1977.

BURCHELL, R. W. and LISTOKIN, D. *The adaptive reuse handbook* New Jersey, Center for Urban Policy Research, 1981.

COUNCIL FOR ENVIRONMENTAL CONSERVATION *Waking up dormant land: community uses for vacant land and buildings*. CO EN CO, 1981.

URBAN LAND INSTITUTE
Adaptive use: development economics; process and profiles. Washington, ULI, 1978.

MOSS, GRAHAM
Britain's wasting acres: land use in a changing society. Architectural Press, 1981.

NABARRO, R. and RICHARDS, D. *Wasteland: a Thames Television report* Thames Television Ltd, 1980.

DRURY, JOLYON *Factories: planning, design and modernisation*. Architectural Press, 1981.

Chapter 2

1 BOLTON REPORT. *op. cit.* Chapter 1 ref 1
2 LONDON BOROUGH OF SOUTHWARK. *op. cit.* Chapter 1 ref 7
3 DRURY, JOLYON. *AJ handbook of factory design.* Series of articles appearing in the AJ from 5 October 1977 – See also: DRURY, J. *Building and planning for industrial storage and distribution*. Architectural Press, 1981.
4 SYMES, M. and DEGW. *Accommodation for entrepreneurs*. DEGW, 1980.
5 REGENERATION/DEGW/URBED 'Brenterprise: an enterprise centre for Brent'. *Regeneration*, 1980.

2 Small enterprises (general)

BOLTON REPORT *Report on the committee of enquiry on small firms* HMSO. 1972.

BOSWELL, J. *The use and decline of small firms* George Allen & Unwin. 1972.

CHARTERMAN, M. *Small businesses* Sweet & Maxwell. 1977.

COMMUNITY BUSINESS VENTURES *Whose business is business*. Calouste Gulbenkian Foundation, 1981

Promotion of small business: a seven country study. Economists

Advisory Group, 1980.
Business in the community: Handbook for action. BIC, 1981.

Chapter 3

1 DEGW. *op. cit.* Chapter 1 Ref 11
2 ELEY, P. and WORTHINGTON, J. 'The management of change.' *In:* MARKUS, A. Thomas. Building conversion and rehabilitation. Butterworth, 1979.

3 Industrial archaeology (general)

HUDSON, K. *Exploring our industrial past* Teach Yourself Books. Hodder & Stoughton. 1975.
COUSINS, N. *BP book of industrial archaeology* David & Charles. 1975
RAISTRICK, A. *Industrial archaeology: an historical survey* Eyre & Methuen. 1972.
RICHARDS, J. M. *The functional tradition in early industrial buildings* Architectural Press. 1958.
PEVSNER, N. *A history of building types* Thames & Hudson. 1976.
MUMFORD, L. *Technics and civilization* Routledge & Kegan Paul. 1934.

Chapter 4

1 FALK, N. Small firms and the inner city. Conference proceedings, Durham Business School, October 1978.
2 CENTRE FOR ADVANCED LAND USE STUDIES *Buildings for industry* College of Estate Management: CALUS Research report, 1979.

4 Building envelope (general)

BURBERRY, P. *AJ Handbook of building for energy conservation.* 1978.
VANDENBERG, M. and ELDER, A. J. *AJ Handbook of building enclosure.* 1974.
LAUNDER, V and BURBERRY, P. 'AJ Handbook of building services and circulation' in AJs 1.10.69 to 7.10.70. AJ Handbook *Design and cleaning of windows and façades* 1973.
TAYLOR, J. E. and COOKE, G. (eds) *The Fire Precautions Act in practice* Architectural Press. 1978.
ALDERSON, L. *Materials for building, Vols 1–4 1972–6* (physical and chemical aspects of matter, water and its effects).
GRATWICK, R. T. *Dampness in buildings, Vols 1 and 2* Crosby Lockwood. 1969.
LAZENBY, D. and PHILLIPS, P. *Cutting for construction* A handbook of methods and applications of handcutting and breaking on site. Architectural Press. 1978.
BOWYER, J. *Guide to domestic building surveys* Architectural Press. Third edition 1984.
MELVILLE, I. A. and GORDON, I. A. *The repair and maintenance of houses* Estates Gazette. 1973.
INSALL, D. *The care of old buildings today. A practical guide* Architectural Press. 1972.
ELLIS, HUTCHINSON, BARTON. *Maintenance and repair of buildings* Newnes Butterworths.
BUILDING RESEARCH ESTABLISHMENT. *Building defects and maintenance* Lancaster MTP Construction. 1974.
BRE Digests related to restoration and preservation of buildings, including building services.
BOWYER, JACK, *Vernacular building conservation.* Architectural Press, 1980.
MILLS, EDWARD. Editor. *Building maintenance and preservation, A guide to design and management.* Butterworths, 1980.
Housing rehabilitation handbook by John Benson *and* others. Architectural Press, 1980.

Chapter 5

1 URBED *Recycling industrial buildings* Capital Planning Information, 6 Castle Street, Edinburgh, 1981.
2 URBED. *Local authorities and industrial development* Urbed, 1978.
3 STAFFORD, F., FRANKLIN, M. and McDONALD, I. 'Rochdale Fights back' and 'Industrial improvement areas' in *Architects' Journal* 18 July and 25 July 1979.
4 TIME FOR INDUSTRY: evaluation of the Rochdale Industrial Improvement area. Report prepared for the DOE, HMSO, 1978.

5 Building materials: history and specification (general)

GLOAG, J. and BRIDGEWATER, D. *A history of cast iron in architecture* Allen & Unwin. 1948.
HUDSON, K. *Building materials* Longmans Industrial Archaeology Series. 1972.
CLIFTON TAYLOR, A. *Pattern of English building* Faber & Faber. 1972.
DAVEY, N. *History of building materials* Phoenix House. 1961.
HURST, J. T. *Elementary principles of carpentry* Thomas Tredgold. Spon. 1904.
McKAY, W. B. *Joinery and carpentry* Longmans. 1969, 1974.
BRUNSKILL, R and CLIFTON TAYLOR, A. *English brickwork* Ward Lock. 1977.
DAVEY, N. *Building stones of England and Wales* Bedford Square Press. 1976.
ASHURST, J. and DIMES, F. *Stone in building: its use and potential today* Architectural Press. 1978.

6 Adaptive reuse of old buildings (general)

CANTACUZINO, S. *New uses for old buildings* Architectural Press. 1975 (out of print).
DOE *Aspects of conservation 1: new life for old buildings* HMSO. 1971. *2: new life in historic areas* HMSO 1972.
KIDNEY, W. C. *Working places* Ober Park Associates Inc. 1976.
SAVE 'Conservation and Jobs' *Built Environment,* September 1976.
STRATTON, J. *Pioneering in the urban wilderness* New York. Urizen Books. 1977.
BOYKIN, J. H. ULI Research Report 21 – *Industrial potential of the central city* Washington DC. The Urban Land Institute. *An investigation of regulatory barriers to the reuse of existing buildings – a team investigation sponsored by the National Bureau of Standards Centre for Building Technology* London. MIT Press. 1978.

LANGENBACH, R. *A future from the past – the case for conservation and reuse of old buildings in industrial communities* Washington DC. US Dept of Housing and Urban Development. 1977.

WALSH, E. D. and Associates *Action plan for North Adams, Massachusetts. The renovation and reuse of industrial space in an older multi-storey mill building* Boston, Massachusetts. E. D. Walsh & Associates. 1978.

MARKUS, T. A. (ed) *Building conversion and rehabilitation – designing for change in building use* Newnes Butterworths. 1978.

Techniques and Architecture No 322 December 1978. Whole journal on conversions.

BRITISH TOURIST AUTHORITY *Britain's historic buildings: a policy for their future use.* BTA, 1981.

STELLA, FRANK. (ed) *Business and preservation: a survey of business conservation of buildings and neighbourhoods.* Inform, 1978.

CANTACUZINO, SHERBAN and BRANDT, SUSAN *Saving old buildings.* Architectural Press, 1980.

GETZELS, JUDITH. *Recycling public buildings.* American Society of Planning Officials, 1976.

New uses for older building in Scotland: a manual of practical encouragement. Edinburgh: HMSO, 1981.

REINER, LAURENCE E. *How to recycle buildings.* McGraw Hill, 1979.

URBED Recycling industrial buildings. Capital Planning Information, 1981.

Chapter 7

General background:

URBED op. cit. chapter 5 ref 1
DEGW op. cit. chapter 1 ref 11

7 *Historical perspective of building construction regulations (general)*

NICHOLSON, P. *The new practical builder* 1828, 1838.
WEALE, J. *Building construction* 1857.
WEAVE, W. R. *Building construction* 1871.
WRAY, H. *Building construction* 1891.
Rivington's notes on building construction 1875, 1915.
Mitchell's building construction from 1890s.
JAGGARD and DRURY, *Architectural building construction* Cambridge University Press. Vol 1 1916, Vol 2 1922, Vol 3 1923.
TREDGOLD, T. *Elementary principles of carpentry* 1820, 1904.
KNOWLES, C. C. and PITT, P. H. *A history of building regulations in London 1189–1972* Architectural Press. 1972.
BURN, R. S. *The builder's practical director* 1860.
TARN, J. N. *Working class housing in nineteenth century Britain* Lund Humphries. AA paper No 7. 1971.
BRUNSKILL, R. W. *Illustrated handbook of vernacular architecture* Faber. 1970.
HALL, Sir R. de Z. *A bibliography of vernacular architecture* David & Charles. 1972.
BARLEY, M. W. *The English farmhouse and cottage* Routledge & Kegan Paul. 1961.
PHYSICK & DARBY *Marble halls* Victoria and Albert Museum. 1973.

Chapter 8

General background:

BERNARD WILLIAMS. *Property Development Feasibility Tables.* Building Economics Bureau, 1977.
Spon's *Architects and Builders Price Book.*
SMITH, ROB 'Building costs' *In: Business Property Manual.* Gower, 1982.

Chapter 13

General background:

'Internal planning: industrial and office'. *In: Business Property Manual.* op. cit. chapter 8.
NEUFERT *Architects data*
OXFORD POLYTECHNIC, BUILDING RESEARCH TEAM. *Small advance factories in rural area.* Series of working papers. Oxford Polytechnic, 1981.
CALUS (Centre for Advanced Land Use Studies) op. cit. chapter 4 ref 2

Statutory regulations

SPEAIGHT, A. and STONE, G. *AJ legal handbook third edition.* London. Architectural Press 1982.
WHITTAKER, C., BROWN, P. and MONAHAN, J. *AJ handbook of environmental powers* Architectural Press 1976.
ELDER, A. J. *Guide to the building regulations* Architectural Press. Seventh edition 1981; see also supplement *Guide to the second amendment* 1981.
McKNOWN, R. *Comprehensive guide to town planning law and procedures* George Godwin (for *The Builder*). Sixth edition 1976.
McKNOWN, R. *Comprehensive guide to factory law* George Godwin (for *The Builder*). Second edition. 1973.
PARLETT, D. S. (ed) *Construction industry* UK House Information Services. 1976.
PITT, P. H. and DUFTON, J. *Building control in inner London* Architectural Press. 1983.
(London Building Acts and Bylaws and their interpretation).
Directory of official architecture and planning George Godwin (for *The Builder*) 21st edition. 1977.
SAVIDGE, REX 'Revise the regs!' *The Architects Journal* on the following dates: 22.2.78 (pp 326–327); 1.3.78 (pp 378–379); 8.3.78 (pp 432–433); 15.3.78 (pp 482–483); 22.3.78 (pp 531–533) 29.3.78 (pp 584–585); 5.4.78 (pp 629–631).
WATERS, BRIAN and ROBINSON, LES 'Making a planning application' *The Architects Journal* 20.9.78 (pp 543–552); 27.9.78 (pp 589–591); 4.10.78 (pp 639–643).
NBA, DOE (Welsh Office) and COI *Planning permission: a guide to industry.* HMSO 1978.
CHARTERED INSTITUTE OF BUILDING SERVICES *Technical memoranda*
No. 2 *Notes on legislation relating to fire and services in buildings.* (1979).
Note. 3. *Notes on legislation relating to the Health and Safety at Work etc, Act, 1974* (1977).
TAYLOR, J. and COOKE, G. *The Fire Precautions Act in practice.* Architectural Press, 1978.

HOME OFFICE AND SCOTTISH HOME AND HEALTH DEPARTMENTS *Guide to the Fire Precautions Act 1971. 2. Factories.* London, HMSO 1977.

HOME OFFICE AND SCOTTISH HOME AND HEALTH DEPARTMENT *Guides to the Fire Precautions Act 1971 3: Offices, shops and railway premises* London: HMSO, 1977.

Houses's guide to the construction industry UK 1981/82 8th edition, 1980.

Directory of official architecture and planning Godwin. 23rd edition.

Fire regulations

DEPARTMENT OF EMPLOYMENT: series *Safety, Health and Welfare*, HMSO.

Fire Protection Association 'Fire protection design guides'.

FIRE OFFICES COMMITTEE *Rules . . . for the construction of buildings.* 1978.

GLC Code of practice: *Means of escape in case of fire.* 1974

GLC 'London building (constructional) by-laws'. 1972 and amendments 1974 and 1979.

HOME OFFICE/SCOTTISH HOME AND HEALTH DEPARTMENT *Guides to the Fire Precautions Act 1971.* HMSO

'Fire Insurance and the Architect' (AJ 16.3.77, pp 489–513)

Index